Neuro-Ophthalmology

Guest Editors

ANDREW G. LEE, MD
PAUL W. BRAZIS, MD

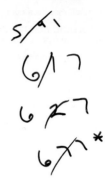

NEUROLOGIC CLINICS

www.neurologic.theclinics.com

Consulting Editor
RANDOLPH W. EVANS, MD

August 2010 • Volume 28 • Number 3

SAUNDERS an imprint of ELSEVIER, Inc.

W.B. SAUNDERS COMPANY
A Division of Elsevier Inc.

1600 John F. Kennedy Boulevard • Suite 1800 • Philadelphia, Pennsylvania 19103-2899

http://www.theclinics.com

NEUROLOGIC CLINICS Volume 28, Number 3
August 2010 ISSN 0733-8619, ISBN-13: 978-1-4377-2467-7

Editor: Donald Mumford

Neurologic Clinics (ISSN 0733-8619) is published quarterly by Elsevier Inc., 360 Park Avenue South, New York, NY 10010–1710. Months of issue are February, May, August, and November. Periodicals postage paid at New York, NY, and additional mailing offices. Subscription prices are $247.00 per year for US individuals, $401.00 per year for US institutions, $124.00 per year for US students, $310.00 per year for Canadian individuals, $482.00 per year for Canadian institutions, $344.00 per year for international individuals, $482.00 per year for international institutions, and $175.00 for Canadian and foreign students/residents. To receive student/resident rate, orders must be accompanied by name of affiliated institution, date of term, and the *signature* of program/residency coordinator on institution letterhead. Orders will be billed at individual rate until proof of status is received. Foreign air speed delivery is included in all *Clinics* subscription prices. All prices are subject to change without notice. **POSTMASTER:** Send address changes to *Neurologic Clinics*, Elsevier Health Sciences Division, Subscription Customer Service, 3251 Riverport Lane, Maryland Heights, MO 63043. **Customer Service: Telephone: 1-800-654-2452 (U.S. and Canada); 314-447-8871 (outside U.S. and Canada). Fax: 314-447-8029. E-mail: journalscustomerservice-usa@elsevier.com (for print support); journalsonlinesupport-usa@elsevier.com (for online support).**

Reprints. For copies of 100 or more of articles in this publication, please contact the Commercial Reprints Department, Elsevier Inc., 360 Park Avenue South, New York, New York, 10010-1710; Tel.: (+1) 212-633-3812; Fax: (+1) 212-462-1935, and E-mail: reprints@elsevier.com.

Neurologic Clinics is also published in Spanish by Nueva Editorial Interamericana S.A., Mexico City, Mexico.

Neurologic Clinics is covered in *Current Contents/Clinical Medicine, MEDLINE/PubMed (Index Medicus), EMBASE/Excerpta Medica, and PsycINFO, and ISI/BIOMED.*

Printed in the United States of America.

Contributors

CONSULTING EDITOR

RANDOLPH W. EVANS, MD
Clinical Professor, Department of Neurology, Baylor College of Medicine, Houston, Texas

GUEST EDITORS

ANDREW G. LEE, MD
Chair, The Department of Ophthalmology, The Methodist Hospital, Houston, Texas; Professor of Ophthalmology, Neurology, and Neurosurgery, Weill Cornell Medical College; Adjunct Professor of Ophthalmology, The University of Iowa Hospitals and Clinics; Clinical Professor of Ophthalmology, University of Texas Medical Branch, Galveston, Texas

PAUL W. BRAZIS, MD
Consultant in Neuro-Ophthalmology and Neurology, Departments of Ophthalmology and Neurology, Mayo Clinic - Jacksonville, Jacksonville, Florida

AUTHORS

REHAN AHMED, MD
Assistant Professor of Ophthalmology, Cullen Eye Institute, Baylor College of Medicine, Houston, Texas

VALÉRIE BIOUSSE, MD
Department of Ophthalmology, Emory Eye Center; Cyrus H. Stoner Professor of Ophthalmology, Professor of Ophthalmology, Department of Neurology, Emory University School of Medicine, Atlanta, Georgia

BEAU B. BRUCE, MD
Assistant Professor of Ophthalmology and Neurology, Departments of Ophthalmology, Neurology and Neurological Surgery, Emory University School of Medicine, Atlanta, Georgia

STEPHANIE S. CHAN, OD
Department of Ophthalmology, Stanford University, Stanford, California

DAVID CLARK, DO
Neurology Resident, Department of Neurology and Ophthalmology, Michigan State University, East Lansing, Michigan

KIMBERLY P. COCKERHAM, FACS, MD
Adjunct Associate Professor, Department of Ophthalmology, Stanford University, Stanford, California

FIONA E. COSTELLO, MD, FRCP
Clinical Associate Professor, Departments of Clinical Neurosciences and Surgery, Foothills Medical Centre, University of Calgary, Calgary, Alberta, Canada

ERIC EGGENBERGER, DO, MS
Professor and Vice Chairman, Department of Neurology and Ophthalmology, Michigan
State University, East Lansing, Michigan

JULIE FALARDEAU, MD
Assistant Professor of Ophthalmology, Casey Eye Institute, Oregon Health and Science
University, Portland, Oregon

ROD FOROOZAN, MD
Assistant Professor of Ophthalmology, Cullen Eye Institute, Baylor College of Medicine,
Houston, Texas

STEVEN L. GALETTA, MD
Van Meter Professor of Neurology, Division of Neuro-Ophthalmology, Department of
Neurology, Hospital of the University of Pennsylvania, Philadelphia, Pennsylvania

KARL GOLNIK, MD, MEd
Professor, Departments of Ophthalmology, Neurology, and Neurosurgery, University
of Cincinnati; Cincinnati Eye Institute, Cincinnati, Ohio

MAYANK GOYAL, MD, FRCP
Professor of Radiology and Clinical Neurosciences, Departments of Clinical
Neurosciences and Radiology; High Field Program, Seaman Family MR Research
Centre, Foothills Medical Centre, University of Calgary, Calgary, Alberta, Canada

PIERRE-FRANÇOIS KAESER, MD
Chief Resident, University Ophthalmology Service, Hôpital Ophtalmique Jules Gonin,
Lausanne, Switzerland

AKI KAWASAKI, MD
Médecin Associé, Neuro-Ophthalmology Unit; Chief, Laboratory of Pupillography, Hôpital
Ophtalmique Jules Gonin, Lausanne, Switzerland

WORKAYEHU KEBEDE, MD
Neuro-Opthalmology Fellow, Department of Neurology and Ophthalmology, Michigan
State University, East Lansing, Michigan

CÉDRIC LAMIREL, MD
Fellow, Department of Ophthalmology, Emory Eye Center, Atlanta, Georgia

TIMOTHY J. MCCULLEY, MD
Director of Ophthalmic Plastic and Reconstruction, Department of Ophthalmology,
University of California San Francisco, San Francisco, California

NANCY J. NEWMAN, MD
Leo Delle Jolley Professor of Ophthalmology, Professor of Ophthalmology and Neurology,
Instructor in Neurosurgery, Department of Ophthalmology, Neurology, and Neurological
Surgery, Emory University School of Medicine, Atlanta, Georgia; Lecturer in
Ophthalmology, Harvard Medical School, Boston, Massachusetts

SASHANK PRASAD, MD
Instructor in Neurology, Division of Neuro-Ophthalmology, Department of Neurology,
Brigham and Women's Hospital, Harvard Medical School, Boston, Massachusetts

NICHOLAS J. VOLPE, MD
Professor of Ophthalmology, Division of Neuro-Ophthalmology, Scheie Eye Institute,
University of Pennsylvania, Philadelphia, Pennsylvania

MICHAEL WALL, MD
Professor of Neurology and Ophthalmology, Department of Neurology and Department of Ophthalmology and Visual Sciences, College of Medicine, University of Iowa, Veterans Administration Medical Center, Iowa City, Iowa

MICHAEL K. YOON, MD
Fellow in Neuro-Ophthalmology and Ophthalmic Plastic and Reconstructive Surgery, Department of Ophthalmology, University of California San Francisco, San Francisco, California

Contents

> Optic neuritis usually presents with painful monocular vision loss in youn-
> ger patients. Spontaneous improvement in vision occurs over weeks, and
> treatment with high-dose intravenous steroids increases the rate but not
> extent of visual recovery. Risk of progression to multiple sclerosis (MS)
> is largely dictated by baseline brain magnetic resonance imaging (MRI).
> Those with a normal MRI finding at the time of optic neuritis diagnosis
> have a lower rate of progression to multiple sclerosis than those with T2
> hyperintense white matter lesions on MRI. High-dose intravenous steroids
> should be considered acutely in optic neuritis, and disease-modifying ther-
> apy should be considered in patients at high risk of MS as defined by MRI.

> Giant cell arteritis is a systemic vasculitis with a wide clinical spectrum,
> and it represents a medical emergency. Visual loss is the most feared com-
> plication, and when it happens, it tends to be profound and permanent.
> Prompt diagnosis and treatment are imperative to minimize potentially
> devastating visual loss and neurologic deficits. A temporal artery biopsy
> should be performed on every patient in whom the diagnosis is suspected.
> The mainstay of therapy remains corticosteroids.

> Idiopathic intracranial hypertension ((IIH) is characterized by increased
> cerebrospinal fluid pressure of unknown cause. It is predominantly a disease
> of women in the childbearing years. Although the cause of IIH remains
> obscure, it has become clear that loss of visual function is common and
> patients may progress to blindness if untreated. Diagnosis should adhere
> to the modified Dandy criteria and other causes of intracranial hypertension
> sought. IIH patient management should include serial perimetry and optic
> disc grading or photography. The proper therapy can then be selected
> and visual loss prevented or reversed. Although there are no evidence-
> based data to guide therapy, there is an ongoing randomized double-blind
> controlled treatment trial of IIH investigating diet and medical therapy.

> Transient monocular visual loss is an important clinical complaint and has
> a number of causes, of which the most common is retinal ischemia. A practical

approach is to perform a careful examination to determine whether there are any eye abnormalities that can explain the visual loss. Despite the transient nature of the symptom, there may be clues to the diagnosis on the examination even after the visual loss has recovered.

Optic atrophy is a clinical term used to describe an optic disc thought to be paler than normal. Optic atrophy is not a diagnosis but an ophthalmoscopic sign. Evidence of visual loss (acuity, color vision, peripheral vision) should be present. Most optic atrophy is diffuse and nonspecific, but historical and examination clues exist that help differentiate the many causes of optic atrophy. Patients with unexplained optic atrophy should be evaluated with magnetic resonance imaging.

Patients with multiple sclerosis commonly describe visual symptoms that result from several eye movement abnormalities that occur from disruption of critical pathways in the brainstem, cerebellum, and cerebral hemispheres. These abnormalities include internuclear ophthalmoplegia, ocular motor palsy, ocular misalignment, pathologic nystagmus, impaired saccades, saccadic intrusions, and impaired pursuit. Detailed knowledge of these problems and their neuroanatomic localization will aid the physician by guiding diagnosis and therapeutic decision making.

Neurologists are frequently consulted because of a pupillary abnormality. An unequal size of the pupils, an unusual shape, white colored pupils, or a poorly reactive pupil are common reasons for referral. A directed history and careful observation of the iris and pupil movements can bear out ocular pathology such as congenital or structural anomalies as the cause of abnormal pupils. Thereafter, it is important to evaluate the neurologic causes of anisocoria and poor pupil function. The first part of this article emphasizes pupillary abnormalities frequently encountered in infants and children and discusses some of the more common acquired iris structural defects. The second part focuses on evaluation of lesions in the neural pathways that result in pupillary dysfunction, with particular attention to those conditions having neurologic, systemic, or visual implications.

Virtually all abnormalities of the orbit can result in neuro-ophthalmic findings: optic neuropathies, motility disorders, and changes in sensation. Subtle orbital disease, presenting with neuro-ophthalmic findings, is frequently overlooked on initial evaluation. By contrast, obvious orbital diseases, such as Graves disease, are also commonly managed by neuro-ophthalmologists, and although they might not come with much of a diagnostic dilemma, may be a challenge to treat. This article focuses on those disorders more commonly encountered or that come with more serious consequences if misdiagnosed. Orbital trauma, hemorrhage, neoplasm, and inflammation are covered in some detail.

Neurologists frequently evaluate patients complaining of vision loss, especially when the patient has been examined by an ophthalmologist who has found no ocular disease. A significant proportion of patients presenting to the neurologist with visual complaints have nonorganic or functional visual loss. Although there are examination techniques that can aid in the detection and diagnosis of functional visual loss, the frequency with which functional visual loss occurs concomitantly with organic disease warrants substantial caution on the part of the clinician. Furthermore, purely functional visual loss is never a diagnosis of exclusion and must be supported by positive findings on examinations that demonstrate normal visual function. The relationship of true psychological disease and functional visual loss is unclear, and most patients respond well to simple reassurance.

Eye movement abnormalities constitute an important clinical sign that can be a manifestation of dysfunction of cranial nerves III, IV, and VI (the 3 ocular motor nerves). Specific motility deficits often have highly localizing value within the neuroaxis, serving to refine a differential diagnosis and guide management. This article reviews the key anatomic concepts, clinical presentation, differential diagnosis, and management of ocular motor nerve palsies. Dysfunction of an ocular motor nerve must be distinguished from other causes of abnormal eye movements, such as myasthenia gravis or thyroid eye disease, which are outside the scope of this article.

THE CLINICS ARE NOW AVAILABLE ONLINE!

Access your subscription at:
www.theclinics.com

Preface

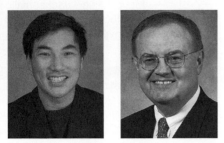

Andrew G. Lee, MD   Paul W. Brazis, MD
Guest Editors

Neuro-ophthalmology is a subspecialty of neurology and ophthalmology that bridges the gap between eye and brain. This issue of *Neurologic Clinics* describes the key features and latest information on topics in neuro-ophthalmology of interest to practicing neurologists and, in particular, highlights areas for which referral might be reasonable to neuro-ophthalmologists.

A quick review of the table of contents for this issue illustrates the depth and breadth of the neurologic topics that fall within neuro-ophthalmology. These include multiple sclerosis, orbital diseases, optic nerve disorders, vascular disorders, neuro-ophthalmic imaging, and ocular motility deficits. We hope that the readers enjoy this issue and are able to recognize, triage, manage, or refer these specific neuro-ophthalmic disorders better.

The editors wish to express gratitude to the article authors for their interesting, educational, and valuable contributions and special thanks also to Don Mumford for his hard work and his guidance throughout the preparation of this issue.

Dr Lee wishes to acknowledge and thank his ever-patient wife, Hilary A. Beaver, MD, for tolerating yet another academic project and his parents, Rosalind Lee, MD, and Alberto C. Lee, MD, for teaching the values of precision, accuracy, and brevity in medical writing.

Dr Brazis wishes to thank his wife, Elizabeth, for her encouragement and support.

Andrew G. Lee, MD
Department of Ophthalmology
The Methodist Hospital
6560 Fannin Street, Scurlock 450
Houston, TX 77030, USA

Neurol Clin 28 (2010) xiii–xiv
doi:10.1016/j.ncl.2010.05.001
0733-8619/10/$ – see front matter © 2010 Elsevier Inc. All rights reserved.

Paul W. Brazis, MD
Departments of Ophthalmology and Neurology
Mayo Clinic - Jacksonville
4500 San Pablo Road
Jacksonville, FL 32224, USA

E-mail addresses:
AGLee@tmhs.org (A.G. Lee)
Brazis.Paul@mayo.edu (P.W. Brazis)

Optic Neuritis

David Clark, DO*, Workayehu Kebede, MD,
Eric Eggenberger, DO, MS

KEYWORDS

- Optic neuritis • Multiple sclerosis • Demyelination • Interferon
- Glatiramer acetate

The authors reserve the term optic neuritis for demyelinating optic neuropathy that is idiopathic or related to multiple sclerosis (MS). An understanding of the typical optic neuritis presentation, differential diagnosis, visual prognosis, and association with MS is essential to proper management of this common condition.

BACKGROUND

The bulk of our understanding of optic neuritis comes from the Optic Neuritis Treatment Trial (ONTT) and the follow-up Longitudinal Optic Neuritis Study (LONS). The inclusion criteria for the ONTT were acute unilateral optic neuritis in those aged 18 to 46 years, visual symptoms that began no more than 8 days before enrollment, a relative afferent papillary defect (RAPD), and visual field defect. Exclusion criteria included those with a prior history of optic neuritis, pallor in the affected eye, or macular exudates; those with painless anterior optic neuropathy (disc edema) with either retinal hemorrhage or an arcuate or altitudinal visual field defect; those with a history of glaucoma, with increased intraocular pressure, on medications known to cause optic neuropathy; and those with fellow eye optic neuritis that had been treated previously with steroids. The study enrolled 448 patients between 1988 and 1991 from 15 centers in the United States.[1] Of participants who were not diagnosed with probable or clinically definite multiple sclerosis (CDMS) at the beginning of the study, 389 were followed up for 15 years to determine the rate of and risk factors for conversion to CDMS. The data collected from these studies have been important in determining the immediate treatment, demographics, and prognosis for visual recovery and progression to CDMS.

EPIDEMIOLOGY

Demyelinating optic neuritis is the most common nonglaucomatous optic neuropathy in young people. Data collected in Olmsted county, Minnesota, show an incidence of 5.1 per 100,000 and a prevalence of 115 per 100,000.[2] The ONTT demonstrated

Department of Neurology and Ophthalmology, Michigan State University, A217 Clinical Center, 138 Service Road, East Lansing, MI 48824, USA
* Corresponding author.
E-mail address: david.clark@hc.msu.edu

Neurol Clin 28 (2010) 573–580
doi:10.1016/j.ncl.2010.03.001
0733-8619/10/$ – see front matter © 2010 Elsevier Inc. All rights reserved.

a female to male ratio of approximately 3:1, with a mean age at onset of 32 years; 85% of subjects were white and 77% were women.[1]

SYMPTOMS

Typically, optic neuritis presents with acute unilateral vision loss progressing to nadir in hours to days. The most common visual symptoms are scotoma (45%) and blur (40%). Pain is present in approximately 92% of patients, may be constant, and is usually worse with eye movement. Pain helps distinguish optic neuritis from other optic neuropathies. In a study of patients with anterior ischemic optic neuropathy, only 5 of 41 (12%) had eye pain in sharp contrast to optic neuritis.[3] Positive visual phenomena, including fleeting colors and flashing lights, are reported in 30% of optic neuritis cases.[1]

SIGNS

Examination features of unilateral optic neuritis typically include an RAPD and may show decreased visual acuity, color perception, and abnormal visual fields. Visual acuity at ONTT entry ranged from 20/20 to no light perception. Dyschromatopsia is common, and patients often report that colors, particularly red, appear less intense in the affected eye. Similarly, light may appear dimmer in the affected eye when compared with the unaffected eye; this is easily assessed during the swinging light test. Various visual field defect patterns can be seen, the most common being diffuse, altitudinal, quadrantanopic, centrocecal, or hemianopic; in general, the nature of the visual field defect in optic neuropathies provides little information regarding the pathophysiology of the optic neuropathy.

The optic disc seems ophthalmoscopically normal acutely in two-third of cases (retrobulbar optic neuritis) and is edematous in one-third of cases (papillitis, bulbar, or anterior optic neuritis). When disc edema is present, the edema is typically mild, nonfocal, and only rarely associated with hemorrhage, retinal exudates, or vitreous cells. When severe edema or hemorrhage is present, the diagnosis of idiopathic optic neuritis is in question. These atypical features also have prognostic value (see later discussion).[1]

CLINICAL COURSE AND PROGNOSIS

Visual symptoms in most patients improve over time whether or not they receive acute steroid therapy. In the ONTT, approximately 80% of patients began improving within the first 3 weeks; if improvement does not begin within the first 5 weeks, the diagnosis of idiopathic optic neuritis should be questioned. Within the ONTT, approximately 95% of patients regained visual acuity of 20/40 or better by 12 months, regardless of treatment assignment. Although most patients note near-normal acuity over time, other optic nerve–related symptoms often remain, albeit mitigated. An RAPD, decreased intensity of light perceived in the affected eye, decreased color saturation, and difficulty with motion perception are common sequelae. Some patients experience transient recurrent blur with increased body temperature (Uhthoff phenomena). Optic atrophy is an end result of optic neuritis (or other optic neuropathy) and can be quantified and followed using optical coherence tomography (OCT).

EVALUATION AND MS CONCERNS

The evaluation of a patient with a first event of optic neuritis is important for diagnostic and prognostic reasons. The diagnosis of optic neuritis is primarily clinical, although ancillary testing may assist in eliminating other entities in the differential diagnosis.

In the ONTT, laboratory testing for inflammatory or infectious diseases (eg, antinuclear antibody, fluorescent treponemal antibody, and angiotensin-converting enzyme) did not change management and is not recommended in typical cases. Cerebrospinal fluid (CSF) samples were obtained in 83 patients within 24 hours of trial enrollment; findings were either normal or consistent with a mild inflammatory process. Glucose was normal in all patients; approximately 10% had protein greater than 50 mg/dL, and a pleocytosis (6–27 white blood cells/mL) was seen in 36% of samples. Of the 83 patients with CSF samples, 13 developed CDMS within 24 months. Oligoclonal bands (OCBs) were seen in 11 of the 13. Of these 11 patients, 9 also had at least one T2 lesion on brain MRI; only 2 of 13 patients who developed CDMS within 24 months had a normal MRI finding and OCBs in CSF. None of the 28 patients with a normal brain MRI finding and without OCBs in CSF progressed to CDMS within 24 months, representing a low-risk cohort.[4]

Optic neuritis is commonly the first demyelinating event in MS. MRI of the brain can help confirm the diagnosis of optic neuritis and helps to stratify the risk of progression to CDMS. In retrobulbar optic neuritis, a fat-suppressed MRI scan obtained within the first several weeks usually demonstrates postcontrast enhancement of the involved optic nerve (**Figs. 1** and **2**). Approximately 50% of patients with optic neuritis harbor white matter T2 hyperintense lesions on MRI (**Figs. 3** and **4**). Those with a normal MRI finding at the time of optic neuritis diagnosis have a 15% risk of progression to CDMS at 5 years, 22% at 10 years, and 25% at 15 years; those with an abnormal brain MRI finding have a 42% risk of progression to CDMS at 5 years, 56% at 10 years, and 72% at 15 years.[5–7]

MRI finding coupled with clinical information aid in identifying those at especially low risk of developing CDMS. Of men with optic disc edema and a normal brain MRI finding, only 1 of 24 (4%) developed CDMS within 15 years. Among the ONTT subcohort with a normal baseline MRI finding, 5 features are associated with very low MS risk (no patients converted to CDMS at 15 years)[6,7]:

1. Painless optic neuritis
2. Severe optic disc edema

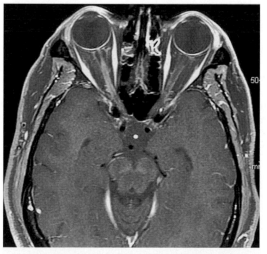

Fig. 1. Axial postcontrast fat -suppressed MRI of the orbits demonstrates enhancement of the right optic nerve.

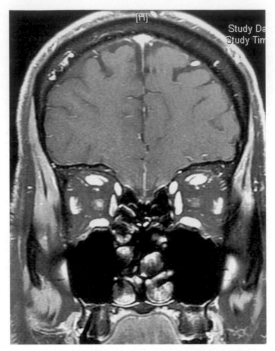

Fig. 2. Coronal image demonstrating the same enhancing optic nerve as seen in **Fig. 1**.

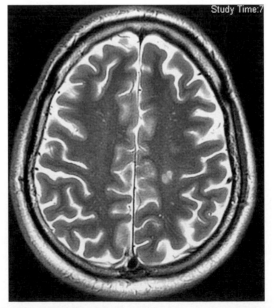

Fig. 3. Axial T2 MRI demonstrating a hyperintense lesion at the left frontoparietal junction.

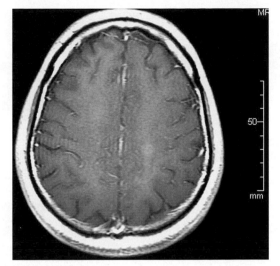

Fig. 4. Axial postcontrast image demonstrates subtle enhancement of the lesion seen in **Fig. 3**.

3. A macular star
4. Optic disc hemorrhage
5. Visual acuity of no light perception.

OCT is a means of quantifying retinal nerve fiber layer (RNFL) thickness and may be useful prognostically in optic neuritis (**Fig. 5**). Costello and colleagues[8] measured RNFL thickness at 1 and 2 years following optic neuritis in 50 patients; 42% of them progressed to CDMS at a mean interval of 27 months. Although RNFL thickness at year 1 and 2 did not distinguish those who progressed to CDMS from those who did not, the MS subcohort showed progressive loss of RNFL between year 1 and 2, whereas the RNFL of those with isolated optic neuritis remained stable.

Thickness of the RNFL measured by OCT correlates with visual recovery. An RNFL of less than 75 μm at 3 to 6 months following optic neuritis is associated with incomplete recovery of visual field.[9] The degree of RNFL loss may help to distinguish neuromyelitis optica (NMO) from MS. In patients with poor visual recovery, RNFL thickness of less than 50 μm, and prominent superior and inferior optic disc quadrant involvement, NMO should be considered.[10]

IMMEDIATE TREATMENT

In the ONTT, patients were randomized to oral prednisone 1 mg/kg/d for 14 days; intravenous methylprednisolone (IVMP) 250 mg every 6 hours for 3 days followed by an oral course; or oral placebo. The rate of visual field, contrast sensitivity, and color improvement was faster in the IVMP group compared with the placebo and oral steroid groups, although the 6-month outcomes were the same; however, those in the oral steroid group had almost twice the rate of recurrent optic neuritis than either placebo or IVMP. Because of the increased recurrence of optic neuritis without enhancement in degree or speed of visual recovery, the 1-mg/kg/d oral steroid regimen has no role in the treatment of optic neuritis.[11] Those who received IVMP

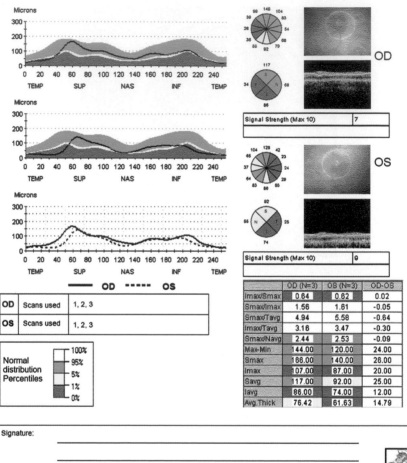

	OD (N=3)	OS (N=3)	OD-OS
Imax/Smax	0.64	0.62	0.02
Smax/Imax	1.56	1.61	-0.05
Smax/Tavg	4.94	5.58	-0.64
Imax/Tavg	3.16	3.47	-0.30
Smax/Navg	2.44	2.53	-0.09
Max-Min	144.00	120.00	24.00
Smax	166.00	140.00	26.00
Imax	107.00	87.00	20.00
Savg	117.00	92.00	25.00
Iavg	86.00	74.00	12.00
Avg.Thick	76.42	61.63	14.79

| OD | Scans used | 1, 2, 3 |
| OS | Scans used | 1, 2, 3 |

Normal distribution Percentiles: 100%, 95%, 5%, 1%, 0%

Signature:

Physician: Michigan State University Neuro-Ophthalmology

Fig. 5. OCT demonstrates bilateral RNFL thinning, most pronounced in the inferior and temporal quadrants.

had a lower rate of progression to CDMS at 2 years than the placebo group. This apparent benefit was no longer present at 5 years.[12]

In the ONTT, IVMP was generally well tolerated. Side effects were usually mild and included weight gain, mood alteration, gastrointestinal upset, and insomnia. Serious side effects of high-dose steroids are rare and include psychosis, avascular necrosis of the femoral head, depression, and pancreatitis. Special attention to blood glucose monitoring and control in patients with diabetes mellitus is warranted. The decision to treat a patient with high-dose steroids is made after taking into account the risks and benefits as well as the side-effect profile, level of visual impairment, and the results of the MRI scan on an individualized, case-by-case basis.

LONG-TERM TREATMENT

Optic neuritis may be the presenting symptom of MS. The Controlled High-Risk Subjects Avonex Multiple Sclerosis Prevention Study (CHAMPS) evaluated patients with clinically isolated syndrome (CIS) or first demyelinating events.[13,14] These included optic neuritis, incomplete transverse myelitis, and a brainstem or cerebellar syndrome. Inclusion criteria included CIS and an MRI scan with at least two T2 hyperintense lesions that were greater than 3 mm. The primary outcome measure was progression to CDMS, and the secondary outcome measure was evidence of T2 or enhancing lesions on MRI. After initial treatment with IVMP for 3 days followed by oral course, patients were randomized to intramuscular interferon beta-1a (IFNa), 30 μg, every week or to placebo. Those on IFNa had a 44% reduction in progression to CDMS. Brain MRI at 6, 12, and 18 months showed fewer T2 or enhancing lesions and smaller T2 lesion volume in the IFNa group. Side effects of IFNa were generally mild, and neutralizing antibodies to the IFNa were present in only 2%.

Similarly, interferon beta-1b (IFNb) and glatiramer acetate (GA) decrease risk of progression to CDMS after CIS. The Betaferon in Newly Emerging Multiple Sclerosis for Initial Treatment (BENEFIT) trial evaluated IFNb in those with CIS.[15] Inclusion criteria were 1 clinical event lasting more than 24 hours plus a brain MRI scan with 2 or more 3-mm white matter T2 lesions. Exclusion criteria include a prior demyelinating event, complete transverse myelitis, bilateral optic neuritis, or prior immunosuppressive therapy. Patients were randomized to either placebo every other day (EOD) or an IFNb titration followed by IFNb, 250 μg, EOD. Analysis at 24 months included 437 of the 468 patients initially randomized. Those in the IFNb group had a 50% lower risk of progression to CDMS than placebo ($P<.0001$). The Patients with Clinically Isolated Syndrome (PreCISe) trial randomized patients with 1 clinical event and a brain MRI scan with 2 white matter T2 lesions of 6 mm to GA, 20 mg, subcutaneous daily or placebo. Those in the GA arm had a 45% lower risk of progression to CDMS at 24 months than placebo.[16] When considering the results of these trials, it is reasonable to discuss starting immunomodulating therapy in all patients who present with optic neuritis and a high-risk MRI finding.

SUMMARY

Optic neuritis usually presents with painful monocular vision loss in younger patients. Spontaneous improvement in vision occurs over weeks, and 95% of patients regain 20/40 vision or better 12 months later. Treatment with high-dose IVMP increases the rate but not extent of visual recovery. Risk of progression to CDMS in optic neuritis is largely dictated by baseline brain MRI. Those with a normal MRI finding at the time of optic neuritis diagnosis have a 15% risk of progression to CDMS at 5 years, 22% at 10 years, and 25% at 15 years; those with an abnormal brain MRI finding have a 42% risk of progression to CDMS at 5 years, 56% at 10 years, and 72% at 15 years. In those with a normal MRI finding, painless optic neuritis, severe disc edema, peripapillary hemorrhage, a macular star, or no light perception visual acuity have a very low risk for progression to CDMS. The appropriate treatment of optic neuritis should be determined on a case-by-case basis. IVMP should be considered immediately in optic neuritis, and disease-modifying therapy should be considered in patients at high risk of MS as defined by MRI.

REFERENCES

1. The clinical profile of acute optic neuritis: experience of the optic neuritis treatment trial. Optic Neuritis Study Group. Arch Ophthalmol 1991;109:1673–8.
2. Rodriguez M, Siva A, Cross SA, et al. Optic Neuritis, a population-based study in Olmsted County, Minnesota. Neurology 1995;45:244–50.

3. Swartz NG, Beck RW, Savino PJ, et al. Pain in anterior ischemic optic neuropathy. J Neuroophthalmol 1995;15:9–10.
4. Rolak LA, Beck RW, Paty DW, et al. Cerebrospinal fluid in acute optic neuritis: experience of the optic neuritis treatment trial. Neurology 1996;46:368–72.
5. The 5-year risk of MS after optic neuritis: experience of the optic neuritis treatment trial. Optic Neuritis Study Group. Neurology 1997;49:1404–13.
6. Optic Neuritis Study Group. High- and low-risk profiles for the development of multiple sclerosis within 10 years after optic neuritis: experience of the optic neuritis treatment trial. Arch Ophthalmol 2003;121:944–9.
7. Optic Neuritis Study Group. Multiple sclerosis risk after optic neuritis: final optic neuritis treatment trial follow-up. Arch Neurol 2008;65(6):727–32.
8. Costello F, Hodge W, Pan Y, et al. Retinal nerve fiber layer and future risk of multiple sclerosis. Can J Neurol Sci 2008;35:482–7.
9. Costello F, Coupland S, Hodge W, et al. Quantifying axonal loss after optic neuritis with optical coherence tomography. Ann Neurol 2006;59:963–9.
10. Naismith RT, Tutlam NT, Xu J, et al. Optical coherence tomography differs in neuromyelitis optica compared with multiple sclerosis. Neurology 2009;72:1077–82.
11. Beck RW, Cleary PA, Anderson MM, et al. A randomized, controlled trial of corticosteroids in the treatment of acute optic neuritis. The Optic Neuritis Study Group. N Engl J Med 1992;326:581–8.
12. Beck RW, Cleary PA, Trobe JD, et al. The effect of corticosteroids for acute optic neuritis on the subsequent development of multiple sclerosis. N Engl J Med 1993; 329:1764–9.
13. CHAMPS Study Group. Interferon β-1a for optic neuritis patients at high risk for multiple sclerosis. Am J Ophthalmol 2001;132(4):463–71.
14. Jacobs LD, Beck RW, Simon JH, et al. Intramuscular interferon beta-1a therapy initiated during a first demyelinating event in multiple sclerosis. (CHAMPS Study Group). N Engl J Med 2000;343:898–904.
15. Kappos L, Polman CH, Freedman MS, et al. Treatment with interferon beta-1b delays conversion to clinically definite and McDonald MS in patients with clinically isolated syndromes. Neurology 2006;67:1242–9.
16. Comi G, Martinelli V, Godegher M, et al. Effect of glatiramer acetate on conversion to clinically definite multiple sclerosis in patients with clinically isolated syndrome (PreCISe study): a randomized, double-blinded, placebo-controlled trial. Lancet 2009;374:1503–11.

Giant Cell Arteritis

Julie Falardeau, MD

KEYWORDS

- Arteritis • Giant cell • Ischemic optic neuropathy • Temporal

Giant cell arteritis (GCA), also known as temporal arteritis, is the most common primary systemic vasculitis in adults. GCA has a predilection for medium and large vessels, especially the extracranial branches of the carotid as well as the aorta and its large branches. Vision loss is the most dreaded complication of GCA, and when it occurs it tends to be profound and permanent. Prompt diagnosis and treatment are imperative to minimize the morbidity associated with visual loss.

EPIDEMIOLOGY

GCA affects almost exclusively Caucasian people over 50 years of age.[1,2] The incidence increases with age, being 20 times more common in the ninth compared with the sixth decade.[3] Women are 2 to 6 times more commonly affected than men.[4] GCA is more common in people of Northern European and Scandinavian descent, irrespective of their place of residence.[3,5]

CLINICAL MANIFESTATION

The spectrum of clinical manifestations associated with GCA encompasses a wide range of symptoms and signs. The onset of symptom can be sudden or may appear insidiously. Permanent vision loss is the best-known and most-feared complication of GCA. Being able to recognize and treat the disease before the onset of visual loss are critical.

Non-ophthalmic Manifestations

Systemic manifestations
The symptoms of systemic inflammation associated with GCA may include anorexia, asthenia, progressive weight loss, fever, arthralgia, myalgia, malaise, night sweats. At least one of these symptoms can be found at presentation in the majority of the patients but some patients have no systemic symptoms ("occult GCA").

Headache, neck, jaw and facial pain
Pain (headache, face, jaw, ear or neck pain) is the most common symptom of GCA and occurs in almost 90% of patients. The new onset of headache in any elderly patient should raise this diagnostic possibility. It is caused by arteritis affecting the carotid arteries and

Casey Eye Institute, Oregon Health and Science University, 3303 South West Bond Avenue, Portland, OR 97239, USA
E-mail address: falardea@ohsu.edu

Neurol Clin 28 (2010) 581–591
doi:10.1016/j.ncl.2010.03.002
0733-8619/10/$ – see front matter © 2010 Elsevier Inc. All rights reserved.

their branches. The location is characteristically temporal, although the headache can be frontal, parietal, or occipital.[6] Scalp tenderness related to tissue ischemia and temporal artery tenderness is also commonly seen. Patients will often report discomfort or pain when brushing or washing their hair. Scalp necrosis is a rare manifestation of GCA but carries a poor prognosis as the incidence of permanent vision loss (67%) and the mortality rate from cerebral or coronary artery occlusion (41%) are both significant.[7]

The presence of jaw claudication is highly specific for GCA but is not very sensitive (being present in less than half of patients at presentation).[6] Jaw claudication manifests as pain occurring after a few minutes of mastication and disappearing with rest. It is related to reduced blood flow to the masseter and temporalis muscles due to vasculitis and occlusive stenosis of the maxillary artery, a branch of the external carotid artery.[6] Less frequently, patients will report symptoms related to ischemia of the tongue, face, or neck.[8]

Neurologic manifestations

The most common neurologic complications from GCA are neuropathies, occurring in up to 14% of patients: peripheral polyneuropathy, cranial neuropathy, mononeuropathy multiplex, cervical radiculopathy, brachial plexopathy, or pure motor neuropathy.[9,10] Cerebrovascular ischemic events occur in 3%–4% of patients and are caused by severe obstruction or occlusion of the vertebral artery, and less commonly of the internal carotid artery.[9,11] With rare exceptions, this systemic vasculitis typically spares the intracranial and intradural arteries.[12]

Large-vessels manifestations

The manifestations of large-vessel involvement reflect the vascular compromise in the upper extremities. The superior branches of the aortic arch, particularly the subclavian and axillary arteries, are affected predominantly.[13] Involvement of the large arteries to the lower extremities occurs very infrequently. Large-vessel arteritis can present with claudication in the upper extremities, arterial bruit, absent or asymmetrical pulses and blood pressure measurements, peripheral paresthesia, Raynaud phenomenon, and rarely tissue gangrene.[14,15] Vasculitic inflammation of the aorta is often clinically silent. However, the presence of aortitis can lead to arterial dilation and aneurysm formation, which in turn can be complicated by aortic valve insufficiency, aortic rupture, or aortic dissection.[16] The diagnosis is often delayed since many patients with large-vessel vasculitis lack the systemic inflammatory symptoms.

Polymyalgia rheumatica

Polymyalgia rheumatica (PMR) is another inflammatory disorder affecting elderly patients but is two to three times more common than GCA.[17] PMR is typically characterized by bilateral aching pain and morning stiffness in the neck, shoulder, and pelvic girdles. Systemic manifestations like low-grade fever, malaise, weight loss, and anorexia can occur in up to 40% of patients with PMR.[18] Over one third of patients with GCA have PMR at presentation, and among patients with pure PMR clinically, the incidence of a positive temporal artery biopsy is 10%–20%.[19–21] Some patients will develop both conditions simultaneously and others will evolve from one condition to the other. Some authors consider PMR and GCA to be on the same spectrum of disease. While PMR and GCA are closely related, the mechanisms by which they are linked remain unknown.

Other non-ophthalmic manifestations

Mesenteric vasculitis resulting in small bowel infarction has only rarely been described with GCA but represents a serious complication. Cranial symptoms are lacking in nearly half of the patients with mesenteric vasculitis.[22,23]

Hearing loss, vertigo, dizziness, and disequilibrium were identified in nearly two thirds of patients with GCA in one study.[24] While vestibular dysfunction appeared responsive to treatment with corticosteroids, improvement of hearing loss was seen in less that 30% of patients.

Ophthalmic Manifestations

Ophthalmic manifestations are commonly seen in patients with GCA. In two large series, ocular signs or symptoms were present at the time of the initial presentation in 26% and 50% of patients, respectively.[25,26] Permanent visual loss is the best-known and most-feared complication of GCA. The visual loss is usually rapid, occurring over only a few days. It can be partial or complete but is typically permanent and devastating, with visual acuities at presentation of count fingers or worse in 54% of affected eyes.[27] Despite the wide use of corticosteroids, severe visual loss may still occur in 14%–20% of patients with GCA.[11,21]

Transient visual loss is a common manifestation of the disease, being reported by 30%–54% of patients with GCA.[25,26,28] It results from hypoperfusion of the optic nerve, retina, or choroid, and precedes permanent visual loss in up to half of untreated patients by an average of 8.5 days.[25,26,29]

Anterior ischemic optic neuropathy (AION) is the most common cause of permanent visual loss related to GCA, and is caused by inflammatory occlusion of the short posterior ciliary arteries resulting in infarction of the laminar or retrolaminar portion of the optic nerve head. Patients typically present with acute, monocular, and often profound vision loss. If untreated, unilateral arteritic AION may become bilateral within days to weeks in 50% of cases.[25,30] The presence of pallid optic disc edema, often described as "chalky white edema," in the acute phase is highly suggestive of GCA but the absence of pallid edema does not exclude GCA. Nerve fiber layer hemorrhages and cotton wool spots are not uncommon. An associated cilioretinal artery occlusion can be found in up to 21% of subjects.[31] Arteritic AION is frequently associated with choroidal ischemia and fluorescein angiography can be very helpful at detecting choroidal hypoperfusion and delayed choroidal filling.[25]

Other causes of permanent visual loss include retinal artery occlusion (central retinal artery occlusion, cilioretinal artery occlusion), occurring in 10%–13% of patients.[32] Less commonly, visual loss can be related to a posterior ischemic optic neuropathy, choroidal infarction, and optic chiasm or postchiasmal pathway ischemia.[29] Cortical blindness related to vertebrobasilar artery involvement is a rare complication of GCA.[26]

Transient or constant diplopia occurs in 5.9%–21% of patients with GCA.[25,26,28] Diplopia is induced by ischemia of the ocular motor nerves or less commonly of the extraocular muscles. Rarely, diplopia can be associated with brainstem ischemia.

GCA can rarely present with a constellation of orbital signs secondary to orbital ischemia or orbital infarction. Signs of orbital involvement include chemosis, ocular injection, proptosis, ophthalmoplegia, lid edema, and visual loss.[33]

It is extremely important to remember that the absence of systemic symptoms in a patient presenting with transient or permanent visual loss or diplopia does not exclude the possibility of GCA. Ocular involvement without the presence of other GCA symptoms occurs in 5%–38% of patients.[34]

DIAGNOSIS

Suspicion for GCA arises from the history, review of systems, and clinical findings, and is supported by abnormal serologic markers of inflammation. A temporal artery biopsy remains, however, the gold standard for diagnosis of GCA and is recommended in all suspected cases of GCA. In 1990 the American College of Rheumatology[35] analyzed 214 patients with GCA (196 proven by positive temporal artery biopsy) and compared them with 593 patients with other forms of vasculitis. If at least three or more criteria of the following five were met, the specificity of diagnosis was 91.2%, and the specificity was 93.5%:

1. Age of onset greater than 50 years
2. Onset of new headache
3. Temporal artery abnormalities (tenderness or reduced pulsation)
4. Elevated erythrocyte sedimentation rate (>50 mm/h using the Westergren method)
5. Positive temporal artery biopsy.

While useful for research purposes, these criteria do not take into account the presence of other important factors such as vision loss, jaw claudication, or elevated C-reactive protein. In addition, although rarely other vasculitic conditions may mimic the pathologic findings of GCA, a positive temporal artery biopsy has extremely high specificity for the diagnosis.

Serologic Markers

An elevated erythrocyte sedimentation rate (ESR) strongly supports a diagnosis of GCA, although ESR is a non-specific marker of inflammation and can be increased in other conditions such as malignancy, infection, trauma, connective tissues disorders, anemia, and hypercholesterolemia. While an elevated ESR is typically found in patients with GCA, a normal ESR does not exclude a diagnosis of GCA.[6] One empiric formula for the upper limit for a normal ESR is defined as the age divided by two for men, and the age plus 10 divided by two for women.[36]

C-reactive protein (CRP) is an acute-phase marker that is not sensitive to age related changes, gender, and hematological factors. CRP has a higher sensitivity for GCA compared with the ESR (97.5% vs 76%–86%). When used in conjunction witthe ESR,the combination of both serologic markers yield a sensitivity of 99%.[37]

Thrombocytosis is a common finding in GCA and has been positively correlated with biopsy-proven GCA. The presence of elevated platelets (>400 × 10³/L) associated with an elevated ESR appears to be highly predictive of GCA.[38,39] Some studies suggested that elevated platelet count (>400 × 10³/L) may be more specific than ESR and CRP in the diagnosis of GCA and in the presence of thrombocytosis, a diagnosis of GCA could potentially be six times more likely.[38,40] A normocytic, normochromic anemia is frequently associated with GCA although its presence is of little predictive value for a diagnosis of GCA.[40]

Several other inflammatory mediators are often elevated in GCA. Many of these are nonspecific markers of inflammation and contribute very little to the diagnosis of GCA. Interleukine-6 however has a potential role as an adjunctive test since it appears to be more sensitive than ESR in indicating disease activity.[41] Fibrinogen is often elevated in GCA and normal in other inflammatory conditions. Thus it can be an interesting additional test in a patient being investigated for GCA.

Temporal Artery Biopsy

Temporal artery biopsy (TAB) is the "gold standard" for the diagnosis of GCA and for most cases is recommended for suspected GCA. Even in the presence of a classic presentation, histologic confirmation is recommended since long-term treatment with corticosteroids is associated with significant complications. An adequate specimen should have a minimum length of 2 cm, and multiple sections should be examined given the possibility of skip lesions. While active arteritis can be detected histopathologically for 4–6 weeks after the initiation of corticosteroids, it is recommended to proceed with the biopsy within the first two weeks of steroid treatment. Although TAB is considered the gold standard test for diagnosis, a negative biopsy may be found in up to 10%–15% of patients with the disease.[42] False negative results can occur secondary to skip lesions or lack of involvement of the artery sampled. If the TAB result is negative and the suspicion of GCA is high, a contralateral biopsy should be performed. It has been shown however that if the first biopsy includes an adequate specimen and is examined adequately, there is virtually no diagnostic yield in doing a second biopsy.[43] Findings that tend to predict a positive biopsy include: presence of jaw claudication, neck pain, CRP > 2.45 mg/dL, ESR > 47 mm/hr, thrombocytosis, pallid optic disc edema, and temporal artery abnormalities.[6]

Histopathologically, the presence of focal areas of intimal hyperplasia, focal areas of fragmentation of inner elastic lamina, focal chronic inflammatory cell infiltrates, or focal concentric scars around the inner elastic lamina are highly consistent with the diagnosis of GCA.[43]

Imaging Studies

Color Doppler ultrasonography

Doppler ultrasonography can identify arterial stenosis and occlusion, as well as hypoechoic "halo" around the affected temporal artery (indicative of an edematous artery) in patients with GCA. In a meta-analysis of 23 studies including 2036 individuals, the overall sensitivity and specificity of the "halo sign" were 69% and 82% respectively compared with biopsy.[44] The sensitivity and specificity of any suggestive vessel abnormality were 88% and 78%, respectively. However, there was significant variation across the individual studies, possibly related to the skill and experience of the operator. In a study of 55 patients suspected of having GCA, the sensitivity of the halo sign was 82% with a specificity of 91% and 100% respectively for unilateral halo and bilateral halos.[45]

In the hands of expert, ultrasonography could be considered as an accurate modality for the diagnosis of GCA. However, it requires a high level of training, and these skills are not yet widespread. Therefore, in general usage, it is not currently considered as a replacement for a TAB. The greatest utility of ultrasonography may be in cases of bilateral halo sign in a patient with a high suspicion for GCA based on presentation, clinical findings, and abnormal serologic markers. Ultrasonography can also play an important role in guiding the biopsy site to avoid skip lesions, finding alternative sites other than the temporal arteries, and as part of the evaluation of the large vessel variant of GCA, in which the aorta and its branches are primarily involved.[44]

Magnetic resonance imaging

Magnetic resonance imaging (MRI) using a contrast-enhanced T_1-weighted sequence with fat saturation has shown to provide useful information for the diagnosis of GCA.[46] High resolution MRI (1.5 or preferably 3 Tesla) can detect increased wall thickness and edema, and mural contrast enhancement in the superficial cranial and extracranial arteries, and additionally in the ophthalmic arteries.[47,48] MRI can also identify mural contrast enhancement and luminal stenosis in patients with suspected aortitis and large vessel GCA.[49] In a series of 64 consecutive patients suspected of GCA, high resolution MRI had a sensitivity of 80.6% and a specificity of 97%.[47] The specificity is sufficiently high that a positive MRI combined with other clinical and laboratory data may be useful in diagnosis GCA. However, given the relatively low sensitivity of the test, a negative MRI would not be sufficient to exclude the diagnosis of GCA.[50]

High resolution MRI can be complemented by a magnetic resonance angiography (MRA) of the cervical and thoracic vasculature to assess the extracranial, large vessel involvement. Such combined high resolution MRI/MRA protocol does not require additional contrast injection and can be performed in less than 45 minutes. MRI/MRA can be useful in diagnostically challenging cases, when suspicion persists in the presence of bilateral negative TAB, and for assessing and monitoring aortitis, which can potentially lead to aortic dissection and aneurysm.[46,51] This costly imaging modality, however, is not ready to replace TAB.

Positron emission tomography

Two prospective studies were published on the value of fluorine-18-fluorodeoxyglucose position emission tomography (FDG-PET) for the diagnosis and monitoring of 35 patients with GCA.[52] Vascular FDG uptake was noted in 83% of patients with biopsy-proven GCA, especially at the subclavian arteries (74%), but also in the thoracic and abdominal aorta (>50%). Vascular FDG uptake is a sensitive marker for large vessel vasculitis. However, FDG-PET has a very limited role in the evaluation of medium-sized and superficial cranial arteries since it cannot evaluate appropriately vessels with diameter inferior to 2–4 mm.[47] In untreated patients with atypical presentations of GCA in whom the vasculitis probably does not involve the temporal arteries, FDG-PET could become the study of choice.[53,54]

TREATMENT
Corticosteroids

Corticosteroids have been the mainstay of treatment of GCA for the past several years and should be initiated immediately and aggressively to prevent visual loss or other ischemic events. There is no consensus on the starting dose, route of administration, and duration of treatment.[27] However, the vast majority of patients respond to a dose of a 1.0 to 1.5 mg/kg/d, or between 60–80 mg/d. Higher doses are suggested (80 to 100 mg/d) for patients with visual or neurologic symptoms of GCA.[27,55] The benefit of intravenous versus oral steroids has been evaluated and there is conflicting evidence over whether initial treatment of GCA with intravenous steroids provides superior preservation of vision as compared with oral steroids alone.[27,56–58] Some studies showed increased chance of visual recovery and reduced risk of contralateral involvement in the IV group.[34,58] However, other studies showed no difference in outcome.[56,59] Visual deterioration occurs in 27% of eyes despite high-dose intravenous methylprednisolone.[31] A recent study by Mazlumzadeh and coworkers[57] found that patients treated with a 3-day-course of IV methylprednisolone at a dose of 15 mg/kg/d could be tapered off steroids more quickly, had a lower frequency of relapse, and lower cumulative steroid doses. Regardless of the route of administration, there is general agreement that the initial treatment for a patient with GCA and new visual symptoms should be high-dose steroids and prompt treatment is paramount to prevent further visual loss and to control symptoms rapidly. Improvement of the headache and constitutional symptoms often begin within hours to days. A gradual steroid taper is considered when the clinical symptoms abate and the laboratory markers normalize. Most patients can discontinue steroids after 1 to 2 years of treatment; however, some patients will require corticosteroids for much longer. Alternate day steroid tapering regimens are not recommended as this practice can lead to relapse.

Other Immunosuppressive Agents

Long term corticosteroids therapy is associated with a number of adverse side effects. Patients with GCA are older and often have multiple co-morbidities. In one cohort, steroid-related adverse effects were seen in 86% of the patients, including fractures (44.6%), diabetes mellitus (10.6%), infection 35.9%, and gastrointestinal bleeding (4.8).[60] Other immunosuppressive drugs may be needed in patients with GCA to reduce the cumulative steroid dose. Methotrexate has been studies the most extensively; however there are conflicting messages from randomized controlled trials of methotrexate as a steroid sparing agent in GCA.[61–63] A recent meta-analysis of three randomized placebo-controlled trials suggests that methotrexate allows a small reduction in the cumulative dose, and a higher probability of steroid discontinuation.[64] Based on this analysis, methotrexate appears as a viable second-line alternative in patients with GCA and severe adverse reactions to steroids or steroid-refractory disease. However, it is unclear at present whether its adverse effects outweigh the adverse effects of prolonged corticosteroid use.

Tumor Necrosis Factor-α Blocking Agents

Granulomatous inflammation is typical of GCA and tumor necrosis factor-α (TNF-α) is important in the formation of granulomata.[65] Therefore, it could be expected that anti-TNF-α therapies potentially hold promise as adjunctive agents; however, current data does not provide much support for their role in the treatment of GCA (Hoffman 2007). The successful use of anti-TNF-α agents has been reported in cases of steroid-resistant GCA.[66] Another report of infliximab in steroid-naïve patients suggested an excellent initial response, but only lasting for 3 months.[67] Furthermore, a small randomized controlled trial of infliximab to maintain remission in newly diagnosed GCA was discontinued early due to inefficacy.[68] A recent randomized, placebo-controlled trial of etanercept in a small group of patients with GCA suggests that this may be a useful steroid-sparing agent, with more steroid discontinuation, and fewer relapses.[69] Further studies with larger groups of patients are needed to demonstrate the efficacy of anti-TNF-α agents in the treatment of GCA.

B-cell Depletion

Rituximab, an anti-CD 20 monoclonal antibody that depletes B cells, has been used in one patient with GCA, with resolution of the arteritis at 4.5 months. However, this patient subsequently developed pneumonia requiring mechanical ventilation.[70]

Aspirin

Aspirin may have protective effect against ischemic events caused by GCA, not only by inhibiting the formation of thrombus but also by virtue of its inhibitory effect on interferon-γ production, which is essential for the development of the inflammatory infiltrate in the vessel wall.[32] The role of aspirin is supported by a recent retrospective study showing low-dose aspirin to be effective in preventing visual loss and stroke in patients with GCA, without increasing hemorrhagic complications.[71] Prospective trials are needed to further evaluate the benefit of aspirin in the treatment of GCA.

PROGNOSIS

Causes of mortality associated with GCA include cardiovascular, neurologic, and gastrointestinal events. Vasculitis of the coronary arteries may result in myocardial infarction or congestive heart failure. The development of aortic aneurysm and aortic dissection are associated with reduced survival rate. Necrotizing segments of bowel are uncommon, but can be fatal. Patients with GCA are more likely than age and gender-matched controls to die within the first 5 years following the diagnosis.[72] Although visual loss does not impact on mortality, it has major complications for the quality of life and independent living. The prognosis for visual recovery is unfortunately poor.

SUMMARY

Giant cell arteritis is a systemic vasculitis of elderly individuals associated with significant morbidity. Vision loss is the most dreaded complication of GCA, and when it occurs it tends to be profound and permanent. Early disease recognition and immediate initiation of high dose steroid therapy is critical to save sight. Temporal artery biopsy remains the diagnostic "gold standard," and ESR, CRP, and platelet count are the primary serologic markers. Imaging studies such as MRI/MRA, FDG-PET, and Doppler ultrasonography are not routinely performed but may provide useful information in diagnostically difficult cases. Corticosteroids are the mainstay of treatment for GCA. Although the search for a safe and effective steroid-sparing agent continues, there is little convincing evidence that any of these agents are really helpful. Low-dose aspirin may be beneficial in preventing ischemic complications of GCA.

REFERENCES

1. Smith Carolyn A, Fidler WJ, Pinals RS. The epidemiology of giant cell arteritis. Report of a ten-year study in Shelby County, Tennessee. Arthritis Rheum 1983; 26:1214–9.
2. Liu NH, LaBree LD, Feldon SE, et al. The epidemiology of giant cell arteritis. Ophthalmology 2001;108:1145–9.
3. Machado EBV, Michet CJ, Ballard DJ, et al. Trends in incidence and clinical presentation of temporal arteritis in Olmstead County, Minnesota, 1950–1985. Arthritis Rheum 1988;31:745–9.
4. Hunder GG. Epidemiology of giant cell arteritis. Cleve Clin J Med 2002;69(Suppl 2): 79–82.
5. Baldursson O, Steinsson K, Bjornsson J, et al. Giant cell arteritis in Iceland. An epidemiologic and histopathologic analysis. Arthritis Rheum 1994;37:1007–12.
6. Hayreh SS, Podhajsky PA, Raman R, et al. Giant cell arteritis: validity and reliability of various diagnostic criteria. Am J Ophthalmol 1997;123:285–96.
7. Campbell FA, Clark C, Holmes S. Scalp necrosis in temporal arteritis. Clin Exp Dermatol 2003;28:488–90.
8. McDonnell PJ, Moore GW, Miller NR, et al. Temporal arteritis. A clinicopathologic study. Ophthalmology 1986;93:518–30.
9. Caselli RJ, Hunder GG, Whisnant JP. Neurologic disease in biopsy-proven giant cell (temporal) arteritis. Neurology 1988;38:352–9.
10. Pfadenhauer K, Roesler A, Golling A. The involvement of the peripheral nervous system in biopsy-proven active giant cell arteritis. J Neurol 2007;254:751–5.
11. Gonzales-Gay MA, Blanco R, Rodriguez-Valverdere V, et al. Permanent visual loss and cerebrovascular accidents in giant cell arteritis: predictors and response to treatment. Arthritis Rheum 1998;41:1497–504.
12. Salvarani C, Giannnini C, Miller DV, et al. Giant cell arteritis: involvement of intracranial arteries. Arthritis Rheum 2006;55:985–9.
13. Brack A, Martinez-Taboada V, Stanson A. Disease pattern in cranial and large-vessel giant cell arteritis. Arthritis Rheum 1999;42:311–7.
14. Klein RG, Hunder GG, Stanson AW, et al. Large artery involvement in giant cell (temporal) arteritis. Ann Intern Med 1975;83:806–12.
15. Levine SM, Hellman DB. Giant cell arteritis. Curr Opin Rheumatol 2002;14:3–10.

16. Nuenninghoff DM, Hunder GG, Christianson TJ, et al. Incidence and predictors of large-artery complication (aortic aneurysm, aortic dissection, and/or large-artery stenosis) in patients with giant cell arteritis: a population-based study over 50 years. Arthritis Rheum 2003;48:3522–31.

17. Smeeth L, Cook C, Hall AJ. Incidence of diagnosed polymyalgia rheumatica and giant cell arteritis in the United Kingdom, 1990–2001. Ann Rheum Dis 2006;65: 1093–8.

18. Salvarani C, Cantini F, Hunder GG. Polymyalgia rheumatica and giant-cell arteritis. Lancet 2008;372:234–45.

19. Dasgupta B, Matteson EL, Maradit-Kremers H. Management guidelines and outcome measures in polymyalgia rheumatica (PMR). Clin Exp Rheumatol 2007;25:S130–6.

20. Hunder GG. The early history of giant cell arteritis and polymyalgia rheumatica: first descriptions to 1970. Mayo Clin Proc 2006;81:1071–83.

21. Salvarani C, Cantini F, Boiardi L, et al. Polymyalgia rheumatica and giant-cell arteritis. N Engl J Med 2002;347:261–71.

22. Annamalai A, Francis ML, Ranatunga SKM, et al. Giant cell arteritis presenting as small bowel infarction. J Gen Intern Med 2007;22:140–4.

23. Scola CJ, Li C, Upchurch KS. Mesenteric involvement in giant cell arteritis. An under-recognized complication? Analysis of a case series with clinicoanatomic correlation. Medicine 2008;87:45–51.

24. Amor-Dorado JC, Llorca J, Garcia-Porrua C, et al. Audiovestibular manifestations in giant cell arteritis: a prospective study. Medicine 2003;82:13–26.

25. Hayreh SS, Podhajsky PA, Zimmerman B. Ocular manifestations of giant cell arteritis. Am J Ophthalmol 1998;125:509–20.

26. Gonzales-Gay MA, Garcia-Porrua C, Llorca J, et al. Visual manifestations of giant cell arteritis: trends and clinical spectrum in 161 patients. Medicine 2000;79(5):283–92.

27. Hayreh SS, Zimmerman B. Management of giant cell arteritis. Our 27-year clinical study: new light on old controversies. Ophthalmologica 2003;217:239–59.

28. Glutz Von Blotzheim S, Borruat FX. Neuro-ophthalmic complications of biopsy-proven giant cell arteritis. Eur J Ophthalmol 1997;7:375–82.

29. Miller NR. Visual manifestations of temporal arteritis. Rheum Dis Clin North Am 2001;27:781–97.

30. Arnold AC. Ischemic optic neuropathy. In: Miller NR, Newman NJ, Biousse V, et al, editors. Clinical neuro-ophthalmology, vol. 1. 6th edition. Philadelphia: Williams & Wilkins; 2005. p. 349–84.

31. Danesh-Meyer H, savino PJ, Gamble GG. Poor prognosis of visual outcome after visual loss from giant cell arteritis. Ophthalmology 2005;112:1098–103.

32. Kawasaki A, Purvin V. Giant cell arteritis: an updated review. Acta Ophthalmol 2009;87:13–32.

33. Lee AG, Tang RA, Feldon SE, et al. Orbital presentations of giant cell arteritis. Graefes Arch Clin Exp Ophthalmol 2001;239:509–13.

34. Liu GT, Glaser JS, Schatz NJ, et al. Visual morbidity in giant cell arteritis. Clinical characteristics and prognosis for vision. Ophthalmology 1994;101:1779–85.

35. Hunder GG, Bloch DA, Michel BA, et al. The American College of Rheumatology 1990 criteria for the classification of giant cell arteritis. Arthritis Rheum 1990;33:1122–8.

36. Miller A, Green M, Robinson D. Simple rule for calculating normal erythrocyte sedimentation rate. Br Med J (Clin Res Ed) 1983;286:266.

37. Parikh M, Miller NR, Lee AG, et al. Prevalence of a normal C-reactive protein with an elevated erythrocyte sedimentation rate in biopsy-proven giant cell arteritis. Ophthalmology 2006;113:1842–5.

38. Foroozan R, Danesh-Meyer H, Savino PJ, et al. Thrombocytosis in patients with biopsy-proven giant cell arteritis. Ophthalmology 2002;109:1267–71.
39. Costello F, Zimmerman B, Podhajsky PA, et al. Role of thrombocytosis in diagnosis of giant cell arteritis and differentiation of arteritic from non-arteritic anterior ischemic optic neuropathy. Eur J Ophthalmol 2004;14:245–57.
40. Niederkohr R, Levin LA. Management of the patient with suspected temporal arteritis. Ophthalmology 2005;112:744–56.
41. Weyand CM, Fulbright JW, Hunder GG, et al. Treatment of giant cell arteritis: interleukine-6 as a biologic marker of disease activity. Arthritis Rheum 2000;43:1041–8.
42. Schmidt WA. Current diagnosis and treatment of temporal arteritis. Curr Treat Options Cardiovasc Med 2006;8:145–51.
43. Zhou L, Luneau K, Weyand CM, et al. Clinicopathologic correlations in giant cell arteritis. Ophthalmology 2009;116:1574–80.
44. Schmidt WA, Kraft HE, Vorpahl K, et al. Color duplex ultrasonography useful for the diagnosis of temporal arteritis. N Engl J Med 1997;337:1336–42.
45. Karahaliou M, Vaiopoulos G, Papaspyrou S, et al. Colour duplex sonography of temporal arteries before decision for biopsy: a prospective study in 55 patients with suspected giant cell arteritis. Arthritis Res Ther 2006;8:R116.
46. Blockmans D, Bley T, Schmidt W. Imaging for large-vessel vasculitis. Curr Opin Rheumatol 2009;21:19–28.
47. Bley TA, Uhl M, Carew J, et al. Diagnostic value of high-resolution MR imaging in giant cell arteritis. AJNR Am J Neuroradiol 2007;28:1722–7.
48. Geiger J, ness T, Uhl M, et al. Involvement of the ophthalmic artery in giant cell arteritis visualized by 3T MRI. Rheumatology 2009;48:537–41.
49. Narvaez J, Narvaez JJ, Nolla JM, et al. Giant cell arteritis and polymyalgia rheumatic: usefulness of vascular magnetic resonance imaging studies in the diagnosis of aortitis. Rheumatology 2005;44:479–83.
50. Khoury JA, Hoxworth JM, Mazlumzadeh M, et al. The clinical utility of high-resolution magnetic resonance imaging in the diagnosis of giant cell arteritis. Neurologist 2008;14(5):330–5.
51. Hall JK. Giant cell arteritis. Curr Opin Ophthalmol 2008;19:454–60.
52. Blockmans D, De Ceuninck L, Vanderschueren S, et al. Repetitive 18F-fluorodeoxyglucose position emission tomography in giant cell arteritis: a prospective study of 35 patients. Arthritis Rheum 2006;55:131–7.
53. De Winter F, Petrovic M, Van de Wiele C, et al. Imaging of giant cell arteritis: evidence of splenic involvement using FDG positron emission tomography. Clin Nucl Med 2000;25:633–4.
54. Janssen SP, Comans EH, Voskuyl AE, et al. Giant cell arteritis: heterogeneity in clinical presentation and imaging results. J Vasc Surg 2008;48(4):1025–31.
55. Fraser JA, Weyand CM, Newman NJ, et al. The treatment of giant cell arteritis. Rev Neurol Dis 2008;5(3):140–52.
56. Chevalet P, Barrier JH, Pottier O, et al. A randomized, multicenter, controlled trial using intravenous pulses of methylprednisolone in the initial treatment if simple forms of giant cell arteritis: a one year follow-up study of 164 patients. J Rheumatol 2000;27:1484–91.
57. Mazlumzadeh M, Hunder GG, Easly KA, et al. Treatment of giant cell arteritis using induction therapy with high-dose corticosteroids: a double-blind, placebo-controlled, randomized prospective clinical trial. Arthritis Rheum 2006;54:3310–8.

58. Chan CCK, Paine M, O'Day J. Steroid management in giant cell arteritis. Br J Ophthalmol 2001;85:1061–4.
59. Hayreh SS, Zimmerman B, Kardon RH. Visual improvement with corticosteroid therapy in giant cell arteritis: report of a large study and review of the literature. Acta Ophthalmol Scand 2002;80:353–67.
60. Proven A, Gabriel SK, Orces C, et al. Glucocorticoid therapy in giant cell arteritis: duration and adverse outcomes. Arthritis Rheum 2003;49(5):703–8.
61. Spiera R, Mitnick H, Kupersmith M, et al. A prospective, double-blind, randomized, placebo controlled trial of methotrexate in the treatment of giant cell arteritis. Clin Exp Rheumatol 2001;19:495–501.
62. Hoffman GS, Cic MC, Hellmann DB, et al. A multicenter, randomized, double-blind, placebo-controlled trial of adjuvant methotrexate treatment for giant cell arteritis. Arthritis Rheum 2002;46:1309–18.
63. Jover JA, Hernandez-Garcia C, Morado I, et al. Combined treatment of giant cell arteritis with methotrexate and prednisone. Ann Intern Med 2001;134:106–14.
64. Marh AD, Jover JA, Spiera RF, et al. Adjunctive methotrexate for treatment of giant cell arteritis: an individual patient data meta-analysis. Arthritis Rheum 2007;56:2789–97.
65. Borg FA, Dasgupta B. Treatment and outcomes of large vessel arteritis. Best Pract Res Clin Rheumatol 2009;23(3):325–37.
66. Cantini F, Niccoli L, Salvarani C, et al. Treatment of longstanding active giant cell arteritis with infliximab. Arthritis Rheum 2001;44(12):2933–5.
67. Andonopoulos AP, Meimaris N, Daoussis D, et al. Experience of infliximab (anti-TNFα monoclonal antibody) as monotherapy for giant cell arteritis. Ann Rheum Dis 2003;62:1116.
68. Hoffman GS, Cic MC, Rendt-Zagar KE, et al. infliximab for maintenance of glucocorticosteroid-induced remission of giant cell arteritis: a randomized trial. Ann Intern Med 2007;146:621–30.
69. Martinez-Taboada VM, Rodriguez-Valverde V, Carreno L, et al. A double-blind placebo controlled trial of etanercept in patients with giant cell arteritis and corticosteroid side effects. Ann Rheum Dis 2007;67(5):625–30.
70. Bhatia A, Ell PJ, Edwards JCW. Anti-CD20 monoclonal antibody (Rituximab) as an adjunct in the treatment of giant cell arteritis. Ann Rheum Dis 2005;64:1099–100.
71. Nesher G, Berkun Y, Mates M, et al. Low dose aspirin and prevention of cranial ischemic complications in giant cell arteritis. Arthritis Rheum 2004;50:1332–7.
72. Crow RW, Katz BJ, Warner JA, et al. Giant cell arteritis and mortality. J Gerontol A Biol Sci Med Sci 2009;64(3):365–9.

Idiopathic Intracranial Hypertension

Michael Wall, MD[a,b,*]

KEYWORDS

• Idiopathic intracranial hypertension • Pseudotumor cerebri
• Papilledema • Visual loss

Idiopathic intracranial hypertension (IIH) is a disorder of increased cerebrospinal fluid (CSF) pressure of unknown cause. Quincke in 1897 reported the first cases of IIH shortly after he introduced the lumbar puncture into medicine. It was named pseudo-tumor cerebri in 1904 but was not well delineated clinically until the 1940s when cerebral angiography was added to pneumoencephalography to identify cases of cerebral mass lesions. Foley coined the term benign intracranial hypertension in 1955 but reports from the 1980s showed a high incidence of visual loss,[1,2] and the term benign is no longer appropriate.

IIH is a syndrome characterized by increased intracranial pressure that usually occurs in obese women in the childbearing years. The signs and symptoms of intracranial hypertension are that the patient maintains an alert and oriented mental state, but has no localizing neurologic findings. There is no evidence of deformity or obstruction of the ventricular system and neurodiagnostic studies are otherwise normal except for increased CSF pressure (>200 mm H_2O, in the nonobese and probably >250 mm H_2O in the obese patient).[3] Neuroimaging signs of increased intracranial pressure include empty sella syndrome, lateral sinus collapse (smooth-walled venous stenoses, **Fig. 1**), flattened globes, and fully unfolded optic nerve sheaths. In addition, no secondary cause of intracranial hypertension can be found. This definition comprises the modified Dandy criteria for IIH.[4]

The symptoms of increased intracranial pressure are headache, pulse synchronous tinnitus (pulsatile tinnitus), transient visual obscurations, and visual loss. Signs are

This study was supported in part by an unrestricted grant to the Department of Ophthalmology from Research to Prevent Blindness, New York, USA, Va Merit Review Support grant and NIH U10 EY017281.

[a] Department of Neurology, College of Medicine, University of Iowa, Veterans Administration Medical Center, Iowa City, IA 52242, USA
[b] Department of Ophthalmology and Visual Sciences, College of Medicine, University of Iowa, Veterans Administration Medical Center, Iowa City, IA 52242, USA
* Department of Neurology, College of Medicine, University of Iowa, Veterans Administration Medical Center, Iowa City, IA 52242.
E-mail address: michael-wall@uiowa.edu

Neurol Clin 28 (2010) 593–617
doi:10.1016/j.ncl.2010.03.003
0733-8619/10/$ – see front matter

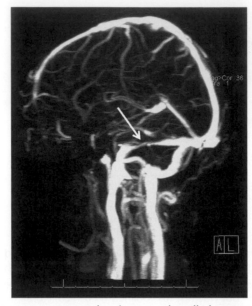

Fig. 1. Magnetic resonance venogram showing smooth-walled venous stenoses of the transverse sinus, characteristic of IIH.

diplopia caused by sixth cranial nerve (CN) paresis and papilledema with its associated loss of sensory visual function. The only major morbidity with IIH is visual loss.

EPIDEMIOLOGY

The annual incidence of IIH is 0.9/100,000 persons and 3.5/100,000 in women 15 to 44 years of age. It is increasing in incidence in parallel with the current epidemic of obesity.[5,6] In obese women aged 20 to 44 years who were 20% (or greater) more than ideal weight, the incidence of IIH was 19 per 100,000.[5] More than 90% of patients with IIH are obese and more than 90% are women of childbearing age. Although symptoms and signs may be recurrent in at least 10%, asymptomatic increased intracranial pressure may persist for years.[7] The mean age at the time of diagnosis is about 30 years.[8]

Studies of conditions associated with IIH are mostly uncontrolled and retrospective. This situation has led to erroneous conclusions because investigators have tried to implicate IIH using chance and spurious associations with common medical conditions and medications. Also, there are a host of case reports of associations with IIH in which the cases do not meet the modified Dandy criteria of IIH.

Box 1 lists the causes of intracranial hypertension that meet the modified Dandy criteria for IIH except when a cause is associated. The highly likely category is a list of cases with many reports of the association with multiple lines of evidence. Probable causes have reports with some convincing evidence. Possible causes have suggestive evidence or are common conditions or medications with intracranial hypertension as a rare association. Also listed are some frequently cited but poorly documented or unlikely causes; 3 case-control studies suggest these associations are not valid.[9–11]

Any disorder that causes decreased flow through the arachnoid granulations or obstructs the venous pathway from the granulations to the right heart is accepted

Box 1	
Differential diagnosis of IIH (cases must meet the modified Dandy criteria of IIH except when a cause is found)	

Highly likely

Decreased flow through arachnoid granulations

    Scarring from previous inflammation (eg, meningitis, sequel to subarachnoid hemorrhage)

Obstruction to venous drainage

    Venous sinus thromboses

        Hypercoaguable states

        Contiguous infection (eg, middle ear or mastoid-otitic hydrocephalus)

    Bilateral radical neck dissections

    Superior vena cava syndrome

    Glomus tumor

    Increased right heart pressure

Endocrine disorders

    Addison disease

    Hypoparathyroidism

    Obesity

    Steroid withdrawal

    Growth hormone use in children

Nutritional disorders

    Hypervitaminosis A (vitamin, liver, or isotretinoin intake and all-*trans* retinoic acid for acute promyelocytic leukemia)

    Hyperalimentation in deprivation dwarfism

Arteriovenous malformations and dural shunts

Probable causes

Anabolic steroids (may cause venous sinus thrombosis)

Chlordecone (kepone)

Ketoprofen or indomethacin in Bartter syndrome

Systemic lupus erythematosus via venous sinus thrombosis

Thyroid-replacement therapy in hypothyroid children

Tetracycline and its derivative

Uremia

Possible causes

Amiodarone

Hypovitaminosis A

Iron-deficiency anemia

Lithium carbonate

Nalidixic acid

Sarcoidosis

Sulfa antibiotics

Causes frequently cited that are unproven and unlikely

Corticosteroid intake

Hyperthyroidism

Menarche

Menstrual irregularities

Multivitamin intake

Oral contraceptive use

Pregnancy

as a cause of intracranial hypertension because of its biologic plausibility. Arteriovenous malformations or dural fistulae with high flow may overload venous return and result in increase of intracranial pressure.

Although steroid withdrawal and Addison disease are clearly associated with IIH,[12–14] as is hypoparathyroidism, links to other endocrine abnormalities remain unproven. For example, corticosteroid use has been associated with many suspected cases of IH; however, none of the cases fulfill the modified Dandy criteria.

Several other purported associations with IIH have been refuted by controlled studies. Pregnancy, irregular menses, and oral contraceptive use have been shown to be simply chance associations.[5,11,15] In case-control studies, no association is found between IIH and multivitamin, oral contraceptive, corticosteroid, or antibiotic use.[10,11] However, case reports associating some drugs seem convincing: nalidixic acid,[16] nitrofurantoin,[17] indomethacin,[18] or ketoprofen in Bartter syndrome,[19] vitamin A intoxication,[20] isotretinoin,[21] thyroid-replacement therapy in hypothyroid children,[22] lithium,[23] and anabolic steroids.[24] Corticosteroid use is not associated with intracranial hypertension, but steroid withdrawal clearly is linked.[12,13]

Arterial hypertension has been associated with IIH.[7,11] However, spuriously increased blood pressure is commonly reported in obese people as a result of the use of standard size rather than oversize sphygmomanometer cuffs and obesity is associated with arterial hypertension. It is unlikely that there is a direct association of arterial hypertension and IIH.

A case-control study has found strong associations between IIH and obesity and with weight gain during the 12 months before IIH diagnosis. In this study, there was no evidence that IIH was associated with any other medical conditions or pregnancy.[11] Other than obesity and recent weight gain, many conditions believed to be associated with IIH are just common disorders of women in childbearing years and are likely chance associations.

PATHOGENESIS

Any hypothesis of pathogenesis of IIH should explain the following observations of patients with the disorder:

1. High rate of occurrence in obese women during the childbearing years
2. Reduced conductance to CSF outflow[25]
3. Normal ventricular size; no hydrocephalus[26]
4. No histologic evidence of cerebral edema.[27]

Changes in cerebral hemodynamics (ie, increased cerebral blood volume and decreased cerebral blood flow) have been reported.[28] However, others have found no significant changes in these factors.[29] The most popular hypothesis is that IIH is a syndrome of reduced CSF absorption. Decreased conductance to CSF outflow may be caused by dysfunction of the absorptive mechanism of the arachnoid granulations or possibly through the extracranial lymphatics.[30] This latter mechanism of an alternative route of drainage along extracranial and spinal nerve roots to the extracranial lymphatics, proposed by Miles Johnston and coworkers,[30] may be an important factor in the mechanism of IIH, because this route may account for a substantial percentage of CSF absorption.

So, regardless of the outflow mechanism, if outflow resistance is increased then intracranial pressure must increase for CSF to be absorbed. Although interstitial and intracellular edema have been reported in brain biopsy specimens,[31] a study with current methods of analysis has concluded that the histologic features of the brain parenchyma are normal and the findings from the initial report are artifactual.[27]

CLINICAL FEATURES

The symptoms of patients with IIH are headache (94%), transient visual obscurations (68%), pulse synchronous tinnitus (58%), photopsia (54%), and retrobulbar pain (44%). Diplopia (38%) and visual loss (30%) are less common accompaniments of IIH; however, some of these symptoms are common in controls (**Fig. 2**).

Headache

The presence of headache is common in patients with IIH and is the usual presenting symptom. The headache profile of the patient with IIH[32] is that of severe daily pulsatile headaches. They are different from previous headaches, may awaken the patient and usually last hours. The headache is often reported as the worst head pain

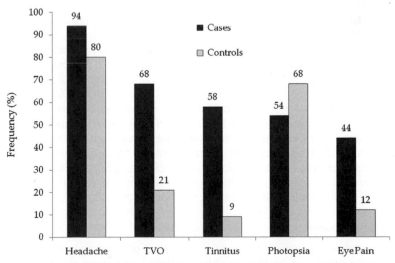

Fig. 2. Frequency in percent of symptoms in IIH and a control group. TVO, transient visual obscurations; ICN, intracranial noises. (*Reprinted from* Giuseffi V, Wall M, Siegel PZ, et al. Symptoms and disease associations in idiopathic intracranial hypertension (pseudotumor cerebri): a case-control study. Neurology 1991;41:239–44; with permission.)

experienced. Associated nausea is common, but vomiting is uncommon. In addition, other headache syndromes frequently coexist such as rebound headache from analgesic or caffeine overuse and require their own therapy.[33]

Transient Visual Obscurations

Visual obscurations are episodes of transient blurred vision that usually last less than 30 seconds and are followed by visual recovery to baseline. Visual obscurations occur in about two-thirds of patients with IIH.[8] The symptoms may be monocular or binocular. The cause of these episodes is believed to be transient ischemia of the optic nerve head related to increased tissue pressure.[34] Although transient visual obscurations are anxiety provoking for the patient, they do not seem to be associated with poor visual outcome.[8]

Pulse-synchronous Tinnitus

Pulsatile intracranial noises or pulse-synchronous tinnitus is common in IIH.[11] The sound is often unilateral, with neither side predominating. In patients with intracranial hypertension, jugular compression or head turning ipsilateral to the sound abolishes it.[35] The sound is believed to be caused by transmission of intensified vascular pulsations by means of CSF under high pressure and turbulence through smooth-walled venous stenoses related to transverse sinus collapse from high CSF pressure (see **Fig. 1**).[36]

The major signs of IIH are papilledema and sixth nerve paresis.

Ophthalmoscopic Examination

Papilledema (optic disc edema caused by increased intracranial pressure) is the cardinal sign of IIH. Optic disc edema either directly or indirectly is the cause of visual loss of IIH. The higher the grade of the papilledema, the worse the visual loss,[37] but, in the individual patient, the severity of visual loss cannot accurately be predicted from the severity of the papilledema. A partial explanation for this situation is that with axonal death from compression of the optic nerve, the amount of papilledema decreases.

Frisén[38] has proposed a useful staging scheme for papilledema with good sensitivity and specificity based on the ophthalmoscopic signs of disturbed axoplasmic transport. It has been modified recently,[39] with a key finding added for each stage or grade. Grade 0 represents a normal optic disc. Grade 1 is characterized by the presence of a C-shaped or reverse C-shaped halo of peripapillary edema obscuring the retina adjacent to the optic disc. The temporal border of the optic disc is spared, presumably because of the fine caliber of these axons (**Fig. 3**). The C-shaped halo becomes circumferential with grade 2 papilledema (**Fig. 4**). In grade 3 papilledema, there is complete obscuration of at least 1 major vessel as it leaves the optic disc (**Fig. 5**). With the increased optic disc edema of grade 4 there is complete obscuration of at least 1 major vessel on the optic disc (**Fig. 6**). Grade 5 is characterized by total obscuration of at least 1 vessel on the disc and leaving the disc and at least partial obscuration of all major vessels leaving or on the disc (**Fig. 7**).

Ocular Motility Disturbances

Horizontal diplopia is reported by about one-third of patients with IIH, and sixth nerve palsies are found in 10% to 20%.[8] Motility disturbances other than sixth nerve palsies have been reported. Some of these reflect erroneous conclusions from the small vertical ocular motor imbalance that is known to accompany sixth nerve palsies. Bell-type palsies of CN VII rarely occur and are usually transient.

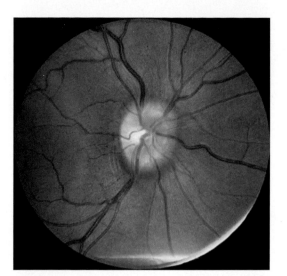

Fig. 3. Characteristic C-shaped halo with a temporal gap surrounding the disc of early of (Frisén grade 1) papilledema.

The common thread here is that the CNs that make nearly a 90° bend (CN II, VI, VII) seem to be susceptible to damage at the site of the bend.[40] The diagnosis of IIH should be viewed with suspicion in patients with ocular motility disturbances other than sixth nerve palsies.

Sensory Visual Function

Visual acuity usually remains normal in patients with papilledema except when the condition is long standing and severe or if there is a serous retinal detachment present and optic disc edema extends to the macula. Snellen acuity testing is insensitive to the

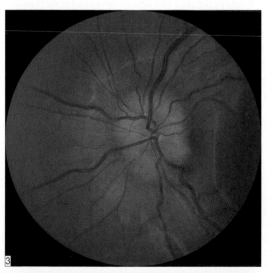

Fig. 4. With grade 2 papilledema the halo becomes circumferential.

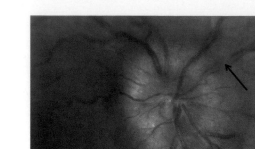

Fig. 5. Grade 3 papilledema is characterized by loss of major vessels as they leave the disc (*arrow*).

amount of visual loss present when compared with perimetry. It is also insensitive to worsening of papilledema grade.[8]

Perimetry

Visual field loss occurs in almost all cases of IIH. In a prospective study of IIH, visual loss in at least 1 eye (other than enlargement of the physiologic blind spot) was found in 96% of patients with Goldmann perimetry using a disease-specific strategy and in 92% with automated perimetry.[8,41] About one-third of this visual loss is mild and unlikely to be noticed by the patient but serves as a marker with which to guide therapy.[8]

The visual field defects found in IIH are the same types as those reported to occur in papilledema resulting from other causes. The most common defects are enlargement of the physiologic blind spot and loss of inferonasal portions of the visual field along with constriction of isopters (**Fig. 8**). Central defects are distinctly uncommon and warrant a search for another diagnosis unless there is a large serous retinal detachment from high-grade optic disc edema spreading toward the macula. The loss of visual field may be progressive and severe, leading to blindness in about 5% of cases. The time course of visual loss is usually gradual; however, acute severe visual loss can occur.

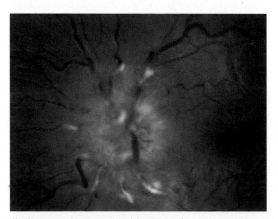

Fig. 6. Grade 4 papilledema is characterized by loss of major vessels on the disc.

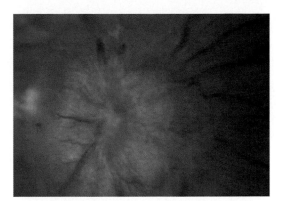

Fig. 7. Grade 5 has the criteria of grade 4 plus partial or total obscuration of all vessels on the disc.

The earliest visual field defect in IIH is often an inferior nasal step defect (see **Fig. 8**) followed by peripheral nasal loss. Arcuate defects may appear next followed by a gradual depression of the entire field, most pronounced peripherally (**Fig. 9**).

Blind spot enlargement is ubiquitous in IIH. Because refraction often eliminates this defect,[42] blind spot enlargement should not be considered significant visual loss unless it encroaches on fixation. Also, because blind spot size is so dependent on refraction, it should not be used to follow the course of therapy.

With treatment there is significant perimetric improvement in about 50% of patients.[8] A study that evaluated a subgroup of patients with worsening of their vision showed that recent weight gain was the only factor significantly associated with decline in vision.[8] Other groups at risk for severe visual loss are black men, those with glaucoma, and patients being rapidly tapered off corticosteroids. The course of IIH is often chronic, with recurrences especially during periods of weight gain.[43]

MECHANISMS OF VISUAL LOSS

The visual field defects found in patients with IIH are optic disc related. They are the type found when nerve fiber bundles are damaged at the level of the optic disk. These types of defects also occur with glaucoma and anterior ischemic optic neuropathy. This finding suggests a common mechanism for the visual loss in these disorders.

Degree of Papilledema and Visual Loss

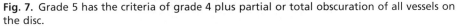

Is visual loss related to degree of papilledema or is the amount of optic disc edema an independent factor? A study of patients with highly asymmetric papilledema was aimed at answering this question.[37] The patients were tested with automated perimetry and a variety of sensory visual function tests. A generalized depression of the visual field in eyes with high-grade papilledema was found. The visual loss increased in magnitude with increasing visual field eccentricity, and although nerve fiber bundlelike defects were frequently observed, visual loss occurred across the visual field. However, this finding was appreciated only when a comparison was made with the low-grade papilledema eye, because the values of the tests of foveal visual function in the high-grade papilledema eye remain in the normal range but are significantly depressed compared with controls or the low-grade eye.

This study and another[44] showed that the amount of visual loss correlates with the severity of disc edema: eyes with more disc edema had more visual loss (**Fig. 10**).

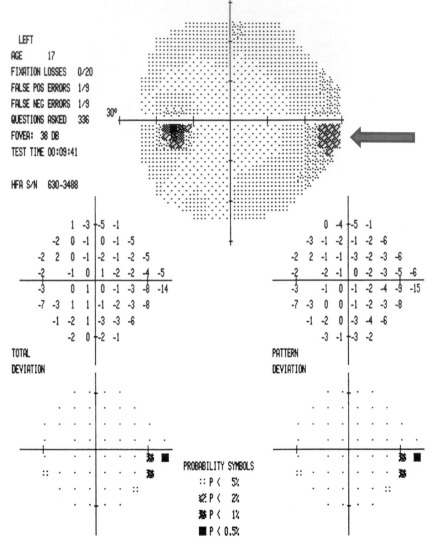

Fig. 8. A typical inferonasal step defect (*arrow*) of early optic disc edema in IIH.

However, there was considerable interindividual variation. That is, some patients with marked optic disc edema appeared to have mild or no visual loss unless a comparison was made with a fellow eye with less disc edema. This relationship of degree of papilledema with visual loss implies that visual loss in IIH occurs because of papilledema (at the optic disc) and not from visual damage occurring posterior to the optic disc.

Factors Interacting with Optic Disc Edema that Lead to Visual Loss

The occurrence of papilledema primarily depends on the relationship of 3 factors: CSF pressure, intraocular pressure, and systemic blood pressure.[45] Increased CSF pressure, low intraocular pressure, or low perfusion pressure can cause axoplasmic flow stasis, optic disc edema, and resultant intraneuronal ischemia.

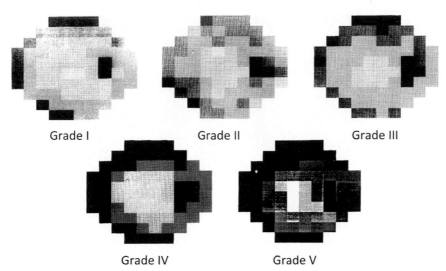

Grade I   Grade II   Grade III

Grade IV   Grade V

Fig. 9. Grades of visual loss in IIH found by grading the visual field examinations and then averaging the values from within each grade.

Hayreh[46] showed the nerve sheath is composed of fibrous tissue and after it unfolds, it cannot expand any further. Optic nerve width is greatest just behind the globe and narrowest within the optic canal. Thick fibrous bands within the canalicular nerve sheath interrupt the subarachnoid space (**Fig. 11**). Hayreh[46] found the number of these bands varied from animal to animal and was sometimes scanty. He observed in monkeys and man that when dye was injected into the optic nerve sheath, fluid usually passed easily into the cranial cavity. The force needed depended on the quality of the fibrous bands within the subarachnoid space. Although the dye usually flowed freely, it concentrated in the subarachnoid space adjacent to the optic canals. There may be differences within individuals in this trabecular meshwork of the optic nerve sheath subarachnoid space contiguous with the optic canal.

Relationship of Papilledema to Visual Loss

As stated earlier, the site of histologic damage in visual loss caused by increased intra-cranial pressure is at the optic disc. Brain parenchyma tolerates generalized raised

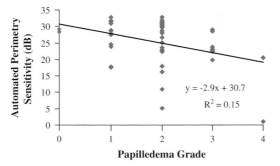

Fig. 10. Relationship of visual field loss by mean threshold value and papilledema grade. *From* Wall M. The morphology of visual field damage in idiopathic intracranial hypertension: an anatomic region analysis. In: Mills RP, Heijl A, editors. Perimetry update 1990/1991. Amsterdam: Kugler Publications; 1991. p. 20–7.

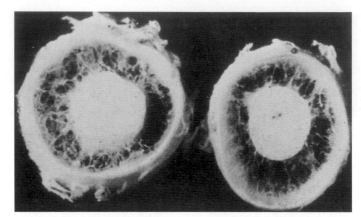

Fig. 11. Gross pathologic specimen of optic nerve (central core), optic nerve sheath, and arachnoid trabeculations in between. Note the well-developed series of arachnoid trabeculations and the fully unfolded optic nerve sheaths. *From* Cogan DG. Neurology of the visual system, ed 6. Springfield (IL): Charles C. Thomas Publisher; 1966; with permission.

intracranial pressure well. Patients do not develop hemianopias. It is unlikely that the intracranial or intraorbital optic nerve is the location of the damage because the visual field defects are not typical and there is no histologic evidence to support this location. There is evidence that the optic nerve head is an important site of damage in this disorder. This finding is based not only on histologic evidence but also because the types of visual field defects seen in patients with IIH are similar to those found in disorders known to affect the optic nerve head: glaucoma and anterior ischemic optic neuropathy. The last site of damage is the retina. Here, there may be either a neurosensory detachment or visual loss from choroidal folds. However, the main location for visual loss in IIH is at the optic disc.

There are 2 leading mechanisms for damage to the optic disc from intracranial hypertension: (1) disruption of axonal transport and (2) intraneuronal optic nerve ischemia. There is considerable evidence that the primary insult to the optic nerve is a slowing of axonal transport.[45,47,48] It is likely that raised intracranial pressure in the subarachnoid space is reflected along the optic nerve sheath. As noted earlier, the health of the optic nerve depends on the harmonious interaction of CSF pressure, intraocular pressure, and systemic blood pressure. Raising intracranial pressure, a drop in intraocular pressure, or a marked decrease of systemic blood pressure can all result in optic disc edema. It is likely that high CSF pressure disturbs the normal gradient between intraocular and retrolaminar pressure and results in increased tissue pressure within the optic nerve. This likely interferes with axoplasmic flow, with resultant stasis involving slow and fast axoplasmic transport resulting in intra-axonal edema.[49]

Another potential mechanism is ischemia of the optic nerve head. Support for this mechanism comes from (1) Hayreh's work showing delays in prelaminar arterial filling with fluorescein angiography and (2) because the visual field defects that occur are similar to those found in other optic neuropathies with ischemic final common pathways as their mechanism of visual loss (glaucoma and anterior ischemic optic neuropathy). It is most likely, however, that the mechanism of visual loss in IIH is through a combination of these 2 mechanisms. High CSF pressure is reflected along and through trabeculations in the subarachnoid space of the optic nerve sheath. This situation results in a disturbance of the pressure gradient across the optic nerve head.

There is resultant axoplasmic flow stasis, intra-axonal swelling, and compression of small arterioles, resulting in intraneuronal ischemic damage to the optic nerve.

DIAGNOSTIC CRITERIA

The accepted criteria initially proposed by Walter Dandy have been modified.[4] Patients who fulfill these criteria are diagnosed as having IIH. These criteria are found in **Box 2**.

Patients with findings on examination other than papilledema, sixth nerve, and rarely seventh nerve paresis should be suspected of having a diagnosis other than IIH. Laboratory evaluation in patients with IIH is normal except for increased intracranial pressure.

There are several issues surrounding the criteria of the measurement and limits of the opening pressure. Whether the patient is supine, prone, or sitting, one must be sure that the reference level for CSF pressure measurement is the level of the left atrium. Next, spuriously high values can occur with Valsalva,[50] and the hypoventilation associated with sedation. The latter is particularly a recurring issue in the pediatric population. Artifactually low values can occur with hyperventilation in the anxious patient from reduction in carbon dioxide levels, and the patient undergoing multiple needle punctures may have falsely low results. CSF pressure fluctuates throughout the day and at times is normal so a single normal CSF measurement does not exclude IIH as the diagnosis.

The normal limits for CSF opening pressure remain controversial. Normal limits are less than 200 mm water in nonobese patients but in obese patients there are conflicting studies. Whiteley and coworkers[51] prospectively recorded CSF opening pressure in 242 adults and measured patients' weights and heights. The 95% reference interval for the CSF opening pressure was 10 to 25 cm CSF. However, neither neck nor hip flexion was altered in their protocol, suggesting some of their patients may have been prone to Valsalva and falsely increased pressures. In addition, the inclusion and exclusion criteria of the study may not have been appropriate.[52] Corbett and Mehta[3] found a cutoff of 250 but their numbers were somewhat small. Bono and coworkers[53] measured CSF pressure in obese and nonobese patients with neck and legs extended and no patients had pressures more than 200 mm water. In summary, the cutoff value for increased intracranial pressure remains unclear. Values between 200 and 250 mm water may be considered borderline with values more than 250 mm water definitely increased.

Box 2
Modified Dandy Criteria for IIH

1. Signs and symptoms of increased intracranial pressure

2. Absence of localizing findings on neurologic examination

3. Absence of deformity, displacement, or obstruction of the ventricular system and otherwise normal neurodiagnostic studies, except for evidence of increased cerebrospinal fluid pressure (>250 mm water). Abnormal neuroimaging except for empty sella turcica, optic nerve sheath with filled out CSF spaces, and smooth-walled non flow-related venous sinus stenosis or collapse should lead to another diagnosis

4. Awake and alert patient

5. No other cause of increased intracranial pressure present (see **Box 1**)

Diagnostic confusion can result from anomalous optic discs in patients with border-line increased intracranial pressure. The main culprit is buried optic nerve drusen, which can cause optic disc edema indistinguishable from low-grade papilledema. Orbital ultrasound (echography) is an excellent test to reveal calcified buried optic disc drusen; the noncalcified variety can be problematic to prove. The authors recommend ultrasound of the optic disc in all cases of IIH with borderline increased CSF pressures and low-grade optic disc edema. Tilted discs, little red discs, and optic discs with anomalous branching and tortuosity can also mimic optic disc edema.

RECOMMENDATIONS FOR EVALUATION

A history tailored to search for the secondary causes of intracranial hypertension is imperative. A series of evaluations can then be selected based on the likelihood of secondary causes (see **Box 1**).

Corbett and Thompson[54] have correctly pointed out that many physicians follow patients with IIH with the wrong tests. Snellen acuity and the visual evoked potential are insensitive methods to detect visual loss in IIH. Repeated measurements of CSF pressure can be misleading because it fluctuates throughout the day and does not correlate well with the clinical state. Patients with IIH should be followed with perimetry with a known sensitive strategy and either serial stereo fundus photographs, drawing-documented indirect ophthalmoscopy, or optic disc grading using the Frisén scheme.[38] Automated perimetry is used for attentive and motivated patients; in others manual perimetry gives more reproducible results.

TREATMENT

Once intracranial hypertension is discovered one should first eliminate presumed causal factors such as excessive vitamin A or tetracyclines and begin a low-sodium weight reduction diet. Therapy aimed at reversing and preventing visual loss should then be instituted. Symptomatic headache treatment can be introduced if this symptom persists in the face of intracranial pressure-lowering agents and procedures. Many medical and surgical treatments have been used for IIH with varying success. All reports to date are anecdotal. Visual loss is the only serious complication and it may occur from the time of first appearance to many years later. We therefore recommend tailoring the treatment primarily to the presence and progression of visual loss.

MEDICAL THERAPY

Medical treatment is aimed at lowering intracranial pressure and treating symptoms directly such as headache. There are no evidence-based data from controlled clinical treatment trials for IIH but such a trial is currently in progress.

Weight Loss

Weight loss has been used to treat IIH for many years. Newborg in 1974 reported remission of papilledema in all 9 patients placed on a low-calorie adaptation of Kemp-ner rice diet. The patients' intake was 400 to 1000 calories per day by fruits, rice, vegetables and occasionally 28 to 56 g of meat. Fluids were limited to 750 to 1250 mL/d and sodium to less than 100 mg/d. All patients had reversal of their papilledema. There was no mention of the patients' visual testing.[55] Others have also documented successful outcomes associated with weight loss[56–58] and it seems only modest degrees of weight loss in the range of 5% to 10% total body weight are needed for reversal of symptoms and signs.[56]

Gastric weight reduction surgery has been used with some success in 24 morbidly obese women with IIH.[59] Symptoms resolved in all but 1 patient within 4 months of the procedure. Two patients regained weight associated with return of their symptoms. There were many significant but treatable complications of this surgery. We reserve this treatment for patients with IIH with morbid obesity.

Because marked recent weight gain is a predictor of visual deterioration[8] and papilledema can resolve with modest weight loss as the only treatment, we strongly encourage our patients to pursue a supervised weight loss program. Institution of a low-salt diet and mild fluid restriction (no forcing of fluids) seem to be beneficial for many patients with IIH. This finding may be especially true in patients who lose only 5% to 10% of their total body mass, yet have resolution of their papilledema. It is not yet clear whether improvement occurs because of weight loss per se or other changes in diet such as fluid or sodium restriction or decrease in the intake of a molecule such as vitamin A.

Lumbar Puncture

Use of repeated lumbar punctures is controversial. Lumbar puncture has only a short-lived effect on CSF pressure[60] with a return of pressure to pretap level after only 82 minutes.[60] Lumbar puncture measures CSF pressure at only 1 point in time. Because CSF pressure fluctuates, this information has only limited clinical use for modifying treatment plans. However, because transverse sinus collapse (smooth-walled venous stenoses) can resolve immediately with lowering pressure,[61] CSF circulatory dynamics may be restored with this procedure and may give temporary relief until the sinus recollapses, usually within weeks.

Corticosteroids

Steroids are still occasionally used to treat IIH but their mechanism of action remains unclear. The side effects of weight gain, striae, and acne are especially unfortunate for these already obese patients. Although patients treated with steroids often respond well, there is usually recurrence of papilledema with rapid tapering of the dose. This effect may be accompanied by marked deterioration of visual function. A prolonged tapering may prevent return of symptoms and signs in some patients. Use of long-term steroids to treat IIH has largely been abandoned. Short-term use may have a role in the preoperative period before a CSF shunting procedure.

Acetazolamide

McCarthy and Reed[62] showed acetazolamide (Diamox) decreases CSF flow but not until more than 99.5% of choroid plexus carbonic anhydrase is inhibited. Gücer and Viernstein[63] used intracranial pressure monitoring before and after treatment in 4 patients with IIH. They monitored acetazolamide treatment in 2 of the patients and showed gradual CSF pressure reduction in both. They reported the dosage in only 1 of the patients (4 g of acetazolamide was needed per day). Apparent efficacy of acetazolamide has also been shown by others[64,65] but we await data from an ongoing multicenter, double-blind, randomized, placebo-controlled study of weight reduction and/or low-sodium diet plus acetazolamide versus diet plus placebo in patients with mild visual loss.

We start with 0.5 to 1 g/d of acetazolamide in divided doses (twice daily with meals) and gradually increase the dosage until either symptoms and signs regress, side effects become intolerable, or a dosage of 3 to 4 g/d is reached. Most patients seem to respond in the 1 to 2 g/d range.

The mechanism of action of acetazolamide is likely multifactorial. It has been found to reduce CSF production; also, it changes the taste of foods and sometimes causes anorexia, aiding in weight loss. Patients nearly always experience tingling in the fingers, toes, and perioral region, and less commonly have malaise. Renal stones occur in a few percent of patients. Metabolic acidosis, indicated by lowered serum bicarbonate, is a good measure of compliance. A rare but serious side effect is aplastic anemia. It occurs in 1 in 15,000 patient years of treatment with acetazolamide and usually occurs in the first 6 months of therapy. Aplastic anemia from acetazolamide has been reported most often in elderly people and is probably less common in younger IIH patients. Because this side effect is so rare and finding the case and stopping the medication does not necessarily cure the patient, repeated blood testing is not usually performed.[66]

Although there are some structural similarities between acetazolamide and sulfa, there is little clinical or pharmacologic evidence to suggest that a self-reported sulfa allergy is likely to produce a life-threatening cross-reaction with acetazolamide or furosemide.[67]

Topiramate (Topomax) has also been used to treat IIH because it has carbonic anhydrase inhibitor activity and weight loss commonly occurs. In studies to date, it seems comparable with acetazolamide.[65,68]

Furosemide

Furosemide has also been used to treat IIH.[7] It has been well documented that furosemide (Lasix) can lower intracranial pressure.[69] It seems to work by diuresis and reducing sodium transport into the brain. We initiate furosemide at a dosage of 20 mg by mouth twice a day and gradually increase the dosage, if necessary, to a maximum of 40 mg by mouth 3 times a day. Potassium supplementation is given as needed.

SURGICAL THERAPY

The surgical forms of therapy now used are various shunting and decompression procedures including stereotactic ventriculoperitoneal shunts and optic nerve sheath fenestration.

Subtemporal or Suboccipital Decompression

Subtemporal or suboccipital decompression was used from the 1940s to the 1960s for patients with visual loss from IIH. These procedures are now infrequently used because of complications, which although rare include seizures, otorrhea, and subdural hematoma. However, long-term success has been reported[70] and this procedure may be underused.

Optic Nerve Sheath Fenestration

Optic nerve sheath fenestration consists of either creating a window or making a series of slits in the optic nerve sheath just behind the globe. This treatment is preferred for the patient with progressive visual loss with mild or easily controlled headaches, although more than 50% of patients with the procedure gain adequate headache control (especially if the headache is frontal). Because improvement in papilledema may occur in the unoperated eye and fistula formation has been reported, the mechanism of action may be local decompression of the subarachnoid space (see **Fig. 11**). Occasional failure of the fellow eye to improve and the asymmetry of papilledema may be explained by the resistance to CSF flow produced by the trabeculations of the subarachnoid space. The mechanism of action may also be closure of the subarachnoid space in the retrolaminar optic nerve by scarring. It is likely that both mechanisms contribute to protection of the optic nerve head.

Many large case series attest to the efficacy of this technique.[71–77] In these series, postoperative visual acuity or perimetry results were as good as or better than preoperative studies in about 90%.[74] However, occasional patients lose vision in the perioperative period (**Table 1**).

CSF Shunting Procedures

Various shunting procedures have been used for the treatment of IIH such as lumbar subarachnoid-peritoneal, ventriculoatrial, ventriculojugular, and ventriculoperitoneal shunts. In general, the indication for a CSF diversion procedure is failed medical therapy or intractable headache. Its use seems to be increasing.[78]

Eggenberger and coworkers[79] studied lumboperitoneal shunt retrospectively in 27 patients with IIH. Although initially successful, 56% required a shunt revision. Rosenberg and colleagues[80] reported on 37 patients with IIH who underwent 73 lumboperitoneal shunts and 9 ventricular shunts with modest success (38% of patients successfully treated after 1 shunting procedure). The most common causes for reoperation were shunt failure in 55% and low-pressure headaches in 21% of patients. The vision of most patients improved or stabilized from the procedure, but 3 who had initially improved later lost vision and 6 had a decrease in vision postoperatively. Serious complications occurred in 3.6%. Other series are similar,[81,82] with the conclusion thet there is initial success but at least half need reoperations. Also, when the procedure is performed primarily for headache relief, long-term success is only about 50%.[83] In-hospital mortality for new shunts is 0.5%, with 0.9% for ventricular shunts and 0.2% for lumbar shunts.[78]

Shunting procedures are successful in selected patients. Shunt occlusion that occurs in about half of those shunted can be accompanied by severe visual loss, limiting the effectiveness of this procedure. **Table 2** summarizes the results of shunting procedures that reported visual outcomes.

Gastric Exclusion Surgery

As discussed earlier, for the morbidly obese patient, successful treatment has been reported using gastric exclusion procedures.[59] This procedure may be especially

Table 1
Case series with visual results from operations for IIH performed with optic nerve sheath fenestration.

Investigators	Year Published	Vision Worse	Vision Not Worse	Total No. of Patients
Hupp et al[96]	1987	6	11	17
Sergott et al[73]	1988	0	23	23
Brourman et al[76]	1988	0	10	10
Kelman et al[97]	1992	1	21	22
Goh et al[71]	1997	3	26	29
Plotnik and Kosmorsky[75]	1993	4	27	31
Acheson et al[72]	1994	3	17	20
Corbett et al[98]	1988	9	31	40
Banta and Farris[99]	2000	10	148	158
Total		36 (11.4%)	314	350

			Shunt	Vision	Vision Not	
	Year	Shunt				
Investigators	Published	Type	Failures	Worse	Worse	Total
Rosenberg et al[100]	1993	LP/VP/V+	20/37	9	28	37
Shapiro et al[101]	1995	LP	0/4	1	3	4
Eggenberger et al[79]	1996	LP	15/27	0	14	14
Burgett et al[81]	1997	LP	19/30	1	29	30
Bynke et al[102]	2004	VP	7/17	0	17	17
Total			61/115	11 (10.7%)	91	102

Table 2
Reported cases with visual results from CSF shunting operations for IIH

useful in treating other conditions comorbid with obesity such as arterial hypertension, diabetes mellitus, and sleep apnea. Complications include major wound infection and stenosis at the gastrojejunal anastomosis.

Venous Sinus Stenting

It has been suggested that the cause of IIH is collapse of the proximal transverse sinus. However, King and colleagues[84] have shown lowering of CSF pressure from a cervical puncture abolishes the pressure gradient. Because this collapse of the transverse sinus, which is ubiquitous in IIH[36] (and occurs in about 7% of normal patients), may obstruct venous return and hence CSF outflow, stents have been placed to keep this portion of the transverse sinus open. This procedure has been reviewed by Friedman,[85] with the conclusion that it can have major morbidity (subdural hematoma), remains unproven, and needs further study.

Treatment Overview

Medical and surgical treatment of patients with IIH is often challenging, requiring integration of the history, examination, and clinical course. Many factors are involved and each is weighted in creating individualized therapy. The most important factor is usually the amount and progression of visual loss. Next in importance is the severity of the patient's symptoms with regard to how much they are disrupting the patient's activities of daily living. Headache is the most problematic symptom but pulse synchronous tinnitus, and diplopia, can be difficult to treat. Also factored in is the degree and change in papilledema grade. The options are summarized in **Fig. 12**.

Patients with mild or no visual loss are treated with modest weight loss and sodium restriction often with the addition of acetazolamide (Diamox). In patients with no visual loss, the decision on whether to add acetazolamide is based on the severity of headache or other symptoms and the degree of papilledema; the greater the grade of papilledema, the greater the risk for visual loss. Patients with mild or no visual loss are usually followed first at 4-month intervals. If their vision improves or papilledema lessens to grade 1 or 0, we use 6-month or 1-year intervals. All patients are encouraged to enter a weight-management program with a goal of 5% to 10% weight loss along with a low-salt diet and modest fluid restriction (drinking only when thirsty rather than forcing fluids as is sometimes done to lose weight).

If the patient presents with moderate to severe visual loss (mean deviation on automated perimetry > −5 dB), the optimal management has yet to be determined. Some advocate early surgery, whereas others give a medical trial. We have seen both approaches work. For maximal medical therapy we start with 1 g/d of Diamox in divided doses and over weeks gradually increase the dose to the maximal tolerated

Treatment of IIH

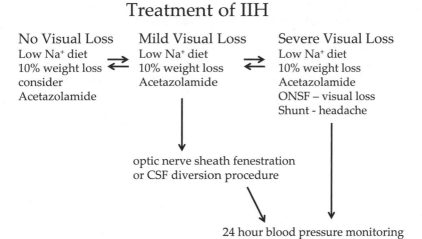

No Visual Loss	Mild Visual Loss	Severe Visual Loss
Low Na⁺ diet	Low Na⁺ diet	Low Na⁺ diet
10% weight loss	10% weight loss	10% weight loss
consider	Acetazolamide	Acetazolamide
Acetazolamide		ONSF – visual loss
		Shunt - headache

optic nerve sheath fenestration
or CSF diversion procedure

24 hour blood pressure monitoring
and sleep study

Fig. 12. Treatment algorithm for IIH. Visual loss does not include enlargement of the blind spot unless it is compromising vision. Optic nerve sheath fenestration is preferred to steroids. Downward arrows show the next step when vision worsens.

dose. We define this the highest dose that does not interfere significantly with activities of daily living. There is some evidence that furosemide (Lasix) can be added in increasing doses to 40 mg by mouth three times a day to further reduce CSF pressure. We use optic nerve sheath fenestration if there is worsening on maximal medical therapy; headache improves in about half of patients, especially if the pain is frontal and worsens with eye movements. This pain is likely caused by distended optic nerve sheaths and pain-sensitive structures are stretched with eye movements. If headache is severe and unresponsive to medical treatments we first make sure the patient does not have rebound headaches from daily analgesics or caffeine. If we believe the headaches are caused by increased intracranial pressure, we proceed with a CSF shunting procedure, although the surgery is successful for headache relief in only about half. We believe stereotactic ventriculoatrial or ventriculoperitoneal shunts are most successful.

Patients who fail to respond to therapy should have repeat neuroimaging, looking for occult meningiomas or other tumors invading the venous sinuses, and a sleep study, looking for obstructive sleep apnea, which should have treatment optimized. Patients with unrelenting visual loss should also have 24-hour blood pressure monitoring to look for periods of hypotension. Hypotension is a strong risk factor for visual loss, especially during surgery. Treatment decisions may be complicated and are further discussed elsewhere.[86]

Headache Treatment

Headache in patients with IIH may improve after a lumbar puncture, but may remain as a management problem even after medications have been given to reduce intracranial pressure. We have had success treating these patients with standard prophylactic vascular headache remedies. However, we try to avoid medications that cause hypotension, such as β-blockers or calcium channel blockers, because they may cause reduced perfusion of the optic nerve head. Tricyclic antidepressants can be problematic because of their side effect of weight gain. We use tricyclics in low doses such as amitriptyline 10 to 25 mg at bedtime. Nonsteroidal antiinflammatory agents, especially naproxen, are used as an adjunct but their use is limited to 2 days per week to prevent the development of rebound headaches. Topiramate may be useful for its migraine prophylaxis, side effect of weight loss, and for carbonic anhydrase inhibition.

Uncommonly, a CSF shunting procedure is needed for persistent headache; but it can produce the hindbrain herniation headache in return. Patients with IIH also have other headache syndromes. Especially in patients with a migraine history, analgesic-rebound or caffeine-rebound headaches may coexist. These patients may require IV dihydroergotamine to treat this troublesome headache syndrome.

IIH IN CHILDREN

The effect of papilledema on vision is the same in children as in adults. Some form of quantitative perimetry can be performed in most children more than the age of 6 years. Excellent reviews of IIH in children can be found.[87–89] These investigators point out differences between adult and childhood forms of IIH. In IIH of childhood up to puberty, the incidence in girls and boys is the same.[90] In addition, obesity does not seem to be an important factor in the pathogenesis or treatment of IIH in prepubertal children. The causes reported only with children are nutritional restoration after malnutrition and thyroid-replacement therapy in hypothyroid children.[22]

IIH IN MEN

Digre and Corbett[9] studied 29 men with IIH using a case-control design and found IIH occurs in men in a similar age distribution to women. They noted that men may require surgical treatment of impending visual loss more often and suggest African American men to be at greater risk to loss of vision. Bruce and colleagues[91] also found men with IIH were 2 times as likely as women to have visual loss.

The issue of IIH in men is complicated by the not infrequent cooccurrence of obstructive sleep apnea.[92] Two studies have documented increased intracranial pressure during apneic periods in these patients.[93,94] Jennum and Borgesen[94] documented the occurrence of increased intracranial pressure during waking hours in the absence of apnea in half their subjects. Because there is a biologically plausible mechanism to explain increased intracranial pressure in sleep apnea and the cooccurrence in men is frequent, we recommend sleep studies in all men and in women with symptoms suggestive of obstructive sleep apnea.

IIH IN PREGNANCY

Digre and colleagues[15] using a case-control design found no increase in obstetric complications in IIH. Visual loss occurred with the same frequency in pregnant and nonpregnant patients with IIH. They concluded that treatment of patients with IIH in pregnancy should be the same as for nonpregnant patients with IIH, except that caloric restriction must be tempered.

The issue of acetazolamide use in the first trimester of pregnancy is complex. Because of potential teratogenic effects in animals and a single case of a sacrococcygeal teratoma in humans, the basis for withholding acetazolamide is not strong. Acetazolamide is a US Food and Drug Authority category C agent and in our experience can be used after appropriate informed consent, discussion with the patient and the obstetrician, and for patients in whom the benefit outweighs the potential risk for treatment.[95]

SUMMARY

IIH is characterized by increased CSF pressure of unknown cause. It is predominantly a disease of women in the childbearing years. Although the cause of IIH remains obscure, it has become clear that loss of visual function is common and patients may progress to blindness if untreated. Diagnosis should adhere to the modified Dandy criteria and other causes of intracranial hypertension sought. IIH patient management should include serial perimetry and optic disc grading or photography. The proper therapy can then be selected and visual loss prevented or reversed. Although there are no evidence-based data to guide therapy, there is an ongoing randomized double-blind placebo controlled treatment trial of IIH investigating diet and acetazolamide therapy.

REFERENCES

1. Corbett JJ, Savino PJ, Thompson HS, et al. Visual loss in pseudotumor cerebri. Follow-up of 57 patients from five to 41 years and a profile of 14 patients with permanent severe visual loss. Arch Neurol 1982;39:461–74.
2. Wall M, Hart WM Jr, Burde RM. Visual field defects in idiopathic intracranial hypertension (pseudotumor cerebri). Am J Ophthalmol 1983;96:654–69.
3. Corbett JJ, Mehta MP. Cerebrospinal fluid pressure in normal obese subjects and patients with pseudotumor cerebri. Neurology 1983;33:1386–8.
4. Smith JL. Whence pseudotumor cerebri? J Clin Neuroophthalmol 1985;5:55–6.
5. Durcan FJ, Corbett JJ, Wall M. The incidence of pseudotumor cerebri. Population studies in Iowa and Louisiana. Arch Neurol 1988;45:875–7.
6. Radhakrishnan K, Ahlskog JE, Cross SA, et al. Idiopathic intracranial hypertension (pseudotumor cerebri). Descriptive epidemiology in Rochester, Minn, 1976 to 1990. Arch Neurol 1993;50:78–80.
7. Corbett JJ. The 1982 Silversides lecture. Problems in the diagnosis and treatment of pseudotumor cerebri. Can J Neurol Sci 1983;10:221–9.
8. Wall M, George D. Idiopathic intracranial hypertension. A prospective study of 50 patients. Brain 1991;114:155–80.
9. Digre KB, Corbett JJ. Pseudotumor cerebri in men. Arch Neurol 1988;45:866–72.
10. Ireland B, Corbett JJ, Wallace RB. The search for causes of idiopathic intracranial hypertension. A preliminary case-control study. Arch Neurol 1990;47:315–20.
11. Giuseffi V, Wall M, Siegel PZ, et al. Symptoms and disease associations in idiopathic intracranial hypertension (pseudotumor cerebri): a case-control study. Neurology 1991;41:239–44.
12. Greer M. Benign intracranial hypertension. II. Following corticosteroid therapy. Neurology 1963;13:439–41.
13. Neville BG, Wilson J. Benign intracranial hypertension following corticosteroid withdrawal in childhood. Br Med J 1970;3:554–6.
14. Walsh FB. Papilledema associated with increased intracranial pressure in Addison's disease. Arch Ophthalmol 1952;47:86.
15. Digre KB, Varner MW, Corbett JJ. Pseudotumor cerebri and pregnancy. Neurology 1984;34:721–9.
16. Deonna T, Guignard JP. Acute intracranial hypertension after nalidixic acid administration. Arch Dis Child 1974;49:743.
17. Mushet GR. Pseudotumor and nitrofurantoin therapy [letter]. Arch Neurol 1977;34:257.
18. Konomi H, Imai M, Nihei K, et al. Indomethacin causing pseudotumor cerebri in Bartter's syndrome [letter]. N Engl J Med 1978;298:855.

19. Larizza D, Colombo A, Lorini R, et al. Ketoprofen causing pseudotumor cerebri in Bartter's syndrome [letter]. N Engl J Med 1979;300:796.
20. Feldman MH, Schlezinger NS. Benign intracranial hypertension associated with hypervitaminosis A. Arch Neurol 1970;22:1–7.
21. Spector RH, Carlisle J. Pseudotumor cerebri caused by a synthetic vitamin A preparation. Neurology 1984;34:1509–11.
22. Van Dop C, Conte FA, Koch TK, et al. Pseudotumor cerebri associated with initiation of levothyroxine therapy for juvenile hypothyroidism. N Engl J Med 1983; 308:1076–80.
23. Saul RF, Hamburger HA, Selhorst JB. Pseudotumor cerebri secondary to lithium carbonate. JAMA 1985;253:2869–70.
24. Shah A, Roberts T, McQueen IN, et al. Danazol and benign intracranial hypertension. Br Med J (Clin Res Ed) 1987;294:1323.
25. Bercaw BL, Greer M. Transport of intrathecal 131-I risa in benign intracranial hypertension. Neurology 1970;20:787–90.
26. Jacobson DM, Karanjia PN, Olson KA, et al. Computed tomography ventricular size has no predictive value in diagnosing pseudotumor cerebri. Neurology 1990;40:1454–5.
27. Wall M, Dollar JD, Sadun AA, et al. Idiopathic intracranial hypertension: lack of histologic evidence for cerebral edema. Arch Neurol 1995;52:141–5.
28. Mathew NT, Meyer JS, Ott EO. Increased cerebral blood volume in benign intracranial hypertension. Neurology 1975;25:646–9.
29. Brooks DJ, Beaney RP, Leenders KL, et al. Regional cerebral oxygen utilization, blood flow, and blood volume in benign intracranial hypertension studied by positron emission tomography. Neurology 1985;35:1030–4.
30. Boulton M, Armstrong D, Flessner M, et al. Raised intracranial pressure increases CSF drainage through arachnoid villi and extracranial lymphatics. Am J Physiol 1998;275(3 Pt 2):889–96.
31. Sahs AL, Joynt RJ. Brain swelling of unknown cause. Neurology 1956;6: 791–803.
32. Wall M. The headache profile of idiopathic intracranial hypertension. Cephalalgia 1990;10:331–5.
33. Friedman DI, Rausch EA. Headache diagnoses in patients with treated idiopathic intracranial hypertension. Neurology 2002;58:1551–3.
34. Sadun A, Currie J, Lessell S. Transient visual obscurations with elevated optic discs. Ann Neurol 1984;16:489–94.
35. Meador KJ, Swift TR. Tinnitus from intracranial hypertension. Neurology 1984; 34:1258–61.
36. Farb RI, Vanek I, Scott JN, et al. Idiopathic intracranial hypertension: the prevalence and morphology of sinovenous stenosis. Neurology 2003;60:1418–24.
37. Wall M, White WN. Asymmetric papilledema in idiopathic intracranial hypertension: prospective interocular comparison of sensory visual function. Invest Ophthalmol Vis Sci 1998;39:134–42.
38. Frisén L. Swelling of the optic nerve head: a staging scheme. J Neurol Neurosurg Psychiatr 1982;45:13–8.
39. Scott CJ, Kardon RH, Lee AG, et al. Diagnosis and grading of papilledema in patients with raised intracranial pressure using optical coherence tomography (OCT) compared to clinical expert assessment using a Clinical Staging Scale. Arch Ophthalmol 2010, in press.
40. Cushing H. Strangulation of the nervi abducentes by lateral branches of the basilar artery in cases of brain tumor. Brain 1910;33:204–35.

41. Wall M, George D. Visual loss in pseudotumor cerebri. Incidence and defects related to visual field strategy. Arch Neurol 1987;44:170–5.
42. Corbett JJ, Jacobson DM, Mauer RC, et al. Enlargement of the blind spot caused by papilledema. Am J Ophthalmol 1988;105:261–5.
43. Shah VA, Kardon RH, Lee AG, et al. Long-term follow-up of idiopathic intracranial hypertension: the Iowa experience. Neurology 2008;70:634–40.
44. Wall M. The morphology of visual field damage in idiopathic intracranial hypertension: an anatomic region analysis. In: Mills RP, Heijl A, editors. Perimetry update 1990/1991. Amsterdam: Kugler Publications; 1991. p. 20–7.
45. Hayreh SS. Pathogenesis of optic disc oedema in raised intracranial pressure. Trans Ophthalmol Soc U K 1976;96:404–7.
46. Hayreh SS. The sheath of the optic nerve. Ophthalmologica 1984;189:54–63.
47. Hayreh SS. Optic disc edema in raised intracranial pressure. V. Pathogenesis. Arch Ophthalmol 1977;95:1553–65.
48. Hayreh SS, March W, Anderson DR. Pathogenesis of block of rapid orthograde axonal transport by elevated intraocular pressure. Exp Eye Res 1979;28:515–23.
49. Tso MO, Hayreh SS. Optic disc edema in raised intracranial pressure. IV. Axoplasmic transport in experimental papilledema. Arch Ophthalmol 1977;95:1458–62.
50. Neville L, Egan RA. Frequency and amplitude of elevation of cerebrospinal fluid resting pressure by the Valsalva maneuver. Can J Ophthalmol 2005;40:775–7.
51. Whiteley W, Al Shahi R, Warlow CP, et al. CSF opening pressure: reference interval and the effect of body mass index. Neurology 2006;67:1690–1.
52. Bono F, Quattrone A. CSF opening pressure: reference interval and the effect of body mass index. Neurology 2007;68:1439–40.
53. Bono F, Lupo MR, Serra P, et al. Obesity does not induce abnormal CSF pressure in subjects with normal cerebral MR venography. Neurology 2002;59:1641–3.
54. Corbett JJ, Thompson HS. The rational management of idiopathic intracranial hypertension. Arch Neurol 1989;46:1049–51.
55. Newborg B. Pseudotumor cerebri treated by rice reduction diet. Arch Intern Med 1974;133:802–7.
56. Johnson LN, Krohel GB, Madsen RW, et al. The role of weight loss and acetazolamide in the treatment of idiopathic intracranial hypertension (pseudotumor cerebri). Ophthalmology 1998;105:2313–7.
57. Kupersmith MJ, Gamell L, Turbin R, et al. Effects of weight loss on the course of idiopathic intracranial hypertension in women. Neurology 1998;50:1094–8.
58. Wong R, Madill SA, Pandey P, et al. Idiopathic intracranial hypertension: the association between weight loss and the requirement for systemic treatment. BMC Ophthalmol 2007;7:15.
59. Sugerman HJ, Felton WL III, Sismanis A, et al. Gastric surgery for pseudotumor cerebri associated with severe obesity. Ann Surg 1999;229:634–40.
60. Johnston I, Paterson A. Benign intracranial hypertension. II. CSF pressure and circulation. Brain 1974;97:301–12.
61. Scoffings DJ, Pickard JD, Higgins JN. Resolution of transverse sinus stenoses immediately after CSF withdrawal in idiopathic intracranial hypertension. J Neurol Neurosurg Psychiatr 2007;78:911–2.
62. McCarthy KD, Reed DJ. The effect of acetazolamide and furosemide on CSF production and choroid plexus carbonic anhydrase activity. J Pharmacol Exp Ther 1974;189:194–201.

63. Gücer G, Viernstein L. Long-term intracranial pressure recording in management of pseudotumor cerebri. J Neurosurg 1978;49:256–63.
64. Tomsak RL, Niffenegger AS, Remler BF. Treatment of pseudotumor cerebri with Diamox (acetazolamide). J Clin Neuroophthalmol 1988;8:93–8.
65. Celebisoy N, Gokcay F, Sirin H, et al. Treatment of idiopathic intracranial hypertension: topiramate vs acetazolamide, an open-label study. Acta Neurol Scand 2007;116:322–7.
66. Zimran A, Beutler E. Can the risk of acetazolamide-induced aplastic anemia be decreased by periodic monitoring of blood cell counts? Am J Ophthalmol 1987; 104:654–8.
67. Lee AG, Anderson R, Kardon RH, et al. Presumed "sulfa allergy" in patients with intracranial hypertension treated with acetazolamide or furosemide: cross-reactivity, myth or reality? Am J Ophthalmol 2004;138:114–8.
68. Shah VA, Fung S, Shahbaz R, et al. Idiopathic intracranial hypertension. Ophthalmology 2007;114:617.
69. Pollay M, Fullenwider C, Roberts PA, et al. Effect of mannitol and furosemide on blood-brain osmotic gradient and intracranial pressure. J Neurosurg 1983;59: 945–50.
70. Kessler LA, Novelli PM, Reigel DH. Surgical treatment of benign intracranial hypertension–subtemporal decompression revisited. Surg Neurol 1998;50:73–6.
71. Goh KY, Schatz NJ, Glaser JS. Optic nerve sheath fenestration for pseudotumor cerebri. J Neuroophthalmol 1997;17:86–91.
72. Acheson JF, Green WT, Sanders MD. Optic nerve sheath decompression for the treatment of visual failure in chronic raised intracranial pressure. J Neurol Neurosurg Psychiatr 1994;57:1426–9.
73. Sergott RC, Savino PJ, Bosley TM. Modified optic nerve sheath decompression provides long-term visual improvement for pseudotumor cerebri. Arch Ophthalmol 1988;106:1391–7.
74. Corbett JJ, Nerad JA, Tse D, et al. Optic nerve sheath fenestration for pseudotumor cerebri: the lateral orbitotomy approach. Arch Ophthalmol 1988;106: 1391–7.
75. Plotnik JL, Kosmorsky GS. Operative complications of optic nerve sheath decompression [review]. Ophthalmology 1993;100:683–90.
76. Brourman ND, Spoor TC, Ramocki JM. Optic nerve sheath decompression for pseudotumor cerebri. Arch Ophthalmol 1988;106:1378–83.
77. Chandrasekaran S, McCluskey P, Minassian D, et al. Visual outcomes for optic nerve sheath fenestration in pseudotumour cerebri and related conditions. Clin Experiment Ophthalmol 2006;34:661–5.
78. Curry WT Jr, Butler WE, Barker FG. Rapidly rising incidence of cerebrospinal fluid shunting procedures for idiopathic intracranial hypertension in the United States, 1988-2002. Neurosurgery 2005;57(1):97–108 [discussion: 97–108].
79. Eggenberger ER, Miller NR, Vitale S. Lumboperitoneal shunt for the treatment of pseudotumor cerebri. Neurology 1996;46:1524–30.
80. Rosenberg M, Smith C, Beck R. The efficacy of shunting procedures in pseudotumor cerebri. Neurology 1989;39:209.
81. Burgett RA, Purvin VA, Kawasaki A. Lumboperitoneal shunting for pseudotumor cerebri. Neurology 1997;49:734–9.
82. Johnston I, Besser M, Morgan MK. Cerebrospinal fluid diversion in the treatment of benign intracranial hypertension. J Neurosurg 1988;69:195–202.
83. McGirt MJ, Woodworth G, Thomas G, et al. Cerebrospinal fluid shunt placement for pseudotumor cerebri-associated intractable headache: predictors of

treatment response and an analysis of long-term outcomes. J Neurosurg 2004; 101(4):627–32.

84. King JO, Mitchell PJ, Thomson KR, et al. Manometry combined with cervical puncture in idiopathic intracranial hypertension. Neurology 2002;58:26–30.

85. Friedman DI. Cerebral venous pressure, intra-abdominal pressure, and dural venous sinus stenting in idiopathic intracranial hypertension. J Neuroophthalmol 2006;26:61–4.

86. Wall M. Papilledema and idiopathic intracranial hypertension (pseudotumor cerebri). In: Noseworthy JH, editor. Neurological theraputics principles and practice. 2nd edition. Abingdon (UK): Informa Healthcare; 2006. p. 1955–68.

87. Cinciripini GS, Donahue S, Borchert MS. Idiopathic intracranial hypertension in prepubertal pediatric patients: characteristics, treatment, and outcome. Am J Ophthalmol 1999;127:178–82.

88. Lessell S. Pediatric pseudotumor cerebri (idiopathic intracranial hypertension). Surv Ophthalmol 1992;37:155–66.

89. Babikian P, Corbett J, Bell W. Idiopathic intracranial hypertension in children: the Iowa experience. J Child Neurol 1994;9:144–9.

90. Balcer LJ, Liu GT, Forman S, et al. Idiopathic intracranial hypertension: relation of age and obesity in children. Neurology 1999;52:870–2.

91. Bruce BB, Kedar S, Van Stavern GP, et al. Idiopathic intracranial hypertension in men. Neurology 2009;72:304–9.

92. Lee AG, Golnik K, Kardon R, et al. Sleep apnea and intracranial hypertension in men. Ophthalmology 2002;109:482–5.

93. Sugita Y, Iijima S, Teshima Y, et al. Marked episodic elevation of cerebrospinal fluid pressure during nocturnal sleep in patients with sleep apnea hypersomnia syndrome. Electroencephalogr Clin Neurophysiol 1985;60:214–9.

94. Jennum P, Borgesen SE. Intracranial pressure and obstructive sleep apnea. Chest 1989;95:279–83.

95. Lee AG, Pless M, Falardeau J, et al. The use of acetazolamide in idiopathic intracranial hypertension during pregnancy. Am J Ophthalmol 2005;139(5): 855–9.

96. Hupp SL, Glaser JS, Frazier-Byrne S. Optic nerve sheath decompression. Review of 17 cases. Arch Ophthalmol 1987;105:386–9.

97. Kelman SE, Heaps R, Wolf A, et al. Optic nerve decompression surgery improves visual function in patients with pseudotumor cerebri. Neurosurgery 1992;30:391–5.

98. Corbett JJ, Nerad JA, Tse DT, et al. Results of optic nerve sheath fenestration for pseudotumor cerebri. The lateral orbitotomy approach. Arch Ophthalmol 1988; 106:1391–7.

99. Banta JT, Farris BK. Pseudotumor cerebri and optic nerve sheath decompression. Ophthalmology 2000;107:1907–12.

100. Rosenberg ML, Corbett JJ, Smith C, et al. Cerebrospinal fluid diversion procedures in pseudotumor cerebri. Neurology 1993;43:1071–2.

101. Shapiro S, Yee R, Brown H. Surgical management of pseudotumor cerebri in pregnancy: case report. Neurosurgery 1995;37:829–31.

102. Bynke G, Zemack G, Bynke H, et al. Ventriculoperitoneal shunting for idiopathic intracranial hypertension. Neurology 2004;63(7):1314–6.

Transient Monocular Visual Loss

Rehan Ahmed, MD, Rod Foroozan, MD*

KEYWORDS

- Transient monocular visual loss • Amaurosis fugax
- Transient monocular blindness

Transient monocular visual loss (TMVL) is the preferred term for the abrupt loss of visual function in one eye that lasts less than 24 hours.[1,2] The terms "amaurosis fugax" (translating from Greek to mean "fleeting blindness") and "translent monocular blindness" are sometimes used by clinicians interchangeably with "transient monocular visual loss." However, "amaurosis fugax" does not specify whether the loss is in one or both eyes, and the term also implies visual loss secondary to ischemic causes.[1,3] As shown in **Box 1**, there are a number of nonischemic causes of TMVL. The term "transient monocular blindness" implies a complete loss of vision, but most episodes of TMVL cause only a partial loss of vision.[2] As TMVL may be nonischemic in etiology, incomplete, and strictly refers only to monocular visual loss, it has been suggested that this term be used in preference to others.[4]

We limit our discussion to conditions that typically cause monocular visual loss. It is crucial to remember, however, that a patient's perception of monocular versus binocular visual loss can be misleading. Patients with binocular hemifield (homonymous) visual loss often localize visual loss only to the eye that lost the temporal visual field.[4] It is important to ask if visual loss was noted in the fellow eye when the affected eye was covered during the episode. In addition, patients with binocular visual loss also tend to have a more pronounced reading impairment, whereas monocular visual loss does not usually impair reading unless the unaffected eye has a prior visual impairment.[2]

Establishing whether the visual loss is monocular or binocular helps to localize the lesion: monocular visual loss results from a lesion anterior to the chiasm (the eye or optic nerve), whereas binocular visual loss may be from lesions to both eyes or optic nerves, or, much more likely, from lesions to the chiasm or retrochiasmal pathways.

The most important step in the clinical evaluation of any patient presenting with transient visual loss (TVL) is to obtain a thorough history. The age of the patient, the duration of visual loss, the pattern of visual loss and recovery, and any associated

Cullen Eye Institute, Baylor College of Medicine, 7200B Cambridge Street, Houston, TX 77030, USA
* Corresponding author.
E-mail address: foroozan@bcm.edu

Neurol Clin 28 (2010) 619–629
doi:10.1016/j.ncl.2010.03.004
0733-8619/10/$ – see front matter © 2010 Elsevier Inc. All rights reserved.

neurologic.theclinics.com

Box 1
Causes of transient monocular visual loss

Typically Associated with Abnormal Eye Examination
Ocular Pathology (nonvascular)
  Blepharospasm
  Tear film abnormalities
  Keratoconus
  Intermittent angle-closure glaucoma
  Vitreous debris
Orbitopathy
  Orbital masses and foreign bodies
Optic Nerve
  Papilledema
  Optic nerve drusen/Congenital optic disc anomalies
  Compressive lesions of the intraorbital optic nerve
  Demyelinating disease
Retina
  Age-related macular degeneration
  Macular disease and photostress
  Retinal detachment
Vascular Disease
  Ocular hypoperfusion (ocular ischemic syndrome)
  Internal/Common carotid artery stenosis
  Embolic phenomenon
    Carotid
    Cardiac
    Great vessels
  Carotid artery dissection
  Vasculitis
  Arterial vasospasm (during acute episode)
  Hypercoagulable state
Typically Associated with Normal Eye Examination
Vascular Disease
  Internal/common carotid artery stenosis
  Hypotension
Neurologic
  Migraine (including retinal migraine)
  Uhthoff's phenomenon (demyelination)
Nonphysiologic visual loss

symptoms or additional signs are all used to formulate a differential diagnosis and initiate an appropriate management plan.

Despite the importance of obtaining a complete history, the approach to TMVL that we have found most useful is determining whether the patient has abnormal eye examination findings that can explain the visual loss.

TMVL WITH AN ABNORMAL EYE EXAMINATION

Patients with abnormalities in the external structures (eg, proptosis), ocular surface, anterior chamber of the eye, vitreous, optic disc, or retina can all present with TMVL.

Anterior Segment Pathology

Blurred vision caused by an irregularity of the corneal tear film may cause moments of visual loss. Patients may complain of pain and ocular irritation. Visual acuity is typically improved with pinhole. Examination using a slit-lamp may reveal an abnormal-appearing tear film and cornea, with punctate keratopathy indicative of dry eyes (sicca syndrome). The visual symptoms may improve with blinking or the application of a tear supplement. Measuring the production of tears with a Schirmer test may confirm poor tear production.[5] Corneal epithelial basement membrane dystrophy can also cause episodes of visual loss, and it is typically associated with pain.[6]

Opacities in the anterior chamber can also cause TMVL. For example, uveitis-glaucoma-hyphema (UGH) syndrome is an uncommon complication of cataract extraction with intraocular lens implantation and presents with a triad of anterior uveitis, glaucoma, and hyphema.[7,8] Typically, the patient has a sudden decrease in vision within minutes, with a resolution of the symptoms over hours to days.[7] This may be associated with pain, and a microhyphema may be seen if the patient is examined during an acute episode. There is not a complete loss of light perception. The patient may also complain of erythropsia (perception of red in the vision) and an ache in the affected eye owing to associated anterior uveitis or raised intraocular pressure (IOP). Episodes of TMVL may correlate with inflammation and recurrent bleeding. Gonioscopy may be required to make the diagnosis. Treatment is required for UGH syndrome if the repeated episodes of visual disturbance are disabling or glaucoma develops. Definitive treatment involves surgical intraocular lens rotation, exchange, or removal.[9]

TMVL accompanied by haloes, pain, and nausea should prompt suspicion for angle-closure glaucoma, although it can rarely occur with painless TMVL.[10] The raised IOP leads to corneal clouding owing to edema and may reduce the perfusion pressure of the eye, thereby impairing blood flow to the retina and optic disc.[11] Intermittent angle closure tends to recur over days to weeks and is usually less severe than acute angle-closure glaucoma. The episodes resolve on their own and between episodes the IOP can be normal, although the presence of glaukomflecken, anterior opacities on the lens surface, may indicate prior episodes of angle closure.

Retinopathy

Transient visual loss or prolonged afterimages following bright light may be suggestive of a macular disorder, such as retinal detachment or age-related macular degeneration.[12] It is thought that in age-related macular degeneration, the retinal pigment epithelium and photoreceptor interaction is anatomically deranged causing abnormal processing of light as it bleaches the rhodopsin in the photoreceptors.[13] Abnormalities in the retina consistent with macular degeneration, such as drusen, would be detected on funduscopy. Performing the photostress test (10 seconds of exposure to a bright light) shows that the return to normal central visual acuity is abnormally prolonged (>45 seconds).[14]

Optic Disc Edema

Optic disc edema is an important cause of TMVL. Patients experience brief (<10 seconds) episodes of "grayouts" or "blackouts" of vision. These episodes, termed transient visual obscurations, are often precipitated by postural changes, although they may occur spontaneously.[4] Dimming of vision lasts for a few seconds, may involve one eye at a time, and resolves completely. Episodes may recur multiple times in the day, are thought to be attributable to transient ischemia of the optic nerve head, and can also occur with optic disc edema that is not related to increased intracranial pressure.[15] Patients may have other symptoms associated with elevated intracranial pressure, such as headache. These obscurations of vision are not a warning sign of impending visual failure.[16] Neuroimaging should be urgently sought to exclude a structural etiology such as a mass lesion, venous sinus thrombosis, or obstructive hydrocephalus. If imaging is normal, patients should undergo lumbar puncture for measurement of opening pressure and cerebrospinal fluid analysis.[16] Treatment is aimed at the underlying cause of elevated intracranial pressure.

Other optic disc anomalies such as optic nerve head drusen can also cause transient visual loss.[17] TMVL or even permanent monocular visual loss owing to optic disc drusen can occur without signs of vascular complications.[18] Nevertheless, it is important that compression by a mass lesion not be overlooked in patients with severe visual loss, especially in patients with loss of central vision.[19] The underlying mechanism of TMVL from optic disc drusen is thought to be similar to causes of optic disc edema.[15] If not directly visible on funduscopy, imaging with ultrasonography or computed tomography (CT) may be required to demonstrate their presence. Funduscopy may also reveal tortuous vessels, and dilated veins that are often present with optic disc drusen. Optic disc drusen can be a harbinger for vascular complications including central retinal artery occlusion and anterior ischemic optic neuropathy.[19]

Orbitopathy

Orbital masses or foreign bodies can cause episodic TMVL in certain fields of gaze, especially downgaze.[20] Clues to the diagnosis may include unilateral proptosis on external examination and restriction in ocular motility. Gaze-evoked episodes most often are the result of intraconal pathology, most commonly optic nerve sheath meningioma and cavernous hemangioma.[21] The common etiology in these patients appears to be compromise of the retinal or optic nerve circulation, either by means of compression of the central retinal artery or disruption of the optic nerve microvasculature.[22] Interestingly, patients may be unaware of positional visual loss and the ability to improve this condition with appropriate surgical therapy suggests that all patients with an orbital disease process should be screened for gaze-evoked visual loss.[20] Testing for gaze-evoked visual loss is performed by having the patient look in all directions of gaze, having the patient hold each eccentric position of gaze for at least 5 seconds, and noting any changes in visual function or pupil reactivity.

Blepharospasm

Patients with blepharospasm who are unable to keep their eyes open may experience moments of visual loss. This is typically easily distinguished from other causes of visual loss. In advanced cases, the eyelids cannot be manually opened during an episode.[23]

Vascular

Emboli

As a result of retinal arteriolar emboli, the patient typically describes a curtain of darkness that descends over one eye, resulting in vision loss lasting 20 to 30 minutes.[24,25] With resolution, the curtain may either ascend or slowly disappear. Emboli that cause TMVL travel and lodge within blood vessels that supply the optic nerve, retina, or choroid. Funduscopy is warranted because the emboli often appear distinctive and can provide clues about the possible site of origin, although the absence of emboli on examination does not exclude them as a cause. The 3 most common types of emboli are cholesterol, platelet-fibrin, and calcium.[26] Their appearance and common sites of origin are reviewed in **Table 1**. Other less common causes include emboli from cardiac tumors (myxoma), fat, sepsis, talc, air, silicone, and depot drugs.[16]

An embolic cause of TMVL requires vascular and cardiac evaluation. Atheroma formation is most common at the bifurcation of the internal and external carotid arteries, but can originate from the heart (eg, in patients with valvular heart disease or atrial fibrillation) and atheromatous plaque in the aortic arch.[27] Emboli may also arise from the common carotid[28] or from carotid dissection.[29] Rarely, emboli may originate from an atrial myxoma,[30] or travel from the systemic venous system to the arterial system via a cardiac septal defect or pulmonary shunt.[31]

Carotid Doppler ultrasound, which allows an estimation of the degree of stenosis, is often used initially to screen for internal carotid artery (ICA) stenosis. The atheroma can remain stationary, become fibrotic, regress, ulcerate, narrow and occlude the lumen, or release emboli. CT and magnetic resonance (MR) angiography are other useful screening tests for ICA stenosis, but catheter angiography remains the gold-standard technique.[32] Echocardiography can identify structural cardiac abnormalities associated with thrombus formation and systemic or paradoxic embolism. In patients with vascular risk factors, initial imaging with carotid Doppler ultrasound and an echocardiogram is typically performed. Regardless of what imaging studies are ultimately pursued, the presence of retinal emboli allows an opportunity to screen for modifiable risk factors such as hypertension, diabetes mellitus, and dyslipidemia.

Table 1 Clinical aspects of common retinal emboli		
Type	**Appearance**	**Source**
Cholesterol	Yellow-orange or copper color Refractile Rectangular Usually located at major vessel bifurcation	Common or internal carotid artery Rarely from aorta or innominate artery
Platelet-fibrin	Dull gray-white color Long, smooth shape Concave meniscus at each end Lodge along course of vessel	From wall of atherosclerotic vessel Heart valves
Calcium	Chalky white Large Round or ovoid Lodge at first or second vessel bifurcation, often overlying disc	From heart or great vessels Rheumatic heart disease Calcific aortic stenosis

Data from Miller N. Embolic causes of transient monocular visual loss. Ophthalmol Clin North Am 1996;9:359–80.

The management of TMVL from retinal embolism is directed at the underlying cause. In patients with a cardiac source, treatment consists of anticoagulation with warfarin and addressing the underlying cardiac disease with careful attention to arteriosclerotic risk factors.[16] In those with ICA stenosis, antiplatelet therapy with aspirin should be initiated and vascular risk factors appropriately addressed.[33] The management of high-grade ICA (70%–99%) stenosis with isolated TMVL remains controversial. The North American Symptomatic Carotid Endarterectomy Trial suggests that 3 or more of the following risk factors should be present to gain a benefit from carotid endarterectomy: age older than 75, male gender, history of hemispheric transient ischemic attack or stroke, history of intermittent claudication, ipsilateral ICA stenosis of 80% to 94%, and absence of intracranial collateral vessels on cerebral angiography.[33] Carotid stenting may produce equivalent long-term outcomes and may be a safer option, but additional data are required.[16]

Retinal vein occlusion

TMVL has also been reported as a symptom of an impending central retinal vein occlusion (CRVO).[34] The episodes can last 2 to 4 hours, longer than is typical for transient arterial retinal ischemia. Patients may complain of cloudiness of vision rather than frank visual loss typically associated with arterial ischemia.[35] On examination, there may be dilated retinal veins; within 2 weeks, the classic ophthalmoscopic appearance of CRVO may be present, which includes scattered intraretinal hemorrhages.[35] Causes of retinal vein disorders include hypercoaguable states, retinal artery occlusion, and arteriosclerosis. In young patients, further laboratory investigation should include anticardiolipin antibody, antiphosphatidyl choline and serine, antinuclear antibody, serum protein electrophoresis, partial thromboplastin time, and protein S and protein C to exclude hyperviscosity and hypercoagulability.[36] In addition, compressive orbitopathies and carotid-cavernous fistulas can cause orbital venous hypertension.[4]

Giant cell arteritis

Among patients with visual manifestations of giant cell arteritis (GCA), a history of transient visual loss is reported 30% to 54% of the time.[37–39] In some patients, transient visual loss may be the only complaint,[40] and precedes the development of acute and permanent visual loss in more than half (50%–64%) of untreated patients by an average of almost 9 days.[38,41] TMVL results from insufficient perfusion of the optic nerve, retina, or choroid. GCA typically causes a relatively short duration of visual loss (<2 minutes), multiple recurrences in the same eye over a short period of time, photopsias or other phenomena during the visual loss, and visual loss with postural change such as standing up or bending down.[40] In addition, a history of headache, jaw claudication, scalp tenderness, polymyalgia rheumatica, or systemic symptoms such as fever, weight loss, or anorexia may suggest the diagnosis. Funduscopic examination may reveal cotton-wool spots, intraretinal hemorrhages, or optic disc edema.[37] Laboratory markers urgently assessed in suspicious cases include erythrocyte sedimentation rate, C-reactive protein, and platelet count.[29] The diagnosis is confirmed with a temporal artery biopsy, characterized by the chief pathologic finding of a panarteritis consisting mostly of lymphocytes and macrophages.[42] Although the temporal artery biopsy is considered the gold-standard test for the diagnosis, it is important to remember that a negative biopsy has been said to occur in up to 10% to 15% of all patients diagnosed clinically as having GCA.[43] TMVL may be a warning symptom for impending anterior ischemic optic neuropathy,[44] and early treatment with corticosteroids may prevent permanent visual loss in patients with TMVL. The optimal dosage and route of corticosteroids remain unclear.

Ocular ischemic syndrome

TMVL can occur from hypoperfusion as a result of stenosis or occlusion of the ipsilateral internal or common carotid arteries. Patients typically describe a dark or black shade that spreads across the visual field that, unlike TMVL from embolic sources, is more gradual in onset and can last for seconds to minutes.[16] It is often precipitated by exposure to bright light,[45,46] but can occur after meals,[47] postural changes,[48] or sexual activity.[49] There also can be signs of the ocular ischemic syndrome, which encompasses a spectrum of findings that result from chronic ocular hypoperfusion. Ocular ischemic syndrome is relatively uncommon, and the diagnosis may be difficult to make because of its variable presentations. A history of TMVL is present in approximately 10% to 15% of patients with ocular ischemic syndrome.[50] The presence of the syndrome implies underlying severe carotid occlusive disease.[51] Anterior segment examination may show dilated conjunctival and episcleral vessels, and signs of an anterior chamber inflammatory reaction.[52] The episcleral injection may be a sign of collateral blood flow from the external carotid artery in the presence of an internal carotid artery occlusion.[53] Chronic ischemia may also cause iris neovascularization that can lead to increased IOP and neovascular glaucoma.[54] Some patients, however, have an IOP in the normal range, or even ocular hypotony owing to ischemia of the ciliary body and reduced aqueous humor production.[55] On funduscopy, the retinal arteries are generally narrowed, and the retinal veins are often irregularly dilated with venous beading.[55] There may be dot and blot hemorrhages in the mid-peripheral retina, microaneurysms, cotton-wool spots, and neovascularization.[54] The episodes of visual loss decrease and the risk of further ischemic damage to the eye is reduced when the stenosis is relieved or the occlusion is bypassed; underlying vascular risk factors should be addressed to prevent future vascular events.[54]

TMVL WITH A NORMAL EYE EXAMINATION
Hypoperfusion

Reduced cardiac output or systemic hypotension may produce TMVL.[4] Although systemic hypotension is typically associated with binocular visual loss, in addition to lightheadedness and confusion, the combination of a hypotensive episode and asymmetric anterior circulation stenosis may cause TMVL alone, particularly orthostatically induced TMVL.[2]

Migraine

Episodes of TMVL designated "retinal migraine" or "ocular migraine" occur in patients with a history or family history of migraine.[56] The International Headache Society diagnostic criteria for retinal migraine require at least 2 attacks of fully reversible monocular-positive visual phenomena such as flashing lights or scintillating scotomas and/or negative symptoms associated with a headache that fulfills diagnostic criteria for migraine without aura.[57] This is in contrast to a typical migraine with aura, which involves the cerebral cortex and is associated with binocular visual phenomena. Retinal migraine affects about 1 of every 200 patients who have migraine, and patients tend to be younger, with most younger than 40 years.[58] Clinically, retinal migraine has a highly variable presentation. Some patients describe visual loss consisting of black, gray, white, or shaded areas of varying size that may progress inward from the peripheral visual field.[56] Most events are transient, lasting from 5 to 20 minutes, and may occur several times a day. When headaches occur in association with the visual changes, they may occur either during or after the visual disturbances.[58] It should be noted, however, that the existence of retinal migraine is a contested issue, and it may remain as a diagnosis of exclusion.[59,60]

Retinal Artery Vasospasm

Similar attacks of TMVL, but without an associated headache, can arise as a result of retinal artery vasospasm, and do not represent the previously mentioned retinal migraine.[61] In the case of retinal vasospasm, the eye examination may be abnormal during an attack of visual loss. A relative afferent pupillary defect may be noted or retinal vasospasm may be observed during funduscopy.[62] Patients report attacks of visual loss that are frequent, recurring many times a day, and often have temporary, complete monocular visual loss rather than loss restricted to the inferior or superior altitudinal visual field.[63] Attacks of transient monocular visual loss attributable to vasospasm may be treated with calcium channel blockers.[63] In either case of retinal migraine or retinal vasospasm, other causes of TMVL should be excluded as part of the diagnostic evaluation.[16]

SUMMARY

TMVL is an important clinical complaint and has a number of causes, of which the most common is retinal ischemia. A practical approach is to perform a careful examination to determine whether there are any eye abnormalities that can explain the visual loss. Despite the transient nature of the symptom, there may be clues to the diagnosis on the examination even after the visual loss has recovered.

REFERENCES

1. Bernstein EF. Amaurosis fugax. New York: Springer-Verlag; 1987.
2. Trobe JD. The neurology of vision. New York: Oxford University Press; 2001.
3. Fisher CM. 'Transient monocular blindness' versus 'amaurosis fugax'. Neurology 1989;39(12):1622–4.
4. Biousse V, Trobe JD. Transient monocular visual loss. Am J Ophthalmol 2005; 140(4):717–21.
5. Tutt R, Bradley A, Begley C, et al. Optical and visual impact of tear break-up in human eyes. Invest Ophthalmol Vis Sci 2000;41(13):4117–23.
6. Reed JW, Jacoby BG, Weaver RG. Corneal epithelial basement membrane dystrophy: an overlooked cause of painless visual disturbances. Ann Ophthalmol 1992;24(12):471–4.
7. Cates CA, Newman DK. Transient monocular visual loss due to uveitis-glaucoma-hyphaema (UGH) syndrome. J Neurol Neurosurg Psychiatr 1998;65(1):131–2.
8. Percival SP, Das SK. UGH syndrome after posterior chamber lens implantation. J Am Intraocul Implant Soc 1983;9(2):200–1.
9. John GR, Stark WJ. Rotation of posterior chamber intraocular lenses for management of lens-associated recurring hyphemas. Arch Ophthalmol 1992;110(7): 963–4.
10. Abe A, Nishiyama Y, Kitahara I, et al. Painless transient monocular loss of vision resulting from angle-closure glaucoma. Headache 2007;47(7):1098–9.
11. Best M, Blumenthal M, Futterman HA, et al. Critical closure of intraocular blood vessels. Arch Ophthalmol 1969;82(3):385–92.
12. Sandberg MA, Gaudio AR. Slow photostress recovery and disease severity in age-related macular degeneration. Retina 1995;15(5):407–12.

13. Dorey CK, Wu G, Ebenstein D, et al. Cell loss in the aging retina. Relationship to lipofuscin accumulation and macular degeneration. Invest Ophthalmol Vis Sci 1989;30(8):1691–9.

14. Glaser JS, Savino PJ, Sumers KD, et al. The photostress recovery test in the clinical assessment of visual function. Am J Ophthalmol 1977;83(2):255–60.

15. Sadun AA, Currie JN, Lessell S. Transient visual obscurations with elevated optic discs. Ann Neurol 1984;16(4):489–94.

16. Thurtell MJ, Rucker JC. Transient visual loss. Int Ophthalmol Clin 2009;49(3): 147–66.

17. Beck RW, Corbett JJ, Thompson HS, et al. Decreased visual acuity from optic disc drusen. Arch Ophthalmol 1985;103(8):1155–9.

18. Meyer E, Gdal-On M, Zonis S. Transient monocular blindness in a case of drusen of the optic disc. Ophthalmologica 1973;166(5):321–6.

19. Auw-Haedrich C, Staubach F, Witschel H. Optic disk drusen. Surv Ophthalmol 2002;47(6):515–32.

20. Otto CS, Coppit GL, Mazzoli RA, et al. Gaze-evoked amaurosis: a report of five cases. Ophthalmology 2003;110(2):322–6.

21. Orcutt JC, Tucker WM, Mills RP, et al. Gaze-evoked amaurosis. Ophthalmology 1987;94(3):213–8.

22. Manor RS, Yassur Y, Hoyt WF. Reading-evoked visual dimming. Am J Ophthalmol 1996;121(2):212–4.

23. Ben Simon GJ, McCann JD. Benign essential blepharospasm. Int Ophthalmol Clin 2005;45(3):49–75.

24. Bruno A, Corbett JJ, Biller J, et al. Transient monocular visual loss patterns and associated vascular abnormalities. Stroke 1990;21(1):34–9.

25. Donders RC. Clinical features of transient monocular blindness and the likelihood of atherosclerotic lesions of the internal carotid artery. J Neurol Neurosurg Psychiatr 2001;71(2):247–9.

26. Miller N. Embolic causes of transient monocular visual loss. Ophthalmol Clin North Am 1996;9:359–80.

27. Russell RW. The source of retinal emboli. Lancet 1968;2(7572):789–92.

28. Hoya K, Morikawa E, Tamura A, et al. Common carotid artery stenosis and amaurosis fugax. J Stroke Cerebrovasc Dis 2008;17(1):1–4.

29. Biousse V, Touboul PJ, D'Anglejan-Chatillon J, et al. Ophthalmologic manifestations of internal carotid artery dissection. Am J Ophthalmol 1998;126(4): 565–77.

30. Bolo-deoku J Jr, Orchard RT, Fison PN. Transient loss of peripheral vision as the presentation of left atrial myxoma. Br J Ophthalmol 1992;76(2):113–4.

31. Nedeltchev K, Arnold M, Wahl A, et al. Outcome of patients with cryptogenic stroke and patent foramen ovale. J Neurol Neurosurg Psychiatr 2002;72(3): 347–50.

32. Wardlaw JM, Chappell FM, Best JJ, et al. Non-invasive imaging compared with intra-arterial angiography in the diagnosis of symptomatic carotid stenosis: a meta-analysis. Lancet 2006;367(9521):1503–12.

33. Johnston SC. Clinical practice. Transient ischemic attack. N Engl J Med 2002; 347(21):1687–92.

34. Shults W. Ocular causes of transient monocular vision loss other than emboli. Ophthalmol Clin North Am 1996;9:381–91.

35. Shuler RK Jr, Biousse V, Newman NJ. Transient monocular visual loss in two patients with impending central retinal vein occlusion. J Neuroophthalmol 2005; 25(2):152–4.

36. Glueck CJ, Goldenberg N, Bell H, et al. Amaurosis fugax: associations with heritable thrombophilia. Clin Appl Thromb Hemost 2005;11(3):235–41.
37. Glutz von Blotzheim S, Borruat FX. Neuro-ophthalmic complications of biopsy-proven giant cell arteritis. Eur J Ophthalmol 1997;7(4):375–82.
38. Hayreh SS, Podhajsky PA, Zimmerman B. Ocular manifestations of giant cell arteritis. Am J Ophthalmol 1998;125(4):509–20.
39. Gonzalez-Gay MA, Garcia-Porrua C, Llorca J, et al. Visual manifestations of giant cell arteritis. Trends and clinical spectrum in 161 patients. Medicine (Baltimore) 2000;79(5):283–92.
40. Kawasaki A, Purvin V. Giant cell arteritis: an updated review. Acta Ophthalmol 2009;87(1):13–32.
41. Font C, Cid MC, Coll-Vinent B, et al. Clinical features in patients with permanent visual loss due to biopsy-proven giant cell arteritis. Br J Rheumatol 1997;36(2):251–4.
42. Nordborg E, Nordborg C, Malmvall BE, et al. Giant cell arteritis. Rheum Dis Clin North Am 1995;21(4):1013–26.
43. Schmidt WA. Current diagnosis and treatment of temporal arteritis. Curr Treat Options Cardiovasc Med 2006;8(2):145–51.
44. Liozon E, Herrmann F, Ly K, et al. Risk factors for visual loss in giant cell (temporal) arteritis: a prospective study of 174 patients. Am J Med 2001; 111(3):211–7.
45. Donnan GA, Sharbrough FW, Whisnant JP. Carotid occlusive disease. Effect of bright light on visual evoked response. Arch Neurol 1982;39(11):687–9.
46. Furlan AJ, Whisnant JP, Kearns TP. Unilateral visual loss in bright light. An unusual symptom of carotid artery occlusive disease. Arch Neurol 1979;36(11):675–6.
47. Levin LA, Mootha VV. Postprandial transient visual loss. A symptom of critical carotid stenosis. Ophthalmology 1997;104(3):397–401.
48. Hollenhorst RW, Kublin JG, Millikan CH. Ophthalmodynamometry in the diagnosis of intracerebral orthostatic hypotension. Proc Staff Meet Mayo Clin 1963;38: 532–47.
49. Kofoed PK, Milea D, Larsen M. Transient monocular blindness precipitated by sexual intercourse. Br J Ophthalmol 2009;93(9):1199–250.
50. Brown GC, Magargal LE. The ocular ischemic syndrome. Clinical, fluorescein angiographic and carotid angiographic features. Int Ophthalmol 1988;11(4): 239–51.
51. Mendrinos E, Machinis TG, Pournaras CJ. Ocular ischemic syndrome. Surv Ophthalmol 2010;55(1):2–34.
52. Blake J, Kelly G. Ocular aspects of internal carotid stenosis. Trans Ophthalmol Soc U K 1975;95(1):194–201.
53. Countee RW, Gnanadev A, Chavis P. Dilated episcleral arteries—a significant physical finding in assessment of patients with cerebrovascular insufficiency. Stroke 1978;9(1):42–5.
54. Chen CS, Miller NR. Ocular ischemic syndrome: review of clinical presentations, etiology, investigation, and management. Compr Ophthalmol Update 2007;8(1): 17–28.
55. Brown GC, Brown MM, Magargal LE. The ocular ischemic syndrome and neovascularization. Trans Pa Acad Ophthalmol Otolaryngol 1986;38(1):302–6.
56. Evans RW, Grosberg BM. Retinal migraine: migraine associated with monocular visual symptoms. Headache 2008;48(1):142–5.
57. Headache Classification Subcommittee of the International Headache Society. The international classification of headache disorders (second edition). Cephalalgia 2004;24(Suppl 1):1–160.

58. Gan KD, Mouradian MS, Weis E, et al. Transient monocular visual loss and retinal migraine. CMAJ 2005;173(12):1441–2.
59. Foroozan R. Visual dysfunction in migraine. Int Ophthalmol Clin 2009;49(3): 133–46.
60. Grosberg BM, Solomon S, Friedman DI, et al. Retinal migraine reappraised. Cephalalgia 2006;26(11):1275–86.
61. Kline LB, Kelly CL. Ocular migraine in a patient with cluster headaches. Headache 1980;20(5):253–7.
62. Burger SK, Saul RF, Selhorst JB, et al. Transient monocular blindness caused by vasospasm. N Engl J Med 1991;325(12):870–3.
63. Winterkorn JM, Kupersmith MJ, Wirtschafter JD, et al. Brief report: treatment of vasospastic amaurosis fugax with calcium-channel blockers. N Engl J Med 1993;329(6):396–8.

Nonglaucomatous Optic Atrophy

Karl Golnik, MD, MEd[a,b,c,d,*]

KEYWORDS

- Optic atrophy • Optic disc • Optic neuropathy • Pallor

DEFINITION

In clinical terms, optic atrophy occurs when the optic disc is thought to be less pink or paler than normal (**Fig. 1**). Thus, optic atrophy is not a diagnosis but simply an ophthalmoscopic sign similar to finding upper extremity weakness; the cause of the weakness must still be determined. Unfortunately, the term "optic disc pallor" is often used synonymously with optic atrophy. A wide range of "normal" optic disc color exists, and thus it can be difficult to be sure if optic atrophy is present. A normal optic disc is often pinker on the nasal side, with relative temporal pallor. The central cup of the disc appears pale because the white lamina cribrosa is visible. Optic discs in patients with axial myopia may appear paler. Furthermore, media opacities such as cataract can impart more color to the disc, and pseudophakia can result in a paler disc appearance. Thus, optic disc pallor should not be used synonymously with optic atrophy. It is essential to compare an individual's optic discs, because they will usually have the same color. If true atrophy (damage) exists, it should be accompanied by visual loss (acuity and/or peripheral vision), decreased color perception (if acuity is compromised), and a relative afferent pupillary defect unless the damage is symmetric. Ophthalmoscopic evaluation of the peripapillary retina may reveal diffuse or segmental nerve fiber layer loss. New technology such as optical coherence tomography can also be helpful in demonstrating axonal loss. Retinal vascular attenuation often occurs after anterior ischemic optic neuropathy (AION).[1] Comparison of vessels from eye to eye helps to confirm this finding and suggests previous ION.

Pathologically, optic atrophy is shrinkage of the optic nerve caused by degeneration of its axons. The axons may degenerate because of damage from anywhere in the ganglion cells in the retina to the point of axonal synapse in the lateral geniculate

---

This work was supported in part by an unrestricted grant from Research to Prevent Blindness, Inc, New York, NY.

a Department of Ophthalmology, University of Cincinnati, Cincinnati, OH, USA
b Department of Neurology, University of Cincinnati, Cincinnati, OH, USA
c Department of Neurosurgery, University of Cincinnati, Cincinnati, OH, USA
d Cincinnati Eye Institute, 1945 CEI Drive,Cincinnati, OH 45242, USA
* Department of Ophthalmology, University of Cincinnati, Cincinnati, OH.
E-mail address: kgolnik@fuse.net

Neurol Clin 28 (2010) 631–640
doi:10.1016/j.ncl.2010.03.005
0733-8619/10/$ – see front matter
neurologic.theclinics.com

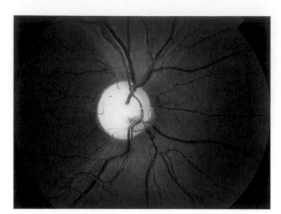

Fig. 1. Nonspecific diffuse optic atrophy.

body. The clinically apparent increase in pallor of the optic disc is not completely understood.[2] Loss of axons with resultant decreased blood supply and gliosis have been proposed causes.[3] Quigley and Anderson[4] proposed that loss of axons affects the normal light transmission and diffusion amongst capillaries and that the light is instead reflected by the remaining white glial tissue. These investigators did not find evidence of astroglial proliferation in atrophic optic nerves. Several investigators have used laser Doppler velocimetry to study optic disc blood flow in patients with atrophy[5,6] and have found diminution of blood flow in such optic discs, but of mild nature. Thus, questions on the exact cause of the pallor observed in optic atrophy still exist.[2]

Rarely, trans-synaptic degeneration from damage to the retrogeniculate visual pathway results in optic atrophy, which occurs primarily in the immature brain (in utero or early infancy).[7] Clinically apparent transsynaptic degeneration does not typically occur in human adults, although it has been demonstrated pathologically in some patients.[8]

DIFFERENTIAL DIAGNOSIS

Anything that damages the retinal ganglion cells or their axons will result in optic atrophy. Most commonly, the atrophy is diffuse and nonspecific, although exceptions do exist (see **Fig. 1**). It is beyond the scope of this article to completely discuss glaucomatous optic atrophy. However, it is important to emphasize the differences between glaucomatous and nonglaucomatous optic atrophy. The hallmark of glaucomatous optic atrophy is a progression in the size of the optic disc cup. The cupping is typically accentuated vertically, thus causing a more vertical than horizontal cup (**Fig. 2**). Focal notching of the disc is also characteristic of glaucoma. Nevertheless, conditions other than glaucoma (eg, compression, ischemia) have been reported to cause an increase in cup-to-disc ratio, but this is usually mild in relation to degree of optic nerve dysfunction.[9,10] Trobe and colleagues[11] had 5 ophthalmologists review 163 fundus stereophotographs of 9 entities as "unknowns." Glaucoma, central retinal artery occlusion, and ION were diagnosed by at least one observer with accuracy greater than 80%. Vertical elongation of the cup was the most important factor in differentiating glaucoma from other conditions. Another important differentiating characteristic was the rim pallor (**Fig. 3**). Thus, even in the presence of definite glaucoma,

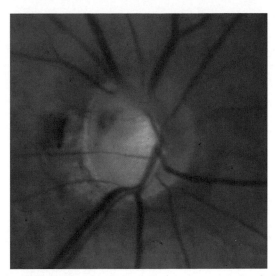

Fig. 2. This optic disc has an elongated vertical cup characteristic of glaucomatous optic atrophy. Note the very thin inferior rim. There is also a hemorrhage on the superior rim at the 10-o'clock position, a finding occasionally seen with glaucoma.

optic disc rim pallor (atrophy) is an important clue to nonglaucomatous optic disc damage and should prompt further evaluation. In the study by Trobe, other optic neuropathies (ie, optic neuritis, compressive, traumatic, and hereditary optic neuropathies) were identified with less than 50% accuracy.[11] Thus, diffuse optic atrophy is a nonspecific finding, only indicating that damage has been done. Vascular changes of arteriolar attenuation and sheathing were somewhat helpful in differentiating ischemic causes from nonischemic ones.

There are several patterns of optic atrophy and other fundoscopic changes that may help narrow the differential diagnosis. Horizontal band (or bow-tie) atrophy may be present with optic chiasmal or retrochiasmal pregeniculate lesions (**Fig. 4**), This

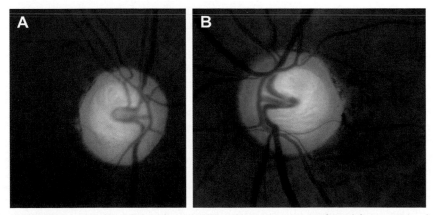

Fig. 3. (A) Right optic disc. (B). Left optic disc. This patient was referred for possible glaucoma because of the large cup/disc ratio. However, the important finding is the relative pallor of the optic disc rim in the right eye (A). This patient had a compressive optic neuropathy from intracranial meningioma.

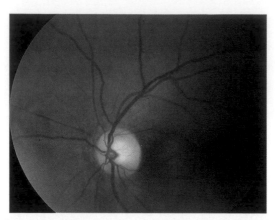

Fig. 4. Bow-tie optic atrophy. Left optic disc of a patient with chiasmal compression. Note the relative pallor of the nasal and temporal portions of the rim versus the superior and inferior portions of the disc.

atrophy occurs because the retinal nerve fibers nasal to the fovea decussate in the chiasm. These fibers include the retinal nerve fibers originating nasal to the optic disc and the nasal retinal fibers between the fovea and optic disc. The latter group of fibers is temporal to the optic disc. Thus, when these decussating fibers are damaged, the nasal and temporal aspects of the optic disc become atrophic. The superior and inferior portions of the optic disc are relatively spared, because the temporal retinal fibers arc around the fovea and enter the optic disc at the upper and lower aspects of the disc. These findings have nothing to do with the underlying cause of the damage but help to determine where the damage occurred. Bilateral temporal optic atrophy is most often associated with conditions that cause symmetric damage to the papillomacular bundle (**Fig. 5**). These conditions are usually hereditary (dominant optic atrophy, Leber hereditary optic neuropathy), nutritional (vitamin B_{12} or folate deficiency), or toxic (ethambutol, methanol). It must be remembered that some degree of relative temporal pallor may be bilaterally present as a normal finding. Superior or inferior altitudinal optic atrophy suggests earlier AION (but is not pathognomonic) (**Fig. 6**).[12] Buncic and colleagues[13] described an "inverse" optic atrophy seen in children with vigabatrin toxicity. The optic disc developed primarily nasal pallor, but this change was associated with retinal atrophy as well. Optociliary collateral vessels may become enlarged and visible when retinal venous outflow is compromised by an optic nerve sheath meningioma (**Fig. 7**). These collateral vessels represent an alternative pathway for blood to escape the eye. Instead of blood flowing back through the central retinal vein, these vessels connect the retinal veins to the choroid, and the blood exits the eye through the vortex veins. These vessels can also be apparent in glaucoma after central retinal artery occlusion or can simply be enlarged as a normal variant. Optic atrophy in the presence of radial choroidal folds may indicate compression of the globe of the eye and optic nerve by a tumor or any mass lesion (**Fig. 8**).

Most optic atrophy is diffuse (see **Fig. 1**) and can be caused by myriad processes, including inflammation (eg, demyelinating optic neuritis, sarcoidosis, systemic lupus erythematosus), infection (eg, syphilis, tuberculosis, Lyme disease), compression (eg, tumor, thyroid eye disease, aneurysm), ischemia (eg, nonarteritic AION [NAION], giant cell arteritis, hypoperfusion related to blood loss, or hypotension), nutritional deficiency, toxins, and heritable conditions.[14–26]

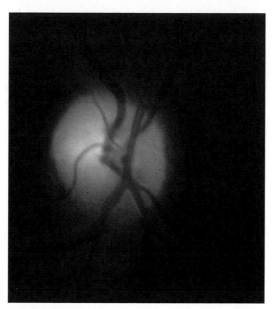

Fig. 5. Superior segmental optic atrophy. Note the relative pallor of the superior portion of the optic disc. This patient presented with sudden visual loss and initially had optic disc swelling. Nonarteritic AION (NAION) was diagnosed and optic atrophy developed over 2 months.

EVALUATION

Optic atrophy is not a diagnosis. The cause of the damage that resulted in the atrophy must be determined. Although the cause of optic atrophy may be elucidated by a thorough history and examination, a definite cause is not always apparent. Ancillary testing is necessary when the cause is not apparent by clinical evaluation. Suggested diagnostic approaches to the patient with optic atrophy are presented in **Table 1**.

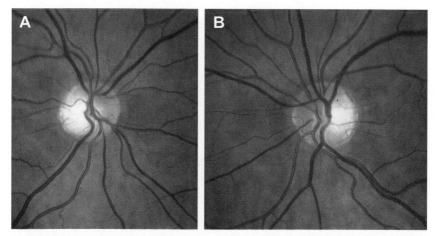

Fig. 6. Bilateral temporal optic atrophy in a patient with dominant optic atrophy. (*A*) Right optic disc. (*B*) Left optic disc.

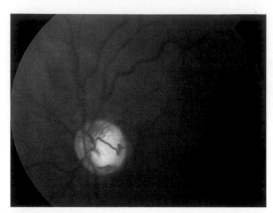

Fig. 7. Cilioretinal collateral vessels. Note the prominent optic disc vessel extending from the center of the disc to the 3-o'clock position. The vessel appears to stop but continues into the choroid. An optic nerve sheath meningioma was compressing the optic nerve and central retinal vein, increasing venous pressure and causing this collateral vessel to become engorged and visible.

History

A complete ophthalmic examination including a comprehensive history will lead to an underlying diagnosis in 92% of cases of optic atrophy.[27] Patients with optic atrophy may or may not be able to specify the date of the onset of their visual loss. In addition, the sudden discovery of monocular visual loss may confound the history. Optic atrophy develops several months after damage, and thus the patient who presents with acute or subacute visual loss (developing in the range of days to several weeks) and optic atrophy must have a more chronic process. A detailed history can provide many diagnostic clues toward an underlying cause of a patient's optic atrophy. The most important causes are the age of the patient, onset of visual loss (sudden vs gradual, static vs progressive), medical history, and other accompanying symptoms.

The most common causes of optic neuropathy, AION, and optic neuritis are also the most common causes of optic atrophy.[27] Optic neuritis typically occurs in young

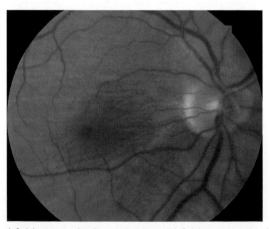

Fig. 8. Radial retinal folds. Note the linear horizontal folds present in this patient with an orbital cavernous hemangioma compressing the globe and optic nerve.

Table 1
Historical features and suggested diagnostic approach

History	Rule Out (Through Diagnostic Approach)
Progressive unilateral or bilateral optic neuropathy	Compressive lesion (MRI with gadolinium of brain and orbits)
Painless, progressive, bilateral, and simultaneous loss of visual acuity and central visual field (eg, central or cecocentral scotomas)	Toxic-nutritional causes (methanol, ethambutol, heavy metals, amiodarone, and deficiencies of vitamin B_{12} or folate).
Bilateral, rapidly sequential optic neuropathy with visual acuity and central visual field loss	Leber hereditary optic neuropathy, neuromyelitis optica
Underlying infectious risk factors (eg, tick bite, cat scratch, sexually transmitted disease, tuberculosis exposure)	Lyme disease, cat-scratch disease (*Bartonella henselae*), syphilis, tuberculosis
Inflammatory symptoms (eg, rash, sinus disease, renal, pulmonary, cardiac, or gastrointestinal dysfunction)	Systemic lupus erythematosus, Behçet disease, Wegener granulomatosis (antinuclear antibody, antineutrophil cytoplasmic antibody, chest radiograph, renal function testing, urinalysis, medicine consultation)
Earlier, acute visual loss; pain with eye movement; and visual recovery suggestive of optic neuritis or prior neurologic symptoms suggesting demyelinating disease	Multiple sclerosis (MRI)
Earlier, acute, static, and painless visual loss in a patient with vasculopathic risk factors (eg, hypertension, diabetes, elevated cholesterol, smoking) or symptoms of scalp tenderness, jaw claudication, malaise	NAION (obtain old records to try and document presence of optic disc edema) Giant cell arteritis (CBC, ESR, CRP)
Steroid-responsive optic neuropathy	Sarcoid (chest radiograph, angiotensin-converting enzyme), other inflammatory optic neuropathies, carcinomatosis (lumbar puncture)
Hereditary optic neuropathy	Dominant optic atrophy, Leber hereditary optic neuropathy (maternal inheritance)

Abbreviations: CBC, complete blood count; CRP, C-reactive protein; ESR, erythrocyte sedimentation rate; MRI, magnetic resonance imaging.

adults (teens to those in their forties), whereas AION usually occurs in older adults (>45 years). Thus, the patient's age can be helpful in differentiating these potential causes. Sudden or subacute visual loss points toward vascular compromise or inflammation, whereas gradual visual loss may indicate a compressive cause. Similarly, static loss of vision favors previous ischemia or trauma, whereas progressive visual loss may indicate continued damage from compression or nutritional deficits. A medical history of diseases such as multiple sclerosis, severe vascular disease, sarcoidosis, pseudotumor cerebri, or malignancy may suggest the cause of the optic atrophy. In addition, systemic diseases such as hypertension, diabetes, or previous myocardial infarction and/or stroke may indicate that an earlier occurrence of AION has led to the optic atrophy. Other associated symptoms may also be helpful. Focal paresthesia and weakness may indicate demyelinating disease or transient ischemia; a history of previous painful visual loss with recovery suggests optic neuritis; and shortness of breath and/or rash may occur with sarcoidosis. Gradual bilateral visual loss in other family members suggests possible dominant optic atrophy, whereas a maternal family history suggests Leber hereditary optic neuropathy. Toxic exposures (methanol), contact with animals (cats, ticks), medications (ethambutol), and vitamin deficiencies (history of alcoholism) may direct diagnostic evaluation.

If old records exist, reviewing these records is an essential part of the history in patients with optic atrophy. The records may document a time course much different from what the patient remembers. Records may indicate that the visual loss was much more gradual than was thought, or they may help to establish that the visual loss was indeed sudden. Documentation of previous optic disc swelling can help to establish that the optic atrophy is due to an earlier AION. In patients with previous optic neuritis, records showing disc swelling and macular exudate indicate neuroretinitis, which has no relationship to multiple sclerosis. **Table 1** lists important historical details in the patient with optic atrophy.

Examination

The ophthalmologic examination can also aid in determining the underlying cause of optic atrophy. Anterior segment examination may reveal evidence of previous trauma such as iris tears. In addition, the presence of active or previous inflammatory cells such as keratic precipitates or active vitreous cells may point toward an infectious or inflammatory cause of optic atrophy such as sarcoid, syphilis, cat-scratch disease, or Lyme disease. Perimetry may detect specific patterns of visual loss helpful in the differential diagnosis. Bilateral central or cecocentral field deficits occur more commonly in nutritional, hereditary, or toxic optic neuropathies. Hemianopic field deficits suggest chiasmal or retrochiasmal damage. Formal perimetry is an important step in documenting current visual function and subsequent deterioration or improvement.

As mentioned earlier, certain optic disc changes may help narrow the differential diagnosis of optic atrophy. Horizontal band (or bow-tie) atrophy may be present with optic chiasmal or retrochiasmal pregeniculate lesions (see **Fig. 4**). Optociliary collateral vessels may become apparent when retinal venous outflow is compromised by an optic nerve sheath meningioma (see **Fig. 7**). Radial retinal folds may indicate compression of the globe (see **Fig. 8**). Examination of the nerve under slit-lamp biomicroscopy is necessary to obtain a good 3-dimensional view and to rule out subtle cupping that might occur in glaucoma. When entertaining a diagnosis of optic atrophy as a sequela of NAION, the examination of the contralateral disc is essential to confirm the presence of the "disc-at-risk"—a small, congested nerve head. Superior or inferior segmental atrophy (see **Fig. 5**) points to a vascular cause, whereas bilateral temporal atrophy (see **Fig. 6**) occurs in conditions that affect the papillomacular bundle (hereditary, nutritional, or toxic).

Ancillary Testing

Laboratory tests such as angiotensin-converting enzyme, fluorescent *Treponemal* antibody absorption test, Lyme titer, and *Bartonella henselae* (cat-scratch) titer also prove useful, but only when history or examination has suggested the possibility of one of these diseases. Similarly, genetic testing may be useful for mitochondrial inherited diseases such as Leber hereditary optic neuropathy or dominant optic atrophy. Indiscriminate broad-spectrum testing for isolated optic atrophy without cause from history or examination is not recommended. Laboratory tests for infectious causes of optic atrophy can produce false-positive results and are not useful without clinical correlation.[28,29] Full-field and multifocal electroretinogram may be helpful when the optic atrophy is unexplained and when one is not sure if the problem is primarily the optic nerve.

Patients with no definite explanation for their optic atrophy should be evaluated with magnetic resonance imaging (MRI). A report from 2 tertiary neuro-ophthalmology centers found 18 of 91 (20%) patients referred with unexplained isolated optic atrophy to have compressive lesion.[27] The MRI should include the brain and orbits. Gadolinium should be administered to increase sensitivity. Fat suppression sequences should be run through the orbits to differentiate enhancing lesions from orbital fat. If previous MR images have been read as "normal," the images should be obtained to determine if the study was of good quality, included gadolinium and fat suppression, and the right places were looked at and interpreted correctly.

SUMMARY

Optic atrophy is a nonspecific finding and should never be considered a diagnosis. Accompanying evidence of visual loss (acuity, color vision, peripheral vision) should be present, which helps to differentiate between true atrophy and normal pallor. A thorough history and examination will determine the underlying cause of optic atrophy in most cases. Laboratory tests are useful only in situations where clinical history or examination points toward a specific diagnosis. For cases of unexplained, isolated optic atrophy, imaging is appropriate. Follow-up of patients with optic atrophy is dictated by the underlying cause. Patients showing signs of progressive optic atrophy may necessitate frequent follow-ups, repeat testing, and re-imaging. If the optic atrophy is unexplained and nonprogressive, follow-up may be gradually discontinued.

REFERENCES

1. Rader J, Feuer WJ, Anderson DR. Peripapillary vasoconstriction in the glaucomas and anterior ischemic optic neuropathies. Am J Ophthalmol 1994;117: 72–80.
2. Sadun AA, Sebag J. Prithee why so pale? Ophthalmology 2004;111:1625–6.
3. Miller NR, Newman NJ. Topical diagnosis of lesions in the visual sensory pathway. In: Miller NR, Newman NJ, editors. Walsh & Hoyt's clinical neuro-ophthalmology. 5th edition. Baltimore (MD): Williams & Wilkins; 1998. p. 237–386.
4. Quigley HA, Anderson DR. The histopathologic basis of optic disc pallor in experimental optic atrophy. Am J Ophthalmol 1977;83:709–17.
5. Sebag J, Delori FC, Feke GT, et al. Effects of optic atrophy on retinal blood flow and oxygen saturation in humans. Arch Ophthalmol 1989;107:222–6.
6. Collignon-Robe NJ, Feke GT, Rizzo JF III. Optic nerve head circulation in nonarteritic anterior ischemic optic neuropathy and optic neuritis. Ophthalmology 2004; 111:1663–72.
7. Miller NR, Fine SL. The ocular fundus in neuro-ophthalmic diagnosis. In: Sights and sounds in ophthalmology, vol. 3. St. Louis (MO): Mosby; 1977. p. 50–3.
8. Beatty RM, Sadun AA, Smith L, et al. Direct demonstration of transsynaptic degeneration in the human visual system. A comparison of retrograde and anterograde changes. J Neurol Neurosurg Psychiatry 1982;45:143–6.
9. Danesh-Meyer HV, Savino PJ, Sergott RC. The prevalence of cupping in end-stage arteritic and nonarteritic anterior ischemic optic neuropathy. Ophthalmology 2001;108:593–8.
10. Bianchi-Marzoli S, Rizzo JF, Brancato R, et al. Quantitative analysis of optic disc cupping in compressive optic neuropathy. Ophthalmology 1995;102:436–40.

11. Trobe JD, Glaser JS, Cassady JC. Optic atrophy. Differential diagnosis by fundus observation alone. Arch Ophthalmol 1980;98:1040–5.
12. Rath EZ, Rehany U, Linn S, et al. Correlation between optic disc atrophy and aetiology: anterior ischaemic optic neuropathy vs optic neuritis. Eye 2003;17:1019–24.
13. Buncic JR, Westall CA, Panton CM, et al. Characteristic retinal atrophy with secondary "inverse" optic atrophy identifies vigabatrin toxicity in children. Ophthalmology 2004;111:1935–42.
14. Ajax ET, Kardon R. Late-onset Leber's hereditary optic neuropathy. J Neuroophthalmol 1998;18:30–1.
15. Alvarez KL, Krop LC. Ethambutol-induced ocular toxicity revisited. Ann Pharmacother 1993;27:102–3.
16. DeBroff BM, Donahue SP. Bilateral optic neuropathy as the initial manifestation of systemic sarcoidosis. Am J Ophthalmol 1993;116:108–11.
17. Cullom ME, Heher KL, Miller NR, et al. Leber's hereditary optic neuropathy masquerading as tobacco-alcohol amblyopia. Arch Ophthalmol 1993;111:1482.
18. Dunn DW, Purvin V. Optic pathway gliomas in neurofibromatosis. Dev Med Child Neurol 1990;32:820–4.
19. Dutton JJ. Optic nerve sheath meningiomas. Surv Ophthalmol 1992;37:167–83.
20. Golnik KC, Schaible ER. Folate-responsive optic neuropathy. J Neuroophthalmol 1994;14:163–9.
21. Jarmouni R, Mouatamid O, El Khalidi AF, et al. Neurosyphilis: 53 cases. Rev Eur Dermatol MST 1990;2:577–83.
22. Smith JL. Syphilitic optic atrophy. J Clin Neuroophthalmol 1983;3:3–4.
23. Amitava AK, Alarm S, Hussain R. Neuro-ophthalmic features in pediatric tubercular meningoencephalitis. J Pediatr Ophthalmol Strabismus 2001;38:229–34.
24. Kumar A, Sandramouli S, Verma L, et al. Ocular ethambutol toxicity: is it reversible? J Clin Neuroophthalmol 1993;13:15–7.
25. Jabs DA, Miller NR, Newman SA, et al. Optic neuropathy in systemic lupus erythematosus. Arch Ophthalmol 1986;104:564–8.
26. Chatterjee PR, Chatterjee D, Chakraborty KS, et al. An unusual presentation of medial sphenoid wing meningioma. J Indian Med Assoc 2004;102:105–6.
27. Lee A, Chau F, Golnik K. The diagnostic yield of the evaluation for isolated unexplained optic atrophy. Ophthalmology 2005;112(5):757–9.
28. Sander A, Posselt M, Oberle K. Seroprevalence of antibodies to Bartonella henselae in patients with cat scratch disease and in healthy controls: evaluation and comparison of two commercial serological tests. Clin Diagn Lab Immunol 1998;5(4):486–90.
29. Bakken L, Callister S, Wand P. Interlaboratory comparison of test results for detection of Lyme disease in 516 participants in the Wisconsin State Laboratory of Hygiene/College of American Pathologists Proficiency Testing Program. J Clin Microbiol 1997;35(3):537–43.

Eye Movement Abnormalities in Multiple Sclerosis

Sashank Prasad, MD[a],*, Steven L. Galetta, MD[b]

KEYWORDS

- Multiple sclerosis • Eye movement abnormalities
- Neuroanatomy • Neuroimaging

Multiple sclerosis (MS) is an inflammatory condition that affects the central nervous system myelin and is capable of causing a host of neurologic deficits Eye movement abnormalities are a common manifestation either at the onset or during the course of the disease.[1] In fact, eye movement abnormalities in MS often correlate with over-all disability from the disease.[2] In this article the authors discuss the disturbances of gaze shifting, gaze holding, and ocular alignment that occur in MS, with an emphasis on underlying neuroanatomic principles and pathologic findings on examination.

Modern neuroimaging has revolutionized the ability to diagnose MS at its earliest stages and to monitor subclinical, silent disease progression. Although MRI has become an indispensible tool in the management of patients with MS, it is not completely sensitive in detecting lesions and therefore does not replace a careful neurologic examination. For example, small lesions in the brainstem may produce overt clinical abnormalities yet fall below the threshold for detection by MRI. This potential dissociation between clinical and radiographic findings further emphasizes the importance of careful clinico-anatomic localization. The proper assessment of subtle visual disturbances often critically impacts rational clinical decisions in the management of patients with MS.

INTERNUCLEAR OPHTHALMOPLEGIA

Internuclear ophthalmoplegia (INO) refers to disruption of rapid, coordinated, horizontal saccades by slowed or limited adduction.[3–6] Conjugate adduction in normal

[a] Division of Neuro-Ophthalmology, Department of Neurology, Brigham and Women's Hospital, Harvard Medical School, 75 Francis Street, Boston, MA 02115, USA
[b] Division of Neuro-Ophthalmology, Department of Neurology, Hospital of the University of Pennsylvania, 3W Gates Building, 3400 Spruce Street, Philadelphia, PA 19104, USA
* Corresponding author.
E-mail address: Sashank.prasad@uphs.upenn.edu

Neurol Clin 28 (2010) 641–655
doi:10.1016/j.ncl.2010.03.006
0733-8619/10/$ – see front matter © 2010 Elsevier Inc. All rights reserved.

neurologic.theclinics.com

horizontal saccades is facilitated by a subset of interneurons within the abducens nucleus. These fibers cross the midline to travel through the contralateral medial longitudinal fasciculus (MLF) from the pons to the medial rectus subnucleus of the ocular motor complex in the midbrain (**Fig. 1**). The MLF is highly myelinated to support the rapid neural transmission necessary for abduction of one eye and adduction of the fellow eye to be nearly synchronous.[7] Even slight impairment of the transmission speeds through the MLF produces symptoms by compromising this synchronicity, causing ocular misalignment during horizontal saccades. Unlike other myelinated tracts in which slight impairment may produce no overt clinical deficits, the system for coordinated horizontal saccades is extremely sensitive to transmission speeds, making INO a frequent manifestation of MS.

The adduction deficit in INO may manifest as slowing during the horizontal duction (adduction lag, ultimately with a full excursion of the eye) or as incomplete adduction producing an incomitant exotropia (**Fig. 2**). Normally, a rapid horizontal saccade is produced by pulse discharges originating in the paramedian pontine reticular formation (PPRF) (see **Fig. 1**). Eccentric gaze following the saccade is maintained by a step function based on inputs from the medial vestibular nucleus and the nucleus prepositus hypoglossus. The step function is derived from velocity information by the process of neural integration, and it serves to maintain gaze holding by overcoming the elastic forces of orbital tissues. Demyelination of the MLF may have greater impact upon the high frequency discharges necessary to produce the rapid saccadic pulse, whereas there may be sparing of the lower frequency discharges required for the step function that ultimately determines the range of adduction.[3] Alternatively, the range of adduction may be spared because of pathways apart from the MLF that possibly mediate a full adducting excursion.[8]

Despite deficient adduction during horizontal saccades, the normal function of the medial rectus in INO can typically be demonstrated by testing convergence of the eyes (**Fig. 3**). Convergence is mediated by separate inputs to the medial rectus subnucleus that are distinct from the inputs arriving via the MLF. The dissociation between limited adduction on horizontal saccades and spared adduction during convergence highlights the supranuclear nature of the adduction deficit in INO, with intact nuclear

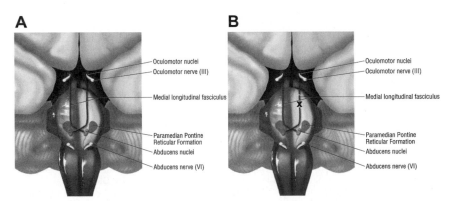

Fig. 1. (*A*) Depiction of the brainstem structures mediating horizontal ductions. Abduction of the ipsilateral eye is mediated by the abducens nerve. Coordinated adduction of the fellow eye is mediated by the oculomotor nerve, once the signal is relayed via the medial longitudinal fasciculus. (*B*) Left internuclear ophthalmoplegia caused by a lesion of the left MLF, would cause limited adduction of the left eye on right gaze. (*Courtesy of* Paul Schiffmacher.)

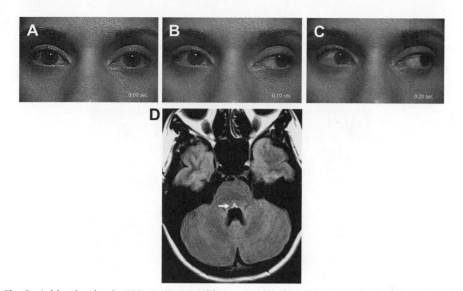

Fig. 2. Adduction lag in INO. A 27-year-old woman developed horizontal diplopia and oscillopsia. Examination revealed bilateral INO, greater on left gaze. (*A*) Primary position (0.0s); (*B*) adduction lag of the right eye on a rapid left saccade (0.10s); (*C*) near-complete adduction of the right eye at the end of the saccade (0.20s). (*D*) Axial FLAIR MRI through the pons, revealing hyper-intensity of the MLF bilaterally (*arrow*).

and infranuclear components of adduction. In some cases, however, dysfunction of the MLF is sufficiently rostral that the medial rectus subnucleus itself is impaired; therefore, impaired convergence will accompany impaired adduction on horizontal saccades. In this setting, referred to as the anterior INO of Cogan, the distinction is blurred between INO and partial third nerve palsy.[9]

Patients with unilateral INO typically do not have significant exotropia in primary gaze, likely because of intact convergence tone. In contrast, bilateral MLF lesions often cause exotropia (see **Fig. 3**). This clinical presentation is described as the WEBINO (wall-eyed bilateral INO) syndrome.

The misalignment produced by INO may cause a variety of ophthalmic symptoms, including visual blurring, diplopia, loss of stereopsis, and asthenopia (eye fatigue).[10] Normally there is cortical sensory suppression during saccades to eliminate blur from retinal slippage, but in INO visual blurring may occur because this mechanism fails to fully suppress inputs from the eye with slowed saccades.[3] Visual symptoms are often proportional to the degree of INO, and patients with mild INO may be essentially asymptomatic. Because use-related fatigue and Uhtoff's phenomenon (worsening symptoms with elevated body temperature) are common in patients with MS, the symptoms caused by INO may fluctuate over the course of the day.

Many patients with INO have normal horizontal pursuit, optokinetic, and vestibulo-ocular responses.[11] These functions may be preserved because they are mediated by lower-frequency neural signals with transmission that is spared despite demyelination of the MLF, or because they are also mediated by alternate connections between the abducens and oculomotor nuclei.

INO is often associated with a dissociated horizontal nystagmus most prominent in the abducting eye (**Fig. 4**). The slow phase of nystagmus is opposite the direction of attempted gaze, with quick saccades in the direction of attempted gaze. The

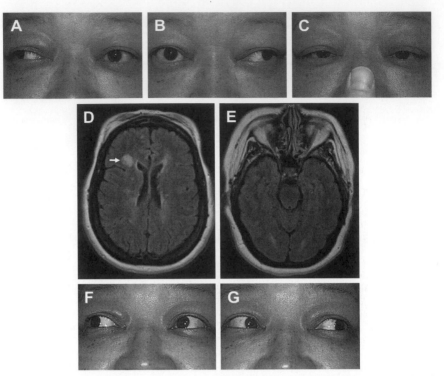

Fig. 3. Bilateral INO. A 47-year-old woman presented with horizontal diplopia. Examination revealed large-angle exotropia and bilateral INO. (*A*) Limited adduction of the left eye on right gaze. (*B*) Limited adduction of the right eye on left gaze. (*C*) Spared convergence of the eyes. (*D*) Axial FLAIR MRI revealed numerous areas of white matter hyper-intensity (for example, *arrow*). (*E*) However, no signal abnormality was detected in the region of the MLF in the pons or midbrain. (*F*) Improvement of INO after 2 months. Improved right eye adduction. (*G*) Full left gaze.

nystagmus has a unique slow phase with an exponentially decaying wave form.[3] With greater excursions, the amplitude or frequency of the nystagmus may increase.[3]

Several mechanisms may account for the abducting nystagmus in INO, and the explanations are not necessarily mutually exclusive. One possibility is that there is a central adaptive response to reduce visual blurring. To attempt to overcome adduction weakness, a compensatory increased saccadic pulse and step could occur (and would affect both eyes by Hering's law of dual innervation).[3,12] Although the adaptive response may improve the adduction of the paretic eye, it would disturb the abduction of the non-paretic eye in two ways. First, amplification of the pulse would lead to saccadic hypermetria; second, pulse-step mismatch would lead to slow post-saccadic drift with exponential decay. According to this account, the phenomenon of abducting nystagmus in unilateral INO is expected to be greatest if patients habitually fixate with the paretic eye, leading to higher demands for central adaptation. On the other hand, if patients fixate with the non-paretic eye, the abducting nystagmus may not be present.[3] In keeping with these predictions, Zee and colleagues[13] demonstrated that in some (but not all) patients with INO, prolonged patching (1–5days) of the paretic eye reduces the abducting nystagmus, whereas patching of the non-paretic eye increases it. On the other hand, temporary patching of one eye (or the performance of horizontal saccades in total darkness) does not mitigate the abducting

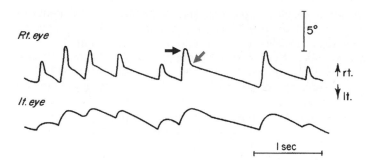

Fig. 4. Eye movement recordings in a patient with left INO demonstrating abducting nystagmus in the right eye while attempting sustained right gaze. Note the cycles of hypermetric abduction (*black arrow*) followed by an exponentially decaying slow waveform back toward primary position (*gray arrow*). The left eye demonstrates lower-amplitude, dysconjugate right-beating nystagmus without overshoots. (*Adapted from* Baloh RW, Yee RD, Honrubia V. Internuclear ophthalmoplegia. I. Saccades and dissociated nystagmus. Arch Neurol 1978a;35:484–9; with permission. Copyright © 1978 American Medical Association. All rights reserved.)

nystagmus, suggesting that the nystagmus is generated not by online target-position error signals but by a stored, long-term adaptive mechanism.[3]

A central adaptive mechanism, however, does not fully account for abducting nystagmus, because not all patients demonstrate the predicted changes following patching.[13] An alternate explanation proposes the disruption of *inhibitory* fibers that travel in the MLF and are postulated to cross in the midbrain to arrive at the antagonist medial rectus of the contralateral eye.[14] By this account, impaired inhibition of these medial rectus motoneurons reduces the abducting step function in that eye and causes a slow movement back from the abducted position. A corrective abducting saccade follows, and the repeating cycle generates abducting nystagmus. This explanation, however, would predict hypometric abducting saccades, rather than the hypermetric abducting saccades commonly seen.[3]

Yet another explanation for abducting nystagmus in INO is that injury to additional structures outside the MLF may directly lead to an asymmetric gaze-holding disturbance, which would manifest with greater severity in the non-paretic eye. By this account, however, the abducting nystagmus would have a typical saw-tooth waveform (in which the slow component has constant velocity directly relating to insufficient gaze-holding mechanisms), rather than the exponentially decaying waveform that is seen.[3]

In severe INO, the affected eye may demonstrate *abduction* slowing in addition to adduction slowing. A potential explanation for reduced abduction velocity is that normal abduction depends upon appropriate inhibition of the antagonist medial rectus of the same eye, which could be compromised by an MLF lesion.[15] An alternative explanation, however, is that patients with INO and abduction slowing in fact have more extensive pontine lesions not limited to the MLF, but also potentially involving the abducens nucleus, fascicle, or other structures.[6,16]

Impaired horizontal saccades are not the only manifestation of an MLF lesion. The MLF also contains fibers mediating many vertical eye movements (pursuit, vestibular, and otolithic pathways); corresponding impairments of vertical gaze therefore frequently accompany INO.[11,17,18] Impaired vertical pursuit may manifest as "staircasing" ductions interrupted by horizontal movements. Patients with bilateral INO may have marked impairment of vertical gaze holding, resulting in primary-position or gaze-evoked vertical nystagmus. In contrast to the exponentially decaying slow waveform of abducting nystagmus, vertical nystagmus in INO has a typical saw-tooth pattern caused by insufficient gaze-holding mechanisms. Impairment of the utricular pathways within the MLF may additionally lead to vertical misalignment of the eyes, in the form of skew deviation or the full ocular tilt reaction (**Fig. 5**).

The precise measurement of eye movements, using methods, such as infrared oculography, allows highly accurate detection and quantification of INO. Furthermore, these methods serve as a gold standard by which the accuracy of the bedside examination can be assessed.[19] Using this method, Frohman and colleagues found that severe INO was accurately detected by virtually all physician observers (regardless of level of training), but that milder INO was missed by many physicians other than trained neuro-ophthalmologists.

Various metrics from eye movement recordings have been used to quantify INO. These include the versional dysconjugacy index (VDI), which compares the peak velocities for abduction in one eye to adduction in the other.[20,21] This measure has the benefit of cancelling intra- and interindividual variations of absolute saccade velocities (caused by fatigue, for example). The VDI has also been assessed by a Z score and histogram analysis, which is a statistical method to better distinguish normal and abnormal results.[22] VDI measures use velocity rather than final amplitude because the extent of final amplitude in INO is often normal. The first-pass amplitude, on the other hand, evaluates the ratio of abducting and adducting eye position at the time that the abducting eye has initially completed its saccade.[23] Finally, recent studies have employed a phase-plane analysis, which plots eye velocity directly as a function of position, removing the effects of temporal variation that arise, for example, from onset latency.[24] Quantified measures of INO may provide a useful way to index the clinical effects of fatigue and Uhtoff's phenomenon, and ultimately may provide a method to objectively assess potential symptomatic treatments.[25]

Patients with INO frequently have a corresponding abnormality in the pons or midbrain that is detectable by MRI.[26] Frohman and colleagues studied 58 subjects with MS and INO and found that the sensitivity of proton density imaging, T2-weighted imaging, and fluid-attenuated inversion recovery (FLAIR) imaging was 100%, 88%, and 48%, respectively. It is not clear from this study, however, how the severity of INO relates to these MRI findings; cases of mild INO may have a higher rate of normal imaging. Furthermore, because patients with MS without INO were not included in this study, the exact specificity of these MRI abnormalities is not known. In some cases, MRI signal abnormality in this region may not have a clinical correlate. Another MRI measure that has been studied in INO is diffusion tensor imaging (DTI), in which the spatial constraints of water diffusion allow assessment of the integrity of white-matter tracts.[27] Fox and colleagues found a modest correlation between INO severity (graded by VDI) and mean white matter diffusivity in the MLF, showing that DTI measures may serve as a surrogate marker of brain-tissue integrity.

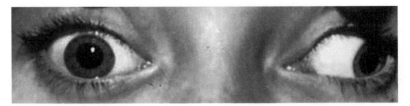

Fig. 5. A 30-year-old woman with MS developed horizontal, vertical, and torsional diplopia. Examination revealed right INO (with incomitant exotropia greatest in left gaze) and skew deviation (with comitant right hypertropia in all directions of gaze). A demyelinating lesion of the right MLF accounts for this pattern of misalignment.

NUCLEAR OR FASCICULAR OCULAR MOTOR PALSY

MS may cause acquired strabismus in the form of nuclear or fascicular palsy of one of the three ocular motor nerves.[16,28,29] In sixth nerve palsy, a fascicular lesion causes impaired abduction of the ipsilateral eye with spared adduction of the fellow eye (**Fig. 6**). A lesion of the sixth nerve nucleus, however, causes ipsiversive *gaze palsy*, consisting of combined deficits of ipsilateral abduction and contralateral adduction. Rarely, a pontine lesion may affect the sixth nerve nucleus (or pontine paramedian reticular formation) and the ipsilateral MLF. The effect of this lesion is a combined ipsiversive gaze palsy and an ipsilateral INO, referred to as a "one-and-a-half" syndrome, and the only spared horizontal eye movement is abduction of the contralateral eye on lateral gaze (see **Fig. 6**).[30,31]

In third nerve palsy, a fascicular lesion may cause partial deficits of elevation, depression, adduction, or lid elevation in the ipsilateral eye.[30] In rare cases, these lesions may be highly selective and cause weakness of a single muscle. Also, a discrete lesion of the third nerve fascicle may mimic superior or inferior divisional third nerve palsy (which more often localizes to the anterior cavernous sinus or orbit).[32] A nuclear third nerve lesion causes bilateral superior rectus weakness (in addition to the ipsilateral deficits), because the superior rectus subnucleus issues fibers that travel through the contralateral nucleus to join the contralateral nerve. In addition, nuclear third nerve palsy often causes bilateral ptosis, because the unpaired central caudal nucleus supplies both levator palpebrae muscles.

Normal eyelid position is maintained by inputs to the levator palpebrae. The motoneurons to both levator palpebrae muscles arise from the unpaired central caudate subnucleus (CCN) of the ocular motor complex. Lesions affecting these fascicles may cause unilateral ptosis, often in addition to other deficits of partial third nerve

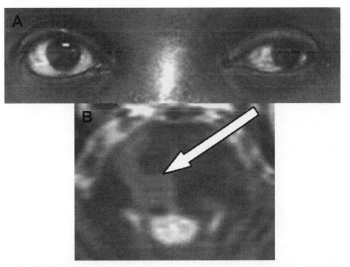

Fig. 6. One-and-a-half syndrome from right pontine lesion in a patient with MS. (*A*) In addition to a complete right gaze palsy (from involvement of the right abducens nucleus), there was deficient adduction of the right eye on attempted left gaze (from involvement of the right MLF). Left eye abduction is the only spared horizontal eye movement. (*B*) Axial T2-weighted MRI revealing a right pontine lesion (*arrow*). (*From* Frohman TC, Galetta S, Fox R, et al. Pearls & Oy-sters: The medial longitudinal fasciculus in ocular motor physiology. Neurol 2008;70:e57–67; with permission.)

palsy. Rarely, isolated unilateral or bilateral ptosis may occur.[33] The CCN is under the control of the nearby M-group cells, which receive tonic inhibitory inputs from the nucleus of the posterior commissure. Disruption of these inputs in the dorsal midbrain causes eyelid retraction (Collier's sign). The M-group cells couple the contractions of the levator palpebrae muscles to those of the vertically acting eye muscles on the basis of inputs from the superior colliculi.[34] Selective lesions in this location may cause abnormal, dissociated lid and eye movements. Blepharospasm (forceful, involuntary contractions of the orbicularis oculi) may occur following MS lesions of the brainstem, possibly caused by denervation supersensitivity of the facial nucleus or disinhibition of facial nerve relexes.[35] Painful, gaze-evoked blepharoclonus that principally involves the orbicularis oculi may also occur in MS, perhaps relating to ephaptic spread of impulses. MRI studies of these patients, however, have not revealed a consistent localization of lesions.[36,37]

A lesion of the fourth nerve nucleus or proximal fascicle causes hyperdeviation of the contralateral eye. Because of the direction of action of the superior oblique muscle, the hyperdeviation of a fourth nerve palsy is greatest in contralateral gaze and with ipsilateral head tilt. Rarely, a solitary lesion may cause combined INO and contralateral fourth nerve palsy, because of the anatomic proximity of the MLF and the fourth nerve nucleus and fascicle (**Fig. 7**).[38]

SKEW DEVIATION

As mentioned earlier, it is possible for skew deviation to accompany INO because the MLF contains utricular pathways maintaining vertical eye position in addition to inter-neurons from the abducens nucleus to the medial rectus subnucleus (see **Fig. 5**). In cases where there is selective damage of the utricular pathways, however, skew deviation will occur in the absence of INO. Imbalance of utricular inputs leads to a cyclo-vertical misalignment of the eyes, typically with a comitant vertical deviation that does not follow a pattern characteristic of third or fourth nerve palsy. With a pontine lesion, the ipsilateral eye is lower, and with a midbrain lesion, the ipsilateral eye is higher. Typically, there is relative intorsion of the higher eye (because intorsion of the higher

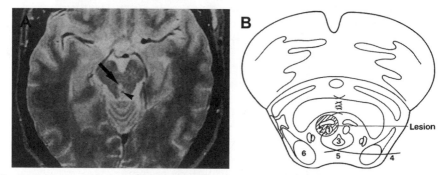

Fig. 7. A 41-year-old man with combined right INO and left fourth nerve palsy. (*A*) Axial T2-weighted MRI revealed a lesion in the right dorsal midbrain (*arrow*), adjacent to the sylvian aqueduct (*arrowhead*). (*B*) Schematic diagram of the lesion location and structures involved, including the right fourth nerve nucleus and fascicle before its decussation (1) and the right MLF (2). Other structures shown are the sylvian aqueduct (3), fourth nerve (4), decussation of the fourth nerve fibers (5), and the inferior colliculi (6). (*From* Vanooteghem P, Dehaene I, Van ZandyckeM, et al. Combined trochlear nerve palsy and internuclear ophthalmoplegia. Arch Neurol 1992;49:108–9; with permission. Copyright © 1992 American Medical Association. All rights reserved.)

eye exceeds extorsion of the lower eye). In the ocular tilt reaction (OTR), the hyperdeviation is accompanied by head tilt away from the higher eye. In addition to diplopia, many patients with skew deviation or OTR describe tilting of the subjective visual vertical.[39]

NYSTAGMUS

Gaze holding is mediated by velocity-position neural integrators; for horizontal gaze, these critical structures are in the medulla (the medial vestibular nuclei and the nucleus prepositus hypoglossus) and for vertical gaze, they are in the midbrain (the interstitial nuclei of Cajal).[40] The superior vestibular nuclei may also influence vertical gaze holding via connections through the MLF. The neural integrators make projections to the cerebellar tonsils (the flocculus and paraflocculus) that function to fine-tune velocity-position coding and maintain normal gaze holding.

Dysfunction of the neural integrators leads to impaired gaze holding and pathologic nystagmus. One common pattern is gaze-evoked nystagmus, which has a jerk waveform in which a slow drift back toward primary position is followed by a quick saccade to re-establish eccentric gaze. More significant gaze-holding impairments lead to primary position jerk nystagmus. Downbeat nystagmus often results from a cerebellar or cervico-medullary lesion that disrupts projections from the posterior semicircular canal, resulting in tonic upward deviation of the eyes with fast downward corrective movements. In contrast, upbeat nystagmus occurs more rarely, following pontomedullary or pontomesencephalic lesions that disrupt projections from the anterior semicircular canal. Rebound nystagmus refers to a transient jerk nystagmus that occurs upon returning from eccentric gaze to primary position, with the fast phase away from the previous direction of lateral gaze. Acquired periodic alternating nystagmus has a shifting null point, with the direction of nystagmus changing every 90 to 120 seconds and an intervening rest period of 5 to 10 seconds.[41,42] This condition may result from damage to the cerebellar centers that maintain velocity storage mechanisms and the stability of the vestibulo-ocular reflex (VOR). An asymmetric, jerk form of see-saw nystagmus, in which there is intorsion and elevation of one eye with synchronous extorsion and depression of the other eye, may follow midbrain lesions that disrupt inputs to vertical gaze-holding centers.[43,44]

Another common pattern is pendular nystagmus, which is often the result of damage to the interconnections between the brainstem neural integrators and the gaze-holding centers of the cerebellar tonsils.[45,46] Demyelination and conduction slowing along these pathways, which is common in MS, sufficiently disrupts their normal function and leads to abnormal, spontaneous firing patterns. The onset of nystagmus may follow the lesion by several months, suggesting that neural deafferentation may contribute to the pathophysiology. Combined pendular nystagmus and palatal tremor often result from a lesion in the Guillain-Mollaret triangle (including the dentate nucleus, superior cerebellar peduncle, red nucleus, central tegmental tract, inferior olive, and finally the inferior cerebellar peduncle).[47,48] There is often inferior olivary hypertrophy, which may be evident on MRI. Monocular visual loss also may contribute to acquired dissociated pendular nystagmus.[49]

Several drugs are available to attempt to dampen nystagmus and may provide symptomatic benefit to patients with MS.[50] Clonazepam, baclofen, gabapentin, and memantine are reasonably well tolerated and are effective in some patients.[51] The aminopyridines have been studied in reducing MS-associated symptoms,[52] and may be specifically helpful in reducing nystagmus. Many forms of pathologic nystagmus are thought to be caused by reduced physiologic inhibition of the vestibular nuclei by cerebellar purkinje fibers, and the aminopyridines are potassium-channel blockers that putatively facilitate action potentials in purkinje cells. Both 4-aminopyridine[53] and 3,4-diaminopyridine[54] have shown efficacy in controlled trials, but side effects including nausea, vomiting, and seizures limit the use of these medications.

SACCADIC ACCURACY

The accuracy of saccadic excursions is under the control of inputs from the posterior fastigial nuclei and dorsal vermis in the cerebellum, which calibrate the size of the saccadic pulse. Dysfunction of these pathways leads to saccadic dysmetria; hypermetric saccades result from damage to the deep nuclei and hypometric saccades result from damage to the vermis alone. Furthermore, dysmetric saccades in one direction of gaze can occur from unilateral lesions.[55] For example, a lesion of the inferior cerebellar peduncle (affecting the climbing fibers) may cause contralateral hypometric saccades, which occurs because of reduced stimulation of the ipsilateral fastigial nucleus, and consequently reduced stimulation of the contralateral PPRF (**Fig. 8**). In contrast, a lesion of the Hook bundle region near the superior cerebellar peduncle will cause contralateral *hypermetric* saccades (**Fig. 9**).[55] The reason for contralateral hypermetric saccades is that fibers from the fastigial nucleus to the

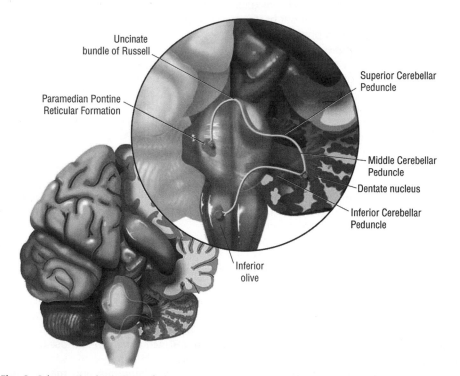

Fig. 8. Schematic depiction of the pathways controlling saccadic accuracy. Fibers arising from the inferior olive ascend through the contralateral inferior cerebellar peduncle and synapse on the dentate nucleus. Then, fibers ascend to traverse the contralateral superior cerebellar peduncle within the uncinate bundle of Russell and reach the paramedian pontine reticular formation. (*Courtesy of* Paul Schiffmacher Medical Illustrator, Thomas Jefferson University.)

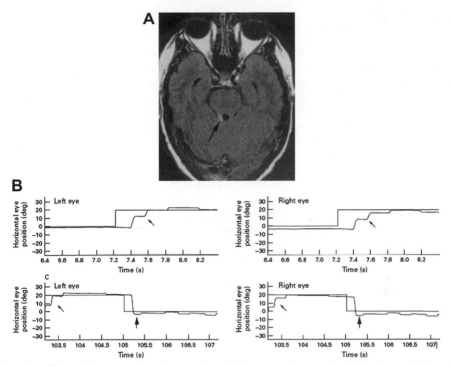

Fig. 9. Ipsilateral hypometric and contralateral hypermetric saccades following a lesion of the Hook bundle region of the superior cerebellar peduncle (SCP) in a patient with MS. (*A*) Axial FLAIR MRI revealed a lesion in the right SCP. (*B*) Eye movement recordings demonstrated hypometric saccades to the left (*small arrows*) and hypermetric saccades to the right (*large arrows*). (*From* Frohman EM, Frohman TC, Fleckenstein J, et al. Ocular contrapulsion in multiple sclerosis: clinical features and pathophysiological mechanisms. J Neurol Neurosurg Psychiatry 2001a;70:688–92; with permission.)

contralateral PPRF first travel across the midline superiorly to circle the superior cerebellar peduncle before descending to the PPRF.[56]

SACCADIC INTRUSIONS

Stable fixation is maintained by pause-cell neurons, which are located in the pontine raphe between the two abducens nuclei. They prevent the occurrence of unwanted saccadic pulses by tonically inhibiting the saccadic premotor burst neurons in the PPRF and the midbrain. Dysfunction of pause cells leads to extraneous saccades interrupting fixation. A square-wave jerk, for example, is a 1- to 5°-movement away from and back to the primary position, with an inter-saccadic latency of 150 to 200 milliseconds. Saccadic interruptions with a larger excursion (up to 10–40°) and a shorter inter-saccadic latency (up to 80 milliseconds) are termed macro square-wave jerks. When large saccadic intrusions occur across the midline in a to-and-fro pattern, they are termed macro-saccadic oscillations. In ocular flutter, back-to-back horizontal saccades occur without an inter-saccadic latency. If the saccadic movements occur in the horizontal and vertical planes, they are termed opsoclonus.[30] In micro-saccadic flutter, low-amplitude, back-to-back saccades occur but are generally seen only on ophthalmoscopy or eye movement recordings.[57]

IMPAIRED SMOOTH PURSUIT AND IMPAIRED SUPPRESSION OF THE VESTIBULO-OCULAR REFLEX

Smooth pursuit movements function to minimize retinal slippage of a moving foveated target. They are generated by cortical and subcortical areas, including V5/MST, the frontal eye fields, the dorsolateral pontine nucleus, the cerebellar flocculus and dorsal vermis, the vestibular nuclei, and ultimately the ocular motor nuclei. Lesions to these pathways are common in MS and often produce low-gain pursuit, in which eye movements are disproportionately slower than the moving target.[58,59] Compensatory catch-up saccades are generated to reestablish visual object tracking.

In natural circumstances, head movements often accompany eye movements to maintain fixation of a moving target. In this situation, the vestibulo-ocular reflex must be suppressed to maintain fixation. Lesions of the cerebellar flocculus commonly impair VOR cancellation, resulting in poor fixation of targets during dynamic head and eye movements. Suppression of the VOR can be assessed by having the subject view the thumb on their own outstretched arm while rotating their chair. If VOR cancellation is deficient, the intact VOR causes the eyes to drift opposite the direction of the head movement, and compensatory catch-up saccades will occur.

SUMMARY

Several eye movement abnormalities occur commonly in MS. The demyelinating lesions of MS can occur quite selectively within critical brainstem and cerebellar pathways that mediate coordinated eye movements, gaze holding, and ocular alignment. Delayed neural transmission in these pathways may lead to INO, ocular motor palsy, ocular misalignment, pathologic nystagmus, impaired saccades, saccadic intrusions, or impaired pursuit. Detailed neuro-ophthalmic examination of patients with MS with visual complaints often yields a diagnosis with highly specific neuroanatomic localization. In turn, a thorough evaluation may suggest targeted symptomatic therapies and enhance the ability to monitor disease progression.

REFERENCES

1. Frohman EM, Frohman TC, Zee DS, et al. The neuro-ophthalmology of multiple sclerosis. Lancet Neurol 2005;4:111–21.
2. Derwenskus J, Rucker JC, Serra A, et al. Abnormal eye movements predict disability in MS: two-year follow-up. Ann N Y Acad Sci 2005;1039:521–3.
3. Baloh RW, Yee RD, Honrubia V. Internuclear ophthalmoplegia. I. Saccades and dissociated nystagmus. Arch Neurol 1978;35:484–9.
4. Paton L. Ocular palsies. Br J Ophthalmol 1921;5:250–69.
5. Sauvineau C. Un nouveau type de paralyse associee des mouvements horizments horizontaux des yeux. Bull Soc Ophtalmol Fr 1895;13:524–34.
6. Zee DS. Internuclear ophthalmoplegia: pathophysiology and diagnosis. Baillieres Clin Neurol 1992;1:455–70.
7. Weidenheim KM, Epshteyn I, Rashbaum WK, et al. Neuroanatomical localization of myelin basic protein in the late first and early second trimester human foetal spinal cord and brainstem. J Neurocytol 1993;22:507–16.
8. Kommerell G. Unilateral internuclear ophthalmoplegia. The lack of inhibitory involvement in medial rectus muscle activity. Invest Ophthalmol Vis Sci 1981; 21:592–9.
9. Cogan DG. Internuclear ophthalmoplegia, typical and atypical. Arch Ophthalmol 1970;84:583–9.

10. Mills DA, Frohman TC, Davis SL, et al. Break in binocular fusion during head turning in MS patients with INO. Neurology 2008;71:458–60.
11. Baloh RW, Yee RD, Honrubia V. Internuclear ophthalmoplegia. II. Pursuit, optokinetic nystagmus, and vestibulo-ocular reflex. Arch Neurol 1978;35:490–3.
12. Abel LA, Schmidt D, Dell'Osso LF, et al. Saccadic system plasticity in humans. Ann Neurol 1978;4:313–8.
13. Zee DS, Hain TC, Carl JR. Abduction nystagmus in internuclear ophthalmoplegia. Ann Neurol 1987;21:383–8.
14. Pola J, Robinson DA. An explanation of eye movements seen in internuclear ophthalmoplegia. Arch Neurol 1976;33:447–52.
15. Feldon SE, Hoyt WF, Stark L. Disordered inhibition in internuclear ophthalmoplegia: analysis of eye movement recordings with computer simulations. Brain 1980; 103:113–37.
16. Bronstein AM, Rudge P, Gresty MA, et al. Abnormalities of horizontal gaze. Clinical, oculographic and magnetic resonance imaging findings. II. Gaze palsy and internuclear ophthalmoplegia. J Neurol Neurosurg Psychiatry 1990;53:200–7.
17. Evinger LC, Fuchs AF, Baker R. Bilateral lesions of the medial longitudinal fasciculus in monkeys: effects on the horizontal and vertical components of voluntary and vestibular induced eye movements. Exp Brain Res 1977; 28:1–20.
18. Ranalli PJ, Sharpe JA. Vertical vestibulo-ocular reflex, smooth pursuit and eye-head tracking dysfunction in internuclear ophthalmoplegia. Brain 1988; 111(Pt 6):1299–317.
19. Frohman TC, Frohman EM, O'Suilleabhain P, et al. Accuracy of clinical detection of INO in MS: corroboration with quantitative infrared oculography. Neurology 2003;61:848–50.
20. Flipse JP, Straathof CS, Van der Steen J, et al. Binocular saccadic eye movements in multiple sclerosis. J Neurol Sci 1997;148:53–65.
21. Ventre J, Vighetto A, Bailly G, et al. Saccade metrics in multiple sclerosis: versional velocity disconjugacy as the best clue? J Neurol Sci 1991; 102:144–9.
22. Frohman EM, Frohman TC, O'Suilleabhain P, et al. Quantitative oculographic characterisation of internuclear ophthalmoparesis in multiple sclerosis: the versional dysconjugacy index Z score. J Neurol Neurosurg Psychiatry 2002;73:51–5.
23. Frohman EM, O'Suilleabhain P, Dewey RB Jr, et al. A new measure of dysconjugacy in INO: the first-pass amplitude. J Neurol Sci 2003;210:65–71.
24. Serra A, Liao K, Matta M, et al. Diagnosing disconjugate eye movements: phase-plane analysis of horizontal saccades. Neurology 2008;71:1167–75.
25. Davis SL, Frohman TC, Crandall CG, et al. Modeling Uhtoff's phenomenon in MS patients with internuclear ophthalmoparesis. Neurology 2008; 70:1098–106.
26. Frohman EM, Zhang H, Kramer PD, et al. MRI characteristics of the MLF in MS patients with chronic internuclear ophthalmoparesis. Neurology 2001;57:762–8.
27. Fox RJ, McColl RW, Lee JC, et al. A preliminary validation study of diffusion tensor imaging as a measure of functional brain injury. Arch Neurol 2008;65: 1179–84.
28. Bronstein AM, Morris J, Du Boulay G, et al. Abnormalities of horizontal gaze. Clinical, oculographic and magnetic resonance imaging findings. I. Abducens palsy. J Neurol Neurosurg Psychiatry 1990;53:194–9.

29. Moster ML, Savino PJ, Sergott RC, et al. Isolated sixth-nerve palsies in younger adults. Arch Ophthalmol 1984;102:1328–30.
30. de Seze J, Vukusic S, Viallet-Marcel M, et al. Unusual ocular motor findings in multiple sclerosis. J Neurol Sci 2006;243:91–5.
31. Frohman TC, Galetta S, Fox R, et al. Pearls & Oy-sters: the medial longitudinal fasciculus in ocular motor physiology. Neurology 2008;70:e57–67.
32. Ksiazek SM, Repka MX, Maguire A, et al. Divisional oculomotor nerve paresis caused by intrinsic brainstem disease. Ann Neurol 1989;26:714–8.
33. Martin TJ, Corbett JJ, Babikian PV, et al. Bilateral ptosis due to mesencephalic lesions with relative preservation of ocular motility. J Neuroophthalmol 1996;16: 258–63.
34. Horn AK, Buttner-Ennever JA. Brainstem circuits controlling lid-eye coordination in monkey. Prog Brain Res 2008;171:87–95.
35. Jankovic J, Patel SC. Blepharospasm associated with brainstem lesions. Neurology 1983;33:1237–40.
36. Jacome DE. Blepharoclonus in multiple sclerosis. Acta Neurol Scand 2001; 104:380–4.
37. Keane JR. Gaze-evoked blepharoclonus. Ann Neurol 1978;3:243–5.
38. Vanooteghem P, Dehaene I, Van Zandycke M, et al. Combined trochlear nerve palsy and internuclear ophthalmoplegia. Arch Neurol 1992;49:108–9.
39. Serra A, Derwenskus J, Downey DL, et al. Role of eye movement examination and subjective visual vertical in clinical evaluation of multiple sclerosis. J Neurol 2003; 250:569–75.
40. Bhidayasiri R, Plant GT, Leigh RJ. A hypothetical scheme for the brainstem control of vertical gaze. Neurology 2000;54:1985–93.
41. Keane JR. Periodic alternating nystagmus with downward beating nystagmus. A clinicoanatomical case study of multiple sclerosis. Arch Neurol 1974;30:399–402.
42. Matsumoto S, Ohyagi Y, Inoue I, et al. Periodic alternating nystagmus in a patient with MS. Neurology 2001;56:276–7.
43. Halmagyi GM, Aw ST, Dehaene I, et al. Jerk-waveform see-saw nystagmus due to unilateral meso-diencephalic lesion. Brain 1994;117(Pt 4):789–803.
44. Sandramouli S, Benamer HT, Mantle M, et al. See-saw nystagmus as the presenting sign in multiple sclerosis. J Neuroophthalmol 2005;25:56–7.
45. Lopez LI, Gresty MA, Bronstein AM, et al. Acquired pendular nystagmus: oculomotor and MRI findings. Acta Otolaryngol Suppl 1995;520(Pt 2):285–7.
46. Averbuch-Heller L, Zivotofsky AZ, Das VE, et al. Investigations of the pathogenesis of acquired pendular nystagmus. Brain 1995;118(Pt 2):369–78.
47. Guillain G. The syndrome of synchronous and rhythmic palato-pharyngo-laryngo-oculo-diaphragmatic myoclonus. Proc R Soc Med 1938;31:1031–8.
48. Revol A, Vighetto A, Confavreux C, et al. [Oculo-palatal myoclonus and multiple sclerosis]. Rev Neurol (Paris) 1990;146:518–21 [in French].
49. Barton JJ, Cox TA. Acquired pendular nystagmus in multiple sclerosis: clinical observations and the role of optic neuropathy. J Neurol Neurosurg Psychiatry 1993;56:262–7.
50. Rucker JC. Current treatment of nystagmus. Curr Treat Options Neurol 2005; 7:69–77.
51. Shery T, Proudlock FA, Sarvananthan N, et al. The effects of gabapentin and memantine in acquired and congenital nystagmus: a retrospective study. Br J Ophthalmol 2006;90:839–43.
52. Solari A, Uitdehaag B, Giuliani G, et al. Aminopyridines for symptomatic treatment in multiple sclerosis. Cochrane Database Syst Rev 2003;2:CD001330.

53. Kalla R, Glasauer S, Schautzer F, et al. 4-aminopyridine improves downbeat nystagmus, smooth pursuit, and VOR gain. Neurology 2004;62:1228–9.
54. Strupp M, Schuler O, Krafczyk S, et al. Treatment of downbeat nystagmus with 3,4-diaminopyridine: a placebo-controlled study. Neurology 2003;61(2):165–70.
55. Frohman EM, Frohman TC, Fleckenstein J, et al. Ocular contrapulsion in multiple sclerosis: clinical features and pathophysiological mechanisms. J Neurol Neurosurg Psychiatry 2001;70:688–92.
56. Solomon D, Galetta SL, Liu GT. Possible mechanisms for horizontal gaze deviation and lateropulsion in the lateral medullary syndrome. J Neuroophthalmol 1995;15:26–30.
57. Ashe J, Hain TC, Zee DS, et al. Microsaccadic flutter. Brain 1991;114(Pt 1B): 461–72.
58. Mastaglia FL, Black JL, Collins DW. Quantitative studies of saccadic and pursuit eye movements in multiple sclerosis. Brain 1979;102:817–34.
59. Sharpe JA, Goldberg HJ, Lo AW, et al. Visual-vestibular interaction in multiple sclerosis. Neurology 1981;31:427–33.

Disorders of Pupillary Structure and Function

Pierre-François Kaeser, MD[a], Aki Kawasaki, MD[b],*

KEYWORDS

- Pupil • Pupillary light reflex • Anisocoria • Miosis
- Mydriasis • Light-near dissociation

ABNORMAL PUPILS IN INFANTS AND CHILDREN

Parents are often the first to notice something odd about their child's pupils. Common concerns include pupils of unequal size, shape, color, or movement. This section emphasizes those congenital anomalies that may be associated with a systemic syndrome as well as specific acquired pupil disorders, which signal more serious underlying pathology or may impair the normal development of vision in infants, mainly through glaucoma or amblyopia.

Pupils of Unequal Size (Anisocoria)

Anisocoria in young subjects is most frequently physiologic and is present in approximately 20% of healthy subjects.[1] Physiologic anisocoria generally measures 1 mm or less, the light reflex is normal as is dilatation dynamics, and there is no associated ptosis or ocular motility disturbance. When physiologic anisocoria is particularly striking, the concern for a pathologic cause arises. In such instances, the clinician is usually worried about an underlying oculosympathetic defect in the child, and pharmacologic testing may be necessary to distinguish between Horner syndrome and physiologic anisocoria (**Fig. 1**). Details on pharmacologic testing for Horner syndrome are given later in this article.

The authors have no proprietary interest in any of the products or instrumentation mentioned in the manuscript.

Funding: none.

Financial disclosure: Dr Kawasaki has received financial compensation from Bayer SpA for advisory work that is unrelated to any of the topics, products, or instruments discussed in this article. Dr Kaeser has nothing to disclose.

Drs Kaeser and Kawasaki discuss the off-label use of topical cocaine, pilocarpine, and apraclonidine in the article.

[a] University Ophthalmology Service, Hôpital Ophtalmique Jules Gonin, Avenue de France 15, Lausanne 1004, Switzerland

[b] Neuro-ophthalmology Unit, Laboratory of pupillography, Hôpital Ophtalmique Jules Gonin, Avenue de France 15, Lausanne 1004, Switzerland

* Corresponding author.

E-mail address: aki.kawasaki@fa2.ch

Neurol Clin 28 (2010) 657–677

doi:10.1016/j.ncl.2010.03.007

0733-8619/10/$ – see front matter © 2010 Elsevier Inc. All rights reserved.

neurologic.theclinics.com

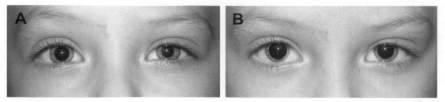

Fig. 1. Young child referred for an acquired anisocoria and ptosis. (*A*) This 6-year-old girl had anisocoria and left lid ptosis 1 day after the removal of a foreign body on the corneal surface. The procedure had been performed under general anesthesia with eyelid forceps. A left Horner syndrome was suspected. (*B*) After instillation of topical cocaine, both pupils dilated to the same size, indicating intact sympathetic innervation on both sides. Anisocoria and ptosis resolved spontaneously over 3 weeks. The relative miosis of the left pupil was attributed to a postsurgical iris sphincter spasm, and the upper lid ptosis was thought to be transient dysfunction of the levator palpebrae superioris muscle from usage of eyelid retractor.

Horner syndrome in infants may be congenital or acquired. Congenital Horner syndrome, defined as present at birth or within the first 4 weeks, is frequently benign, related to stretching of the oculosympathetic fibers in and around the brachial plexus during difficult birth (breech position, use of forceps).[2] It is only rarely associated with a severe pathologic condition such as neuroblastoma.

On the contrary, acquired Horner syndrome in older infants and children without a surgical history is associated with a potentially serious condition in more than half of cases, the most feared being neuroblastoma (**Fig. 2**). Despite being a congenital tumor, neuroblastoma is usually not clinically evident at birth and most present before 5 years of age, nearly all before 10 years of age. An isolated Horner syndrome is the initial presentation in 2% of cases with neuroblastoma.[2] Iris heterochromia is often stated to be a clue to congenital Horner syndrome, but sympathetically mediated melanocyte migration and iris pigmentation continue until 2 years of age. Thus, heterochromia irides cannot be relied on as a sign of benignity.

What is the evaluation of infants and children with Horner syndrome? One study recommends that every child presenting with Horner syndrome be investigated, even if there is a history of difficult delivery because birth trauma and neoplasm may, albeit rarely, occur concurrently.[2] The investigation includes a general physical examination including palpation of the neck, axilla, and abdomen; spot urine testing with quantitative high-performance liquid chromatography for the catecholamine

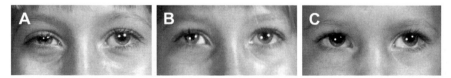

Fig. 2. Right Horner syndrome in a teenager due to prior tonsillectomy. (*A*) A 16-year-old girl requested cosmetic repair of a longstanding right upper lid ptosis. Examination and cocaine testing revealed a Horner syndrome on the right side. Investigation revealed no obvious causes. (*B*) Review of serial school photographs showed appearance of anisocoria and ptosis at 9 years of age. Lower lid ptosis is also seen. More detailed history revealed that the patient had had an uncomplicated tonsillectomy several months before the photograph was taken. (*C*) All photos before 9 years of age showed no evidence of either anisocoria or ptosis. Photograph of patient at 4 years of age is shown. The Horner syndrome was attributed to tonsillectomy.

metabolites, homovanillic acid or vanillylmandelic acid; and MRI of the head, neck, and chest. Despite such a workup, a specific cause is not identified in about one-third of the children with Horner syndrome.[2]

A poor light reflex is never present with physiologic anisocoria. If the child has a large, poorly reactive pupil, considerations include iris anomalies, tonic pupil, pharmacologic mydriasis, and oculomotor (third) nerve palsy. Pupil abnormalities are present in 60% to 78% of pediatric oculomotor nerve palsies and include a large pupil size, a poor reaction to light and accommodation, or constriction evoked by eye movement due to aberrant regeneration (pupil gaze synkinesis).[3] The diagnosis of oculomotor nerve palsy is straightforward when mydriasis is accompanied by ipsilateral ptosis and ophthalmoplegia. In cases of early or partial palsy, motor findings and asymmetry of the pupillary light reflex are subtle or difficult to appreciate in very young children. To avoid overlooking an acquired palsy that presents mostly as an anisocoria in a child, formal orthoptic examination may be necessary.

In pediatric patients, it is useful to remember that the relative frequency of causative agents is different when compared with adults: 20% to 43% of oculomotor nerve palsies are congenital, and trauma and tumors (most commonly a brainstem glioma) are the most frequent causes of acquired palsy.[3,4] Special considerations in management of pediatric third nerve palsy include prevention of strabismic and/or deprivation (ptosis) amblyopia as well as support of binocular function.[4]

Pupils with an Unusual Shape (Dyscoria)

One of the most frequent congenital causes of dyscoria is iris coloboma. Dyscoria occurs when the fetal fissure fails to close properly between the fifth and seventh weeks of gestation and typically manifests as an inferonasal notch in the iris, the so-called keyhole pupil (**Fig. 3**).[5] When the defect is only partial, the pupil appears ovoid. Iris coloboma is frequently associated with coloboma of more posterior ocular structures (choroid, optic nerve) and microphthalmia. Although iris coloboma can occur as an isolated anomaly, it is important to recognize its association with multisystem anomalies, as in the CHARGE syndrome (ocular Coloboma, Heart defects, which can be lethal, choanal Atresia, Retardation of growth and/or development, Genital abnormalities, and Ear anomalies [abnormal pinnae or hearing loss]).[5] CHARGE syndrome is associated in two-third of cases with *CHD7* gene mutations.

Other causes of congenital dyscoria or corectopia (displacement of the pupil from its normal location—slightly inferonasal to iris center) include diffuse or sectorial iris hypoplasia, ectopia lentis et pupillae (in which corectopia is associated with lens subluxation), persistent pupillary membrane (residue of embryonic anterior segment vascularization), anterior segment dysgenesis syndrome (eg, Axenfeld-Rieger syndrome), and iridocorneal endothelial (ICE) syndrome (see **Fig. 3; Fig. 4**).[6] True polycoria, that is, multiple pupils with distinct functional sphincters, occurs rarely.

Iris defects and the resulting abnormalities in pupil shape and position produce no major threat to visual function but can cause photophobia. Most treatments are undertaken for cosmetic reasons. Treatment relies on fitting colored cosmetic contact lenses or suturing the coloboma with nonabsorbable material. If the iris defect is large, a prosthetic iris can be implanted. Surgical correction of iris defects is generally performed only if another intraocular surgery in indicated.

White Colored Pupils (Leukocoria)

Leukocoria is caused by reflection of incident light off the retinal lesion within the pupillary area when the fundus is directly illuminated.[7] Parents frequently notice leukocoria on flash photography (**Fig. 5**). Leukocoria is a red flag for a serious pathologic condition

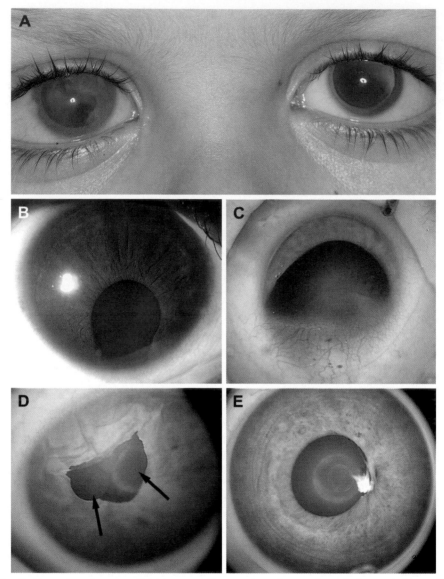

Fig. 3. Examples of congenital iris anomalies causing abnormal pupil size and shape. (*A*) Patient with bilateral aniridia. The striking red reflex is due to complete absence of iris tissue. (*Courtesy of* F. Majo, MD, Lausanne, Switzerland.) (*B*) Inferonasal iris coloboma of the right eye, forming a "keyhole" pupil. (*C*) Large coloboma involving most of the inferior iris. Opacification and neovascularization of the inferior cornea are seen. (*D*) Dyscoria secondary to a big iris cyst located superiorly. The scalloped margin of the pupil is due to smaller cystic lesions of the pigmented ruff (*arrows*). (*E*) Dyscoria secondary to synechia between the iris and a sectoral lens capsule fibrosis. (*B–E: Courtesy of* Professor F. Munier, MD, Lausanne, Switzerland.)

because it is caused by retinoblastoma in nearly 50% of cases.[7] Other causes include congenital cataract, persistent hyperplastic primary vitreous, posterior coloboma, Coats disease, ocular toxocariasis, retinopathy of prematurity, retinal hamartomas (tuberous sclerosis, von Recklinghausen disease), congenital falciform fold, organized vitreous hemorrhage, and persistent pupillary membrane (see **Fig. 5**). Early diagnosis is vital in retinoblastoma management, thus any child with leukocoria, by history or examination, needs a dilated retinal examination, even if general anesthesia is required.

Pupils Too Large

Relatively large pupils are physiologic in premature neonates until 29 weeks of gestation (mean pupil diameter 4.7 mm for a corneal diameter of 7.0 mm at 26 weeks, 3.5 mm at 29 weeks), and pupillary light response does not develop until 32 weeks of gestational age. Fixed mydriasis should then not be considered suggestive of blindness or central nervous system disorder until 32 weeks of gestational age.[8]

The most extreme case of congenitally large pupils is aniridia, which literally means "absence of iris" (see **Fig. 3**). The incidence is between 1:64,000 and 1:100,000. Two-third of cases are familial, and one-third is sporadic.[9] Aniridia is secondary to mutations in *PAX6* gene on band p13 of chromosome 11.[9] Because *PAX6* has a central role in the organization of the developing eye, aniridia is associated with various other ocular anomalies (corneal lesions, glaucoma, cataract, optic nerve, and foveal hypoplasia). Lack of an iris causes symptoms of decreased visual acuity, glare, and photophobia. Symptomatic treatment includes use of colored cosmetic contact lenses, corneal tattooing, and the implantation of artificial iris.[9]

It is critically important to recognize aniridia because of its strong association with Wilms tumor (nephroblastoma), and aniridia may be the first clue to the diagnosis of this renal tumor.[9,10] Wilms tumor is the second most common extracranial malignancy in children (after neuroblastoma).[10] Children with aniridia have a 30% to 50% risk for developing Wilms tumor, which is bilateral in 20%.[10] Wilms tumor can be associated with sporadic aniridia or be part of the WAGR syndrome through the simultaneous deletion of both *PAX6* and *WT1* genes on chromosome 11p13.[10] The WAGR syndrome consists of Wilms tumor, bilateral sporadic Aniridia, Genitourinary abnormalities, and mental Retardation. It is recommended that children with aniridia undergo chromosomal analysis for the Wilms tumor gene defect.

Familial iridoplegia is a very rare condition in which the dilated pupil is due to sphincter muscle aplasia, with otherwise normal-appearing iris. The condition may be unilateral or bilateral. The pupil neither reacts to light, accommodation, or convergence nor does it constrict with pilocarpine. Unlike aniridia, familial iridoplegia is an isolated and otherwise benign condition.

Acquired defects of the iris in children are usually due to trauma, intraocular inflammation or infection, ICE syndrome (see **Fig. 4**), or anterior segment dysgenesis. Large pupils can also result from a tonic pupil (detailed later). Tonic pupil may be a sequela of chickenpox and is usually unilateral. Children with unilateral tonic pupil, may be at risk of anisometropic amblyopia caused by loss of accommodation in the affected eye, should be closely monitored and given an appropriate bifocal refractive correction.[11]

Finally, pharmacologic mydriasis must be considered. Inadvertent contact with plants containing parasympatholytic substances (eg, *Atropa belladonna*) or with a topical medication is the most common scenario in children.

Pupils Too Small

Congenital miosis (microcoria) is a developmental ocular anomaly in which affected pupils are generally smaller than 2 mm, may be eccentrically placed, are

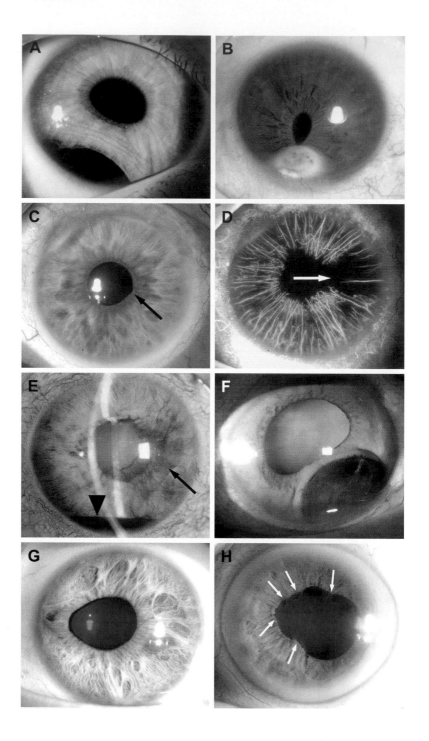

nonresponsive to light or accommodation, and dilate poorly with topical mydriatics. Microcoria can result from absence or malformation of the dilator pupillae muscle, contracture of fibrous material on the pupil margin, remnants of the tunica vasculosa lentis, or anomalies of neural crest cells. It can be unilateral or bilateral, sporadic or hereditary, and cases associated with congenital rubella have been described. It can occur in association with various ocular pathologic conditions, namely glaucoma and myopia.

Acquired miosis in infants and children can result from traumatic iris paralysis, post-uveitis synechiae between iris and lens, Horner syndrome, or topical medication.

Paradoxic Pupillary Reaction

Pupillary constriction to darkness is a rare phenomenon seen in patients with retinal diseases such as cone dysfunction syndromes, congenital stationary night blindness, congenital achromatopsia, Leber congenital amaurosis, retinitis pigmentosa, Best disease, macular dystrophy, and albinism. The mechanism of this phenomenon is still unknown, but one hypothesis is that malfunctioning cones permit an unusually strong "bleaching signal" to be sent by the rods during passage from strong illumination to darkness.[12] An electroretinogram should be obtained in patients with a paradoxic pupillary reaction.

ACQUIRED STRUCTURAL DEFECTS OF THE IRIS

The iris consists of 2 layers, an anterior stroma and a posterior pigmented epithelium. The anterior surface of the iris is uneven, with the alternance of crypts and interlinked trabeculae. The posterior layer is opaque and limits the amount of light that enters the eye.

◄───

Fig. 4. Examples of acquired defects of the iris causing pupillary distortion and dysfunction. (*A*) A 6-year-old girl complained of light sensitivity and monocular diplopia after a blunt ocular trauma. Examination revealed inferior iridodialysis causing pseudopolycoria. (*B*) Dyscoria in a 9-year-old boy, caused by inferior iridocorneal synechia. Careful history revealed a forgotten ocular trauma that occurred several years back. (*Courtesy of* F. Majo, MD, Lausanne, Switzerland.) (*C*) A subtle deformity of the pupil (*arrow*) in a patient with known Fuchs heterochromia. The pupil was also noted to demonstrate sectoral palsy. (*D*) Iris angiography in the same eye revealed a sectoral vascular atrophy (*arrow*) typical of Fuchs heterochromia and corresponding to the area of sphincter dysfunction. (*E*) A very sluggish pupillary reaction in a 56-year-old patient. Close examination revealed small red lines on the iris surface (neovascularization) (*arrow*) and blood level in the anterior chamber (*arrowhead*). This patient had poorly controlled diabetes mellitus with no regular ophthalmologic follow-up. The cause of his poor pupillary light reflex and iris neovascularization was ocular ischemia. (*F*) Dyscoria and sluggish pupillary reaction with sectoral palsy in a 63-year-old patient. A pigmented mass is obvious on gross examination. Review of old pictures suggested a progressively enlarging tumor. Patient was diagnosed with iris melanoma. (*C–G*: *Courtesy of* Professor L. Zografos, MD, Lausanne, Switzerland.) (*G*) 38-year-old patient with dyscoria, incidentally discovered by his wife. Review of old pictures revealed that the dyscoria was acquired. Ultrasound studies revealed an underlying iris cyst. Slit-lamp examination revealed associated corneal endothelial lesions. Patient was diagnosed with ICE syndrome. ICE syndrome is a progressive nonhereditary abnormality of corneal endothelium, in which abnormal corneal endothelial cells grow across the angle and iris, inducing corneal edema, glaucoma, and iris distortion. (*H*) Dyscoria in a 35-year-old patient who reported an episode of eye pain, redness, and photophobia 3 months back. Numerous synechiae between the iris and lens are present (*arrows*), mechanically restricting the pupil in these sectors. (*Courtesy of* J. Vaudaux, MD, Lausanne, Switzerland.)

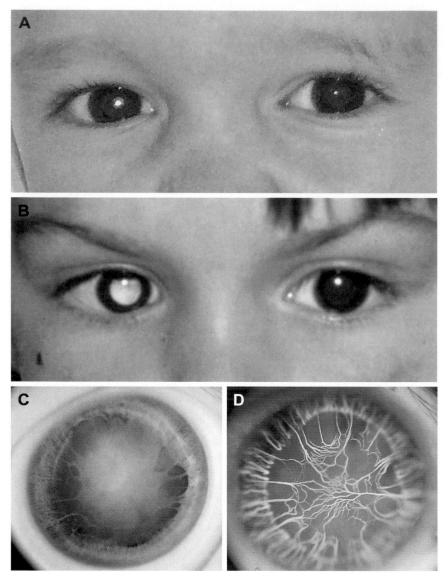

Fig. 5. Examples of leukocoria. (*A*) Example of normal bilateral red reflexes. (*B*) Leukocoria of the left eye, discovered on this picture taken by the child's parents. Investigations revealed a retinoblastoma (*Courtesy of* A. Balmer, MD, Lausanne, Switzerland.) (*C*) Example of a persistent pupillary membrane blocking the red reflex and causing leukocoria. (*D*) Fluorescein angiography in the same eye showing the persistent vascularization of the membrane. (*Courtesy of* Professor F. Munier, MD, Lausanne, Switzerland.)

The color of iris is linked to the melanin content of the melanocytes, which are present in both stroma and posterior epithelium. At the pupillary margin, the pigmented epithelium (ruff) is very close to the lens anterior capsule and can easily form adhesions (iris-lens synechia) during inflammation. The iris contains 2 muscles (sphincter and dilator pupillae), which regulate the movements of the pupil.[13]

Microscopic iris structure is best appreciated with a slit-lamp biomicroscope, which is often neither available nor familiar to neurologists. Nevertheless, careful examination with a magnifying glass can sometimes reveal an iris defect. Certain symptoms elicited during history are suspicious for acquired ocular pathologic conditions. For example, repeated episodes of eye redness, pain, and photophobia should raise concern for recurrent uveitis (see **Fig. 4**).

There is a rare but dramatic pupil condition called Urrets-Zavalia syndrome. This syndrome is characterized by a fixed mydriatic pupil that appears after an uncomplicated anterior segment surgery, most frequently penetrating keratoplasty and even routine cataract extraction. The pupil does not react to light, accommodation, or pilocarpine. Iris atrophy and transient glaucoma are most often present. Proposed mechanisms of injury include iris ischemia, toxic reaction of iris to topical agents, intraoperative iris trauma, abnormalities in the sympathetic nervous system, and relative pupil block.[14]

AUTONOMIC PATHWAYS AND THE PUPIL

Pupillary movement is under control of the autonomic nervous system. The parasympathetic pathway innervates the iris sphincter, which causes pupillary constriction, whereas the sympathetic pathway mediates pupillary dilation via the radially oriented dilator muscle. In general, the motor signal to the iris muscles is distributed evenly so that both pupils constrict and dilate in symmetric fashion. A unilateral lesion along either the parasympathetic or sympathetic pathway to the eye disrupts this balance and thus results in unequal pupil sizes, or anisocoria.[15] In such a case, the dysfunctional pupil can usually be determined by observing the magnitude of anisocoria in different lighting conditions. If anisocoria is most apparent in bright room light, this suggests that the larger pupil is faulty, that is, not constricting as well as the fellow pupil. A relative mydriasis, particularly notable under light stimulation, diminished or sluggish pupillary light reflex, and absence of pupil constriction to near effort are signs of parasympathetic pupillary dysfunction. Conversely, an anisocoria that is more apparent in dim illumination suggests relative failure of the smaller pupil to dilate and an oculosympathetic defect. Although a damaged iris (caused by trauma or inflammation) can cause mydriasis or miosis, iris supersensitivity to dilute topical agonists is specific to neurologic denervation.

Bilateral lesions of either the parasympathetic or sympathetic pathway to the eye are difficult to detect because both pupils are affected, often symmetrically, and so anisocoria does not appear. Such patients may simply note that their pupils seem unusually large or rather small. Diagnosis usually depends on quantitative measures of dynamic pupillary function in conjunction with topical agents, which test for denervation supersensitivity of the iris.[16]

Finally, it is worth remembering that mixed sympathetic and parasympathetic deficits can occur in the same eye. For example, an expanding lesion in the cavernous sinus can cause Horner syndrome and loss of the pupillary light reflex in the ipsilateral eye. This condition occurs because postganglionic sympathetic fibers on the wall of the carotid artery and preganglionic parasympathetic fibers located peripherally in the oculomotor nerve are both vulnerable to compression. Mixed autonomic deficits in both eyes can occur with most autonomic neuropathies. The following sections focus on unilateral lesions of the autonomic pathways to the eye because these are commonly recognized clinical syndromes (oculomotor nerve palsy, tonic pupil, Horner syndrome) and then discuss the autonomic neuropathies as pertinent to the pupil.

Preganglionic Oculoparasympathetic Defect: Oculomotor Nerve Palsy

The preganglionic oculoparasympathetic fibers originate in the Edinger-Westphal subnucleus of the oculomotor nerve complex and travel alongside the ocular motor fibers in the oculomotor nerve and at the ciliary ganglion in the orbit. Oculomotor nerve palsy does not always include pupillary dysfunction, and in cases of minimal palsy, either ptosis or weakness of a single extraocular muscle has been reported (**Fig. 6**).[17] On the other hand, rarely ever is isolated mydriasis a manifestation of oculo-motor nerve palsy. In rare case descriptions, a pupil abnormality was the only clinical sign of oculomotor nerve dysfunction, which is caused by schwannoma, arachnoid cyst, and midbrain hemorrhage.[18,19] Accompanying motor deficits typically appear within days or weeks. During transtentorial herniation, a dilated and poorly reactive pupil is a sign of third nerve compression, but it is possible that other manifestations of oculomotor nerve dysfunction are not demonstrable because the examination is limited due to the patient's decreased consciousness. In an alert patient, careful examination always reveals the lid and eye movement deficits that confirm a diagnosis of oculomotor nerve palsy. An acute oculomotor nerve palsy with pupillary involve-ment is considered a neurologic emergency, and diagnoses to consider include aneu-rysm, pituitary apoplexy, cavernous sinus lesion, skull base pathology, and meningitis.

Postganglionic Parasympathetic Pupil Palsy: Tonic Pupil

A tonic pupil is caused by postganglionic parasympathetic pupillomotor damage,[20] and the site of the lesion is in the orbit, either in the ciliary ganglion or in the short ciliary nerves (**Fig. 7**A).[20] In the acute phase of a tonic pupil, the iris sphincter and ciliary muscles are freshly paralyzed. The pupil is widely dilated and poorly reactive. Patients complain of photophobia and blurry vision at near (loss of accommodation). Because nerve injury is typically incomplete, there is sectoral paralysis of the sphincter, which is best observed with a slit lamp. The iris crypts stream toward the area of normal sphincter function, bunching up along the pupillary border in areas of normal function, and remain loose and thin in the areas of paralysis (see **Fig. 7**B). It is a powerful clinical finding because, in the absence of structural iris damage, sectoral sphincter palsy is diagnostic of postganglionic oculoparasympathetic damage and effectively rules out oculomotor nerve palsy and pharmacologic mydriasis.

Within a few weeks after denervation, supersensitivity develops. Dilute pilocarpine (0.125% or less) is the pharmacologic agent most often used to test for cholinergic

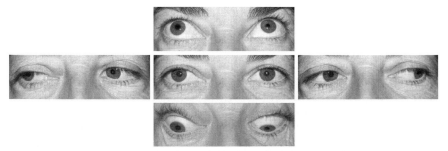

Fig. 6. Eye movements in a patient with partial third nerve palsy and dilated pupil on the right side. The eyes appear aligned in upgaze and right gaze. There is a slight adduction deficit in left gaze, but only in downgaze is a deficit of ocular motility clearly revealed. It is emphasized that careful testing of motility in all gaze positions is critical in patient who has an unilateral, dilated, and poorly functioning pupil.

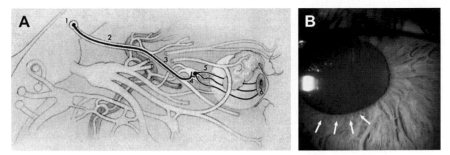

Fig. 7. (*A*) Parasympathetic pathway to the iris and ciliary body. (1) Edinger-Westphal and anterior median nuclei of the dorsal midbrain. (2) Oculomotor nerve. (3) Branch to the inferior oblique muscle. (4) Motor root of the ciliary ganglion. (5) Short ciliary nerves. (6) Iris sphincter and ciliary muscle. (*From* Miller N, Newman NJ, Biousse V, et al, editors. Walsh and Hoyt's clinical neuro-ophthalmology. 6th edition. Baltimore (MD): Lippincott, Williams and Wilkins; 2004. p. 670; with permission.) (*B*) Sectoral sphincter palsy due to idiopathic (Adie) tonic pupil. Close direct examination of the iris reveals normal architecture in segment between the 12-o'clock and 4-o'clock positions. There is a pigmented pupillary ruff, and the iris stroma is compactly stacked as radially aligned rows. The architecture is disrupted in the segment between the 4-o'clock and 9 o'clock positions and is seen as absence of the pupillary ruff, a flattened pupillary margin, and loosening of the iris stroma (*arrows*).

denervation supersensitivity of the iris sphincter. Supersensitivity is present if the larger pupil demonstrates greater constriction to dilute pilocarpine when compared with the unaffected, normal pupil.[21] Despite its popular use, this pharmacologic test is neither specific nor particularly sensitive for tonic pupil. The presence of cholinergic supersensitivity is also found with oculomotor nerve palsy.[21] The absence of cholinergic supersensitivity does not rule out tonic pupil because only about 80% of cases demonstrate this finding.

The subacute and chronic phases of tonic pupil is characterized by nerve regeneration. Resprouting accommodative fibers reinnervate the ciliary muscle but can also mistakenly innervate the iris sphincter.[20] The result is a misdirection synkinesis in which pupillary constriction occurs with near effort because of the aberrant reinnervation of the iris sphincter, but the constriction, as well as the redilation after a near effort, is slow and delayed or tonic. The pupillary light reflex, however, never recovers and in some cases, gets worse. The combination of a poor light reflex with a better near response is termed light-near dissociation and is discussed later in this article (**Fig. 8**).

Over time, tonic firing in the accommodative fibers innervating the sphincter reduces the baseline size of a tonic pupil. Such a small, chronic tonic pupil may be, at first glance, confused for a Horner pupil but is readily distinguished by its poor light reflex, light-near dissociation, and sectoral sphincter palsy.[22]

A unilateral tonic pupil in an intact eye in an otherwise healthy person requires little investigation. Typically, a blood sample for determining blood count, glucose level, syphilis serologies, antinuclear antibodies, and angiotensin-converting enzyme level is sufficient. Evaluation of sedimentation rate and C-reactive protein level is added if the patient is older than 60 years to investigate the possibility of giant cell arteritis.

Oculosympathetic Defect: Horner Syndrome

Dilation of the pupil to abrupt darkness or an alerting stimulus is mediated by the sympathetic pathway to the eye. A lesion anywhere along this 3-neuron pathway leads to a small pupil, ipsilateral ptosis, and anhidrosis and is clinically known as Horner

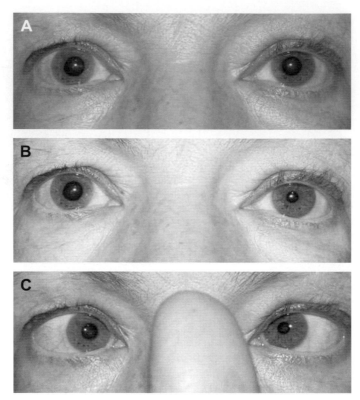

Fig. 8. Patient with a right tonic pupil. (*A*) In dim illumination, both pupils are large and fairly symmetric in size. A slight deformation of the right pupil is seen at the 8-o'clock position. (*B*) Under bright light, an obvious anisocoria manifests due to failure of the right pupil to constrict to light. (*C*) The right pupil, however, constricts mildly to near effort, thus demonstrating light-near dissociation.

syndrome (**Fig. 9**A). The extent of anhidrosis depends largely on the site of the lesion. A central lesion tends to cause hemianhidrosis of the entire face and body, whereas a sympathetic lesion distal to the carotid bifurcation causes anhidrosis only in a patch of ipsilateral forehead and side of nose, if at all. Other less-appreciated findings include lower lid ptosis (an upward shifting of the resting position of the lower lid because of weakness of the inferior tarsal muscle), conjunctival hyperemia, harlequin sign from hemifacial flushing, iris heterochromia (the affected eye has a pale blue iris if denervation occurred in infancy), and pupillary dilation lag in darkness.[15,23] The most consistent of these is the pupil defect, such that in some patients Horner syndrome manifests primarily as an anisocoria (see **Fig. 9**B).

Because the clinical findings or sympathetic denervation of the head and eye are variably present, a firm diagnosis of Horner syndrome often requires pharmacologic confirmation. At present, topical cocaine and topical apraclonidine are most widely used for this purpose (**Fig. 10**).[24] Cocaine is an indirect-acting sympathomimetic agent that blocks presynaptic uptake of released norepinephrine at the terminal synapse. In a healthy subject, topical cocaine causes vasoconstriction of conjunctival vessels, lid retraction, and pupillary dilation. The patient with a sympathetic lesion, however, lacks sufficient norepinephrine in the terminal synapse for cocaine to have a clinically

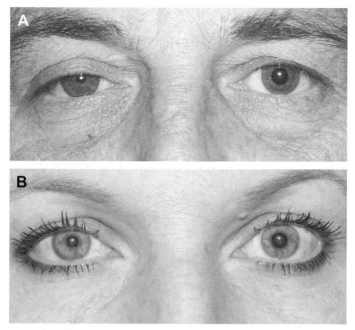

Fig. 9. Two examples of Horner syndrome. (*A*) Patient with a right Horner syndrome. Classic clinical findings of miosis, moderate upper lid ptosis, and lower lid ptosis (elevation of the lower lid obscuring the inferior corneal margin) are seen. (*B*) Patient was referred for evaluation of anisocoria. Ptosis on the right side is so minimal that it was overlooked.

observable effect, thus the ptosis and miosis remain generally unchanged (see **Fig. 10**A).[25] Apraclonidine uses a different mode of action for detecting oculosympathetic insufficiency. Apraclonidine is a weak, direct-acting alpha1-agonist that does not typically cause observable ocular changes in most healthy eyes. The patient

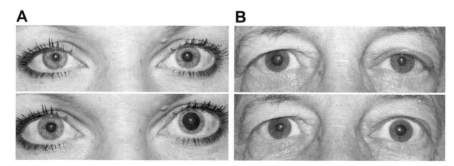

Fig. 10. Pharmacologic testing for confirmation of Horner syndrome. (*A*) Testing with cocaine. The top image shows the patient from **Fig. 9**B 45 minutes after instillation of 2 drops of 4% cocaine in each eye; the right pupil has not dilated to the same degree as the left pupil, indicating absence of sympathetic neurotransmitter at the terminal synapse and confirming Horner syndrome on the right side. (*B*) Testing with apraclonidine. The top image shows a patient with anisocoria and left ptosis. After administration of 1 drop of 1% apraclonidine in each eye, the left pupil is dilated to the point where the anisocoria is now reversed. In addition, the left upper lid is retracted and the conjunctiva is blanched. These findings are consistent with adrenergic supersensitivity to apraclonidine, confirming Horner syndrome on the left side.

with a sympathetic lesion, however, develops supersensitivity to adrenergic agonists and demonstrates pupillary dilation and lid retraction to apraclonidine. A reversal of anisocoria after apraclonidine use is considered diagnostic for Horner syndrome (see **Fig. 10B**).[26] Apraclonidine is not recommended for use in infants due to potential central effects.

The causes of Horner syndrome are numerous, because the sympathetic pathway to the eye follows a long and circuitous route (**Fig. 11**). The differential diagnosis can be narrowed if the location of the lesion is known or suspected.[23] A simple way to localize Horner syndrome is to note the extent of anhidrosis and the presence of accompanying symptoms or signs. Hemianhidrosis, vertigo, ataxia, sensory deficits, swallowing difficulty, or upper cervical cord syndrome point to a lesion of the central, or first order, sympathetic neuron. Brainstem infarcts are the most common cause of

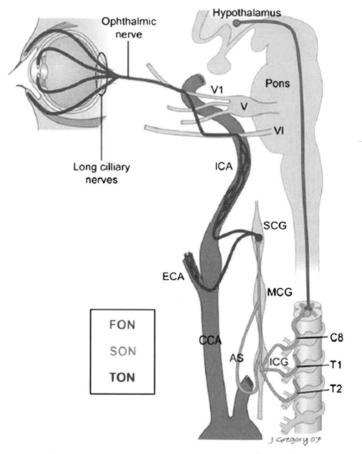

Fig. 11. Anatomy of the oculosympathetic pathway. *Abbreviations:* AS, ansa subclavia; ECA, external carotid artery; FON, first order neuron; ICA, internal carotid artery; ICG, inferior cervical ganglion; MCG, middle cervical ganglion; SCG, superior cervical ganglion; SON, second order neuron; TON, third order neuron. (*From* Reede DL, Garcon E, Smoker WRK, et al. Horner's syndrome: clinical and radiographic evaluation. Neuroimag Clin N Am 2008;18:370; with permission.)

a central Horner syndrome. Hemifacial anhidrosis, a scar or mass in the anterior neck, new shoulder or arm pain, hand weakness, or past history of central venous catheterization suggest a lesion of the second order neuron (also called the preganglionic neuron). Tumor or trauma is the most common cause of a preganglionic Horner syndrome. Absence of anhidrosis or a new, ipsilateral headache suggests damage of the postganglionic, or third order, neuron. The most common conditions are internal carotid artery dissection, parasellar lesion, and cluster headache. Loss or distortion of taste is a peculiar accompanying symptom, presumably due to involvement of the chorda tympani, and has been described with lesions of the internal carotid artery including dissection.[27] **Table 1** gives a more comprehensive list of the causes of Horner syndrome.

Acute, painful Horner syndrome is a specific category that warrants emphasis because this may be the presenting manifestation of an acute carotid dissection.[28] The pain is acute, usually in a focal area of the face or head ipsilateral to the side of the dissection. Other sites of pain include the neck, jaw, pharynx, and ear. Tinnitus and pulsatile sounds are frequent. Urgent evaluation is necessary because the risk of ischemic complication to the retina or brain is highest in the first few weeks of an acute dissection.

Table 1
Etiologies of Horner syndrome

Central (First Order Neuron)	Preganglionic (Second Order Neuron)	Postganglionic (Third Order Neuron)
Infarction Brainstem Hypothalamus	Tumor Neuroblastoma Lymphoma Paraganglioma Sympathetic chain schwannoma Apical lung cancer Thyroid carcinoma	Internal carotid artery Pathology Dissection Agenesis or malformation Tumor Thrombosis Inflammation
Trauma Vertebral artery dissection	Trauma Cord trauma Anterior neck trauma Lower brachial plexus injury	Cluster headache
Demyelinating disease	Cervical spine disease Cervical spondylosis Cervical rib	Tumor Cavernous sinus meningioma Pituitary adenoma Paraganglioma Nasopharyngeal carcinoma at skull base
Hypothalamic tumor	Subclavian aneurysm	Cavernous carotid aneurysm
Cervical syrinx	Iatrogenic Chest tube placement Internal jugular vein cannulation Subclavian vein cannulation Epidural anesthesia Infection Pneumonia Thyroid hydatid cyst Mediastinitis	Inflammation Tolosa-Hunt syndrome Giant cell arteritis Raeder syndrome Otitis media Retropharyngeal abscess Iatrogenic Tonsillectomy Parapharyngeal surgery Endarterectomy

Finally, mention is made of bilateral Horner syndrome. It is difficult to detect because anisocoria is typically absent. It is usually part of the syndrome of diabetic polyneuropathy but may also result from pathologic conditions of the upper cervical cord, such as syringomyelia, thyroidectomy, epidural anesthesia, and rarely, bilateral carotid artery tumors.

Autonomic Neuropathies and the Pupil

Generalized peripheral polyneuropathies cause clinical or subclinical evidence of autonomic dysfunction. When small and unmyelinated fibers are selectively or disproportionately damaged, autonomic dysfunction is the dominant clinical picture. Features associated with autonomic neuropathy include the impairment of cardio-vascular, gastrointestinal, urogenital, thermoregulatory, and sudomotor function.[29] Pupillomotor dysfunction is also present in many of these autonomic neuropathies. The pupil abnormality takes the form of mixed parasympathetic and sympathetic deficits, ranging from mild to severe. As mentioned earlier, clinical detection is difficult without quantitative pupillometry or topical pharmacologic agents due to the bilateral and symmetric nature of the neuropathy. Most patients are asymptomatic.[16]

Herein are discussed those autonomic neuropathies in which pupil involvement is an early and constant feature or the pupil abnormality is a particularly distinctive one. Knowing the disorders that tend to affect the pupil can aid the differential diagnosis and in some cases, secures a diagnosis.

Diabetic polyneuropathy is the most common cause of neuropathy. The development of autonomic dysfunction occurs late in the course of the disease and is associated with increased mortality and sudden death.[29] The prevalence of pupillary abnormalities is 75% among diabetic patients with neuropathy. The most common abnormality is small pupils with intact light reflexes. Exaggerated mydriasis to weak, direct-acting adrenergic agonists, such as apraclonidine or 1% phenylephrine, suggests damage or decreased functioning of the sympathetic pathway, which seems to be more susceptible to diabetes than the parasympathetic fibers.[30] Some diabetic patients with small pupils also demonstrate incomplete mydriasis to standard dilating eye drops, which may reflect a local effect of dilator dysfunction (eg, the sticky iris) rather than a neurologic deficit.

In contrast to diabetes, certain infections (Epstein-Barr virus, Coxsackie virus, herpes simplex virus, *Streptococcus*), connective tissue disorders (systemic lupus erythematosus, Sjögren syndrome, scleroderma), paraneoplastic conditions, and Guillain-Barré syndrome can sometimes cause an acute or subacute autonomic neuropathy in which the autonomic signs are the sole or predominant manifestations. These signs include orthostatic hypotension, anhidrosis, constipation, bladder atony, impotence, secretomotor paralysis, blurry vision due to impaired accommodation, and poor pupillary light reflexes. Typically, both the sympathetic and parasympathetic divisions of the autonomic nervous system are involved.

The Miller Fisher syndrome is a disorder characterized by acute onset of ophthalmoplegia, ataxia, and areflexia, which frequently follows a flulike illness. Pupillary abnormalities, typically mydriasis with poor or no light reflexes, are noted in about half of cases and manifest early in the disease course. Some patients demonstrate a transient light-near dissociation as well. The disorder is self-limiting, and within several months, most clinical signs including those involving the pupils are significantly improved.[31]

Botulism is caused by a bacterial toxin, which interferes with the release of acetylcholine at the neuromuscular junction and in the cholinergic autonomic nervous system.

Although several different subtypes of the toxin exist and routes of human infection can vary (food-borne, wound, gastrointestinal tract colonization), clinical manifestations are similar. Almost 90% of patients with botulism complain of acute blurring of vision, especially for reading, due to paralysis of accommodation. This blurring appears within the first few days of illness, and in some cases, accommodative failure is the initial and sole sign of nervous system involvement. Concomitantly or shortly thereafter, there is impairment of the pupillary light reflex although this is less severely affected than accommodative function for unclear reasons.[15] Other manifestations include progressive descending skeletal muscle weakness, ocular motor palsies, bulbar paralysis, and cardiovascular lability. Recognition of the clinical syndrome is critical because respiratory failure can result in mortality rates of up to 20%.

LIGHT-NEAR DISSOCIATION

Reflex pupillary constriction is caused by 2 stimuli: light and accommodation. Accommodation serves to put close objects into focus and occurs synchronously with pupillary constriction and convergence. This triad is called the near reflex. In the physiologic state, a bright light stimulus causes greater, or at least equal, pupillary constriction than a near stimulus. Light-near dissociation is a pathologic state in which the near reflex evokes greater pupillary constriction than the light reflex. Light-near dissociation appears when the light reflex pathway is damaged but the near reflex pathway has remained intact.

The afferent influences for the near reflex are not precisely established but likely arise from various supranuclear areas (occipital lobe, cerebellum) and are under both reflex and volitional control.[13] Therefore, decreased mental status, inattention, or simply unwillingness to cooperate lead to a poor near response. An encouraging tone by the clinician and several attempts to get a patient to focus a near object are helpful maneuvers for obtaining an adequate near response.

Light-Near Dissociation Due to an Afferent Lesion

Light-near dissociation associated with visual loss is caused by a lesion of the optic nerve or chiasm. Such a lesion interrupts light signal coming from the retina and does not involve the afferent signals mediating the near reflex. Although optic neuropathy may be the most common cause of light-near dissociation, this pupil finding is clinically overshadowed in this setting by the more readily observable relative afferent pupillary defect in the bad eye. The most obvious example of light-near dissociation caused by an afferent lesion occurs in the patient who is blind (or nearly so) from bilateral optic neuropathy. The light reflex from either eye is absent, yet a brisk near reflex can be initiated by simply asking the patients to attempt to focus on their own nose.

Central Light-Near Dissociation

The 2 pretectal olivary nuclei in the dorsal midbrain receive the retinal afferent information mediating the pupillary light reflex and relay it to the Edinger-Westphal subnuclei. The close proximity of these paired nuclei to one another and their exiting fibers permit a single lesion in the dorsal midbrain to interrupt the pupillary light reflex signals to both eyes. The near reflex is spared because its afferent connections approach the Edinger-Westphal subnuclei from the ventral aspect. Thus, in a patient with no known optic neuropathy, bilateral light-near dissociation must be considered due to a dorsal midbrain lesion, until proven otherwise. The dorsal midbrain syndrome (also known as pretectal syndrome or Parinaud syndrome) refers to central light-near dissociation accompanied by other neurologic deficits, such as vertical gaze palsy, lid retraction, accommodative paralysis or spasm, and convergence-retraction nystagmus.[15,32] Common lesions causing central light-near dissociation and the dorsal midbrain syndrome are ischemic stroke, hemorrhage, tectal tumor, demyelinating disease, and acute hydrocephalus. Sometimes, the earliest clinical indication of shunt malfunction in treated hydrocephalus is the combination of light-near dissociation and a subtle upgaze palsy.

Miotic pupils that demonstrate light-near dissociation are classically attributed to neurosyphilis. They are called Argyll Robertson pupils. It is speculated that inflammatory damage in the region around the sylvian aqueduct in the rostral midbrain damages light reflex fibers as they course toward the Edinger-Westphal subnuclei yet spares the more ventrally located near reflex fibers.[33] The presence of miosis is considered an essential feature of Argyll Robertson pupils, as there must be a unique mechanism that maintains such small pupillary size in the presence of impaired light reflexes, because with dorsal midbrain lesions, the pupils are typically moderate to large in size. One proposed mechanism of syphilitic miosis is that periaqueductal inflammation also damages supranuclear inhibitory pathways that converge at the Edinger-Westphal subnuclei.

Probably a more common cause of small pupils with light-near dissociation is bilateral, chronic tonic pupil, or "little old Adie pupil." These pupils can usually be distinguished from Argyll Robertson pupils by their slow, tonic movement during and after near effort, the presence of sectoral palsy of the iris sphincter, and cholinergic supersensitivity of the iris sphincter.[22]

Peripheral Light-Near Dissociation

Peripheral light-near dissociation represents a form of misdirection synkinesis occurring after peripheral nerve injury, either damage to the oculomotor nerve or to the short ciliary nerves. Peripheral light-near dissociation is usually unilateral and the most common example is idiopathic tonic (Adie) pupil (see **Fig. 8**). It can also occur following other types of injury to the ciliary ganglion or the short ciliary nerves, notably orbital trauma or ocular surgery such as optic nerve sheath decompression, laser iridectomy, or retinal detachment repair. Occasionally, light-near dissociation is noted in a patient with chronic oculomotor nerve palsy from a compressive lesion. Presumably there is cross talk of signals between accommodative and pupillary constrictor fibers. If the pupillary constriction occurs whenever the eye moves in adduction, either attempted lateral gaze or attempted convergence, then it is not truly the near effort that evokes the pupil response but rather a synkinesis between medial rectus muscle and iris sphincter muscle. This pupil-gaze synkinesis is called a "pseudo" light-near dissociation.

TRANSIENT ANISOCORIA

An alert patient in no acute distress who reports episodes of transient anisocoria not accompanied by another neurologic deficit is not likely to harbor serious intracranial pathologic conditions such as tumor or aneurysm. It is, however, critical to ensure that pupillary function in light and dark is normal between episodes. If pupillary function is normal then physiologic anisocoria or benign episodic mydriasis may be the cause of transient anisocoria. Physiologic anisocoria can fluctuate from day to day and can seem to go away in sunlight. Distinction from Horner syndrome is important in these patients. Benign episodic mydriasis is a descriptive term for recurrent episodes of isolated unilateral mydriasis occurring in young adults, usually migrainous women.[34] The mydriasis typically appears in the same eye but can alternate sides. It may occur during a migraine or may be independent of headache. The duration of mydriasis is usually several hours but may persist for days. The mechanism of benign episodic mydriasis is not established, and it is a clinical diagnosis of exclusion.

In some patients, pupil dysfunction occurs only in conjunction with a headache. Anisocoria during a migraine attack is a well-described association, but the mechanism is not fully established and is likely multifactorial. In some patients, migrainous vasospasm causing local and reversible ischemia of the ciliary ganglion leads to a dilated, poorly reactive pupil and accommodative palsy. In some other patients, sympathetic dysregulation, occurring either as increased or decreased activity and may be unilateral or bilateral and asymmetric, has been described.

If the patient reports visual blur, haloes around light, ocular pain, and redness during an episode of anisocoria, intermittent subacute angle-closure glaucoma must be suspected (**Fig. 12**). This ocular disorder occurs in patients with a structurally narrow anterior chamber angle, which may be a primary defect or a secondary complication from ocular inflammation, trauma, or ischemia. When the anterior chamber angle closes, the normal outflow of aqueous humor is acutely blocked and intraocular pressure increases rapidly. Periocular pain and sometimes excruciating headache develops. The pupil becomes mildly dilated and fixed. Such a clinical presentation may be mistaken for an acute neurologic state, such as intracranial hemorrhage. Precipitating factors include prone position, dark or dim lighting, prolonged near work, stress, sneezing, pharmacologic mydriasis, and certain anesthetic agents. Patients can have repeated self-limited episodes of subacute angle closure before a full-blown attack. Ophthalmologic examination is necessary for confirmation of diagnosis. Failure to recognize this cause of intermittent mydriasis can lead to permanent visual loss.

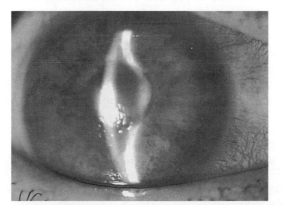

Fig. 12. An eye with acute angle-closure glaucoma and secondary corneal decompensation. The patient complained of several prior episodes in which the eye became painful and red and haloes seen around lights. This episode did not resolve spontaneously, and the patient went to the emergency room for pain control. Anisocoria was noted. The pupil in this eye did not respond well to light stimulation. On direct palpation, the painful eye felt hard like a stone. Intraocular pressure was measured at 50 mm Hg, and slit-lamp examination revealed iridocorneal angle closure. The pressure was lowered with systemic and topical drugs, and a YAG laser iridotomy was subsequently performed in both eyes.

SUMMARY

In summary, disorders of the pupil range from benign or congenital anomalies to life-threatening intracranial pathologic conditions. The clinician should have a systematic approach for examining pupillary movements, iris structures, and neurologic status of the patient and be familiar with commonly used pharmacologic agents, which assess neural integrity to the iris. Aniridia, iris coloboma, Horner syndrome, oculomotor palsy with pupillary involvement, and bilateral light-near dissociation with preserved vision are disorders of the pupil, which may signify a more serious underlying pathologic condition.

REFERENCES

1. Lam BL, Thompson HS, Corbett JJ. The prevalence of simple anisocoria. Am J Ophthalmol 1987;104(1):69–73.
2. Mahoney NR, Liu GT, Menacker SJ, et al. Pediatric Horner syndrome: etiologies and roles of imaging and urine studies to detect neuroblastoma and other responsible mass lesions. Am J Ophthalmol 2006;142(4):651–9.
3. Kodski SR, Younge BR. Acquired oculomotor, trochlear, and abducent cranial nerve palsies in pediatric patients. Am J Ophthalmol 1992;114(5):568–74.
4. Schumacher-Feero LA, Yoo KW, Solari FM, et al. Third cranial nerve palsy in children. Am J Ophthalmol 1999;128(2):216–21.
5. Onwochei BC, Simon JW, Bateman JB, et al. Ocular colobomata. Surv Ophthalmol 2000;45(3):175–94.
6. Idrees F, Vaideanu D, Fraser SG, et al. A review of anterior segment dysgeneses. Surv Opthalmol 2006;51(3):213–31.
7. Balmer A, Munier F. Differential diagnosis of leukocoria and strabismus, first presenting signs of retinoblastoma. Clin Ophthalmol 2007;1(4):431–9.
8. Isenberg SJ, Molarte A, Vazquez M. The fixed and dilated pupils of premature neonates. Am J Ophthalmol 1990;110(2):168–71.
9. Lee H, Khan R, O'Keefe M. Aniridia: current pathology and management. Acta Ophthalmol 2008;86(7):708–15.
10. Kurli M, Finger PT. The kidney, cancer, and the eye: current concepts. Surv Ophthalmol 2005;50(6):507–18.
11. Orssaud C, Roche O, El Dirani H, et al. Delayed internal ophthalmoplegia and amblyopia following chickenpox. Eur J Pediatr 2006;165(10):728–47.
12. Ben Simon GJ, Abraham FA, Melamed S. Pingelapese achromatopsia: correlation between paradoxical pupillary response and clinical features. Br J Ophthalmol 2004;88(2):223–5.
13. Kardon R. Anatomy and physiology of the autonomic nervous system. In: Miller N, Newman NJ, Biousse V, et al, editors. Walsh and Hoyt's clinical neuro-ophthalmology. 6th edition. Baltimore (MD): Lippincott, Williams and Wilkins; 2004. p. 649–714.
14. Fournié P, Ponchel C, Malecaze F, et al. Fixed dilated pupil (urrets-zavalia syndrome) and anterior subcapsular cataract formation after descemet stripping endothelial keratoplasty. Cornea 2009;28(10):1184–6.
15. Kawasaki A. Disorders of pupillary function, accommodation and lacrimation. In: Miller N, Newman NJ, Biousse V, et al, editors. Walsh and Hoyt's clinical neuro-ophthalmology. 6th edition. Baltimore (MD): Lippincott, Williams and Wilkins; 2004. p. 739–805.
16. Bremner F, Smith S. Pupil findings in a consecutive series of 150 patients with generalized autonomic neuropathy. J Neurol Neurosurg Psychiatr 2006;77(10): 1163–8.

17. Bartleson JD, Trautmann JC, Sundt TM. Minimal oculomotor nerve paresis secondary to unruptured intracranial aneurysm. Arch Neurol 1986;43(10): 1015–20.
18. Shuaib A, Israelian G, Lee MA. Mesencephalic hemorrhage and unilateral pupillary deficit. J Clin Neuroophthalmol 1989;9(1):47–9.
19. Ashker L, Weinstein JM, Dias M, et al. Arachnoid cyst causing thrid cranial nerve palsy manifesting as isolated internal ophthalmoplegia and iris cholinergic supersensitivity. J Neuroophthalmol 2008;28(3):192–7.
20. Kardon RH, Bergamin O. Adie's pupil. In: Levin LA, Arnold AC, editors. Neuroophthalmology, the practical guide. New York: Thieme; 2005. p. 325–39.
21. Jacobson DM, Vierkant RA. Comparison of cholinergic supersensitivity in third nerve palsy and Adie's syndrome. J Neuroophthalmol 1998;18(3):171–5.
22. Kardon RH, Corbett JJ, Thompson HS. Segmental denervation and reinnervation of the iris sphincter as shown by infrared videographic transillumination. Ophthalmology 1998;105(2):313–21.
23. Reede DL, Garcon E, Smoker WRK, et al. Horner's syndrome: clinical and radiographic evaluation. Neuroimaging Clin N Am 2008;18(2):369–85.
24. Mughal M, Longmuir R. Current pharmacologic testing for Horner syndrome. Curr Neurol Neurosci Rep 2009;9(5):384–9.
25. Kardon RH, Denison CE, Brown CK, et al. Critical evaluation of the cocaine test in the diagnosis of Horner's syndrome. Arch Ophthalmol 1990;108(3):384–7.
26. Brown SM, Aouchiche R, Freedman KA. The utility of 0.5% apraclonidine in the diagnosis of Horner syndrome. Arch Ophthalmol 2003;121(8):1201–3.
27. Mokri B, Silbert PL, Schievink WI, et al. Cranial nerve palsy in spontaneous dissection of the extracranial internal carotid artery. Neurology 1996;46(2):356–9.
28. de Bray J-M, Baumgartner R, Guillon B, et al. Isolated Horner's syndrome may herald stroke. Cerebrovasc Dis 2005;19(4):274–5.
29. Freeman R. Autonomic peripheral neuropathy. Lancet 2005;365(9466):1259–70.
30. Bremner FD, Smith SE. Pupil abnormalities in selected autonomic neuropathies. J Neuroophthalmol 2006;26(3):209–19.
31. Nitta T, Kase M, Shinmei Y, et al. Mydriasis with light-near dissociation in Fisher's syndrome. Jpn J Ophthalmol 2007;51(3):224–7.
32. Wilhelm BJ, Wilhelm H, Moro S, et al. Pupil response components: studies in patients with Parinaud's syndrome. Brain 2002;125(10):2296–307.
33. Thompson HS, Kardon RH. The Argyll Robertson pupil. J Neuroophthalmol 2006; 26(2):134–8.
34. Jacobson DM. Benign episodic unilateral mydriasis. Clinical characteristics. Ophthalmology 1995;102(11):1623–7.

Orbital Disease in Neuro-Ophthalmology

Michael K. Yoon, MD, Timothy J. McCulley, MD*

KEYWORDS

• Orbit • Fracture • Traumatic optic neuropathy
• Orbital inflammatory disease • Orbital hemorrhage

Virtually all abnormalities of the orbit can result in neuro-ophthalmic findings: optic neuropathies, motility disorders, and changes in sensation. Subtle orbital disease, presenting with neuro-ophthalmic findings, is frequently overlooked on initial evaluation. By contrast, obvious orbital diseases, such as Graves disease, are also commonly managed by neuro-ophthalmologists, and although they might not come with much of a diagnostic dilemma, may be a challenge to treat.

Comprehensive coverage of all orbital diseases is beyond the scope of this article. The focus is on disorders more commonly encountered or that come with more serious consequences if misdiagnosed. **Table 1** catalogs orbital diseases and abnormalities based on presenting symptoms. However, the remainder of the article is structured around the specific orbital disease, as opposed to working from a given symptom. Graves disease, covered in article by Cockerham and Chan elsewhere in this issue, is not specifically addressed. Orbital trauma, hemorrhage, neoplasm, and inflammation are covered in some detail.

ORBITAL TRAUMA

Traumatic injury of the bony orbit and its contents can result in any number of neuro-ophthalmologic abnormalities. Sensation can be affected by injury to any of the sensory branches coursing the orbit. The most commonly injured is the infraorbital nerve, a terminal branch of the second division of the trigeminal nerve.[1] This nerve is a fairly reliable mark of an orbital floor fracture because the bony canal through

Financial support: none.
Proprietary interest: The authors have no affiliations with or involvement in any organization or entity with a direct financial interest in the subject matter or materials discussed in the article.
Department of Ophthalmology, University of California San Francisco, 10 Koret Way, K-301, San Francisco, CA 94143-0730, USA
* Corresponding author.
E-mail address: mcculleyt@vision.ucsf.edu

Table 1
Orbital disease associated with neuro-ophthalmic findings

Finding	General Category	Specific Disease
Motility abnormality	Enophthalmos	Traumatic fracture
		Silent sinus syndrome
		Sagging eye sunken brain syndrome
	Inflammatory	Graves disease
		Diffuse orbital inflammatory syndrome
		Myositis
		Infectious cellulitis
	Myopathy	Chronic progressive external ophthalmoplegia
		Congenital fibrosis syndrome
	Neoplastic	Adjacent neoplasm with extension to muscle
		Metastasis to muscle
		Primary neoplasm of muscle
	Neuropathy	Neoplasm (usually with apical compression)
		Iatrogenic (post surgical)
	Trauma	Mechanical effect of hematoma/edema
		Contused muscle
		Entrapped muscle
		Neuropathy
Optic neuropathy	Compressive	Neoplastic
		Graves disease
	Inflammatory	Perioptic neuritis
		Related to systemic disease (eg, sarcoidosis)
	Neoplastic	Intrinsic to nerve
		Adjacent with compression
		Metastasis and lymphoproliferative
	Trauma	Indirect traumatic optic
		Direct traumatic injury (fracture or penetrating)
Pain	Inflammatory	Idiopathic orbital inflammatory disease
		Related to systemic disease (eg, sarcoidosis)
	Neoplastic	Primary (eg, adenoid cystic carcinoma)
		Perineural spread (eg, squamous cell carcinoma)
	Neurogenic	Trigeminal neuralgia
		Cluster headache
		Paroxysmal hemicrania

which the nerve runs is often damaged with these fractures, which frequently results in hypesthesia of the lower eyelid and adjacent cheek extending inferiorly to the upper lip and teeth. Injury to the infraorbital nerve is generally of little clinical consequence, as sensation returns within 6 months in the majority of cases.[2] More concerning are motility abnormalities and loss of vision via a "traumatic optic neuropathy." Before discussing these separately, a brief overview of fractures is needed.

Orbital Fractures

Orbital fractures can loosely be classified in 1 of 3 categories: orbital rim fractures, comminuted orbital wall fractures, and trapdoor orbital wall fractures. Fractures of the rim come in pairs. If the rim breaks at one point there will almost always be a second fracture site on which the displaced bone pivoted. This site might be on the same rim with a posteriorly dislodged piece, which most commonly occurs when the rim is struck focally with a hard object, such as a golf ball. More commonly, the fractures involve more than one rim. A "tripod" or "zygomatic complex" fracture

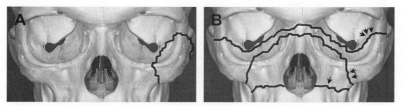

Fig. 1. Complex orbital rim fractures. (*A*) Tripod fractures involve the inferior and lateral orbital rims as wall as the zygomatic arch. (*B*) There are 3 types of LeFort fractures distinguished by specific location of the fracture. Type I (*single arrow*) does not involve the orbits at all. Type II (*double arrow*) extends through both the medial and inferior orbit walls. Type III (*triple arrow*) extends from the medial wall to the lateral wall via the floor of the orbit.

involves the inferior and lateral orbital walls as well as the zygomatic arch (**Fig. 1**A). This fracture is the most common type to involve the orbit rims. LeFort fractures, characterized by posterior extension through the pterygoid plates, are more extensive. There are 3 types, but only LeFort fracture types 2 and 3 involve the orbital walls (see **Fig. 1**B). Complex fractures of this nature are unlikely to be overlooked, and further discussion of their management is beyond the scope of this article and is deferred.

Comminuted wall fractures comprise the vast majority of isolated orbital fractures. These fractures are characterized by displaced chips of bone (**Fig. 2**). The classic "blowout" fracture occurs when pressure on the eye and surrounding soft tissue is transmitted to the orbit, causing outward fracturing of the wall. The wall may also "buckle" when sufficient force is applied to the rim. Pure forms of "blowout" and "buckling" fractures exist, but a large number are likely due to a combination of the 2 means.[3–5] Regardless of mechanism, motility abnormalities may occur. Extraocular muscles can be displaced within the defect or "hung up" on the edge of fractured bone, either of which may cause dysfunction of the muscle. Fortunately, there is no hurry in repairing such fractures. Numerous studies have suggested that equivalent

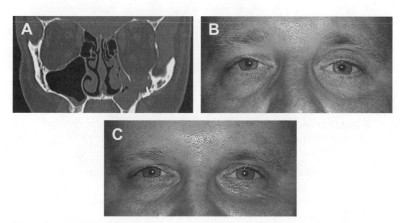

Fig. 2. Comminuted orbital wall fracture. (*A*) Computed tomography of a large complex fracture, including a large comminuted fracture of the orbital floor. (*B*) External photo 1 year after injury, without proper repair. (*C*) Postoperative appearance following fracture repair more than 1 year after initial injury.

results are achieved with urgent (with a few days) or late (up to months following injury) repair.[6–8]

The final category, trapdoor fractures, is in need of particular attention because if missed, delaying repair to such fractures may result in permanent diplopia. A trapdoor fracture with an entrapped muscle is also the most likely scenario to be mistaken for a cranial neuropathy (**Figs. 3** and **4**). Trapdoor fractures result from an acute transient increase in orbital pressure causing a linear orbital wall fracture with outward displacement of adjacent bone, which immediately returns to its original position, potentially incarcerating orbital soft tissue.[9–14] This mechanism is dependent on ample bone elasticity, characteristic of children. In contrast, the less elastic nature of adult bone leads to the frequently seen comminuted fractures.[15] Not surprisingly, trapdoor fractures are encountered almost exclusively in children.[9–14] However, several reports have described trapdoor type fractures in adults (see **Fig. 4**).[16,17] Kum and colleagues[17] described a patient with a well documented trapdoor fracture at 37 years of age. Although the vast majority of published cases of trapdoor fractures with muscle incarceration have involved the orbital floor, trapdoor fractures of the medial wall occur as well.[14]

Jordan and colleagues coined the term "white-eyed blowout fracture" to describe trapdoor fractures. This term emphasizes the common lack of external signs of trauma, which may decrease the clinician's level of suspicion of serious injury.[11] This, along with additional characteristics of trapdoor fractures, makes them likely

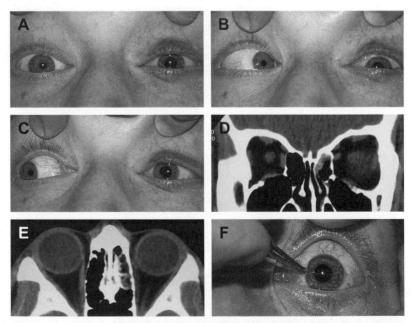

Fig. 3. Trapdoor orbital wall fracture. This young man was initially given the wrong diagnosis of an abducens nerve palsy. He was orthophoric in primary gaze (*A*) with markedly limited abduction (*B*) as well as moderately reduced adduction (*C*). Computed tomography was misread as normal. Although the orbital wall is not displaced, the medial rectus muscle appears abnormal. On the coronal image (*D*) the left medial rectus muscle is smaller and misshapen relative to that of the fellow eye. On the axial image (*E*) the muscle is poorly visualized. Forced duction testing (*F*) confirms muscle entrapment.

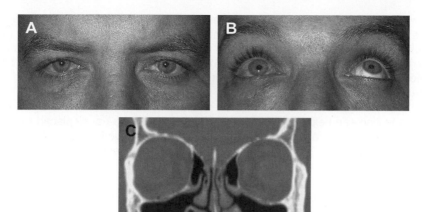

Fig. 4. An adult male with the right inferior rectus entrapped within an inferior trapdoor fracture with limited vertical motility (*A*, *B*). Computed tomography (*C*) with a nondisplaced inferior orbital floor fracture evidenced only by several small pockets of air adjacent to the inferior rectus muscle.

to evade recognition. Radiologic evidence of injury may also be minimal; attention should be directed at the location and appearance of the muscles themselves, as there may be no obvious bone abnormality (see **Figs. 3** and **4**). Lastly, the presence of an oculocardiac reflex with associated nausea may decrease cooperation, making thorough ocular motility evaluation difficult in a child.[12]

Several reports have suggested that a superior outcome is achieved when surgical intervention is performed within days of injury. Egbert and colleagues[9] demonstrated more rapid resolution of diplopia with early intervention. Although they reported a trend toward a decrease in persistent long-term diplopia, this difference was not statistically significant. Bansagi and Meyer[13] found that time to surgical intervention was critical, with earlier surgical repair yielding better clinical outcomes. Jordan and colleagues[11] similarly reported improved outcomes with early intervention. Taken together, improved short- and long-term outcomes have been well established with early (within a few days of injury) surgical repair of muscle entrapment in trapdoor fractures.

Management of Diplopia Following Orbital Trauma

Abnormal ocular motility following blunt orbital trauma can result from numerous causes including muscle contusion, cranial nerve palsy, the mass effect of soft tissue edema and hemorrhage, globe malposition, and muscle malposition or entrapment. It is important to appropriately assess and recognize the specific cause of abnormal motility following blunt trauma. This assessment is imperative not only to guide appropriate therapy but, more importantly, to avoid unnecessary surgery.

Ocular misalignment and/or pain on eye movement are very common immediately following an orbital wall fracture. In most case it relates to tissue edema and hemorrhage, is self-limited, and requires no intervention. The clinician's task is to determine in which patients the misalignment is due to the fracture and will require surgery.

Identifying muscle entrapment can be a challenge that is ultimately a clinical diagnosis. Orbital computed tomography should be obtained in all patients with abnormal extraocular motility following trauma. Although very helpful in assessing a fracture, muscle entrapment cannot be definitively diagnosed or excluded based on imaging alone. A rectus muscle herniating into the adjacent sinus through an orbital defect does not necessarily predict abnormal motility. In contrast, patients with the most severe motility limitations often have little to no radiographic evidence of a fracture, as in trapdoor fractures. Soft tissue adjacent the rectus muscles may contain the intermuscular or other fibrous septum, and if incorporated into the fracture, profound restriction in motility may result.[18]

Clinical findings should be correlated with radiography. In some cases forced duction testing can help identify and entrapped muscle. If a nondisplaced trapdoor fracture with muscle entrapment is suspected, forced ductions can be used to confirm the diagnosis (see **Fig. 3**). Unfortunately, when there is severe soft tissue swelling, forced duction testing is difficult to interpret, as edema alone can alter forced ductions.

The use of steroids in patients with orbital fractures is controversial. There is limited data suggesting that better outcomes in motility are achieved with their use.[19] Admittedly, there is insufficient evidence to the contrary. However, given the lack of sound evidence in support of steroid use, most orbital surgeons do not believe that there are any long-term benefits to steroid use. Steroids do have the benefit of more rapid resolution of pain and swelling;[19] this is helpful not only in terms of patient comfort but also in sorting out the cause of abnormal motility. Orbital congestion alone can limit ocular motility and by more quickly eliminating it from the equation, one can better assess whether other factors such as a cranial nerve palsy or an entrapped muscle are the source of diplopia. A common regimen would be a 1-week course of oral prednisone (1 mg/kg) followed by a rapid taper.

In patients with a comminuted fracture, tissue edema or hemorrhage, and abnormal motility, observation is a reasonable option. If the motility fails to resolve after resolution of the edema, alternative causes are considered, leaving 2 possibilities: a cranial nerve palsy or muscle entrapment. These diagnosis should be easily differentiated, based the pattern of abnormal motility. If the pattern is that of restriction, with a radiographic correlate, fracture repair can be undertaken. The argument against this approach is, in some clinicians' opinion, the difficulty of performing surgery later. However, several studies have suggested that the ultimate motility outcome is not dependent on the time of fracture repair.[6–8] The patient depicted in **Fig. 2** had definitive repair more than a year after injury, with marked improvement in extraocular motility. The downside to delaying repair is the formation of scar tissue, making tissue planes less distinct and surgery more difficult. For this reason, in larger fractures with significant tissue displacement likely to cause a motility disturbance, repair within a week or two of injury might be preferable.[20]

Enophthalmos

Enophthalmos, another common consequence of orbital fractures, is also an indication for surgical repair. When severe, extraocular motility may be affected, resulting in diplopia. Enophthalmos is also cosmetically unacceptable in most patients' opinion. As with the management of diplopia in the setting of an orbital fracture, there are 2 schools of thought. Some recommend repair of every "large fracture," usually defined as greater than 50% of the area of the orbital floor. However, based on the size of the fracture alone it is impossible to predict which patients will develop troublesome enophthalmos. Moreover, there is evidence that delaying repair does not negatively impact outcome. Therefore, it can be reasonably argued that patients should be observed, reserving surgery for those who develop enophthalmos that is of either functional or cosmetic concern.

Traumatic Optic Neuropathy

Traumatic optic neuropathies have been classically separated into 2 categories. The first is direct injuries resulting from orbital or cerebral trauma that transgress normal tissue planes to disrupt the anatomic integrity of the optic nerve. The second and more common are indirect injuries, caused by forces transmitted from a distance to the optic nerve. Direct injury is usually not subtle and is unlikely to go undetected. Direct injury can result from penetrating injury (eg, foreign body or stab wound) or from a displaced piece of bone directly cutting the nerve near to or within the optic canal. Such injuries usually result in severe visual loss and have limited therapeutic options.

An indirect traumatic optic neuropathy occurs when tissue planes are not disrupted, with visual loss occurring due to optic nerve injury remote to the point of impact. Although indirect injury may occur anywhere along the length of the nerve, the most common site of injury is the bony optic canal.[21,22] Injury is presumed to occur by impact force transmission through the bones. This belief is largely based on laser interferometer study of cadaver crania devoid of soft tissue, which demonstrated external impact causing significant force concentration and deformation of the sphenoid bone and optic canal.[23] Theoretically this causes contusion necrosis of the nerve by disrupting axons and/or vasculature. Although this may explain occurrences of optic canal fractures and associated nerve damage, alternative mechanisms might be considered when the integrity of the bone surrounding the optic nerve is preserved. Indirect optic neuropathies are almost always the result of deceleration injury, with the point of impact being the forehead.[24] A frontal blow would result in an anterior to posterior propagation of a shock wave within the soft tissues of the orbit. As the wave propagates though the conically shaped orbit, it would be concentrated/amplified at the orbital apex, where the optic nerve enters its bony canal.[25] This situation is consistent with indirect traumatic optic neuropathy occurring almost exclusively with frontal impact, as opposed to lateral or posterior cranial impact. It would also explain why the optic canal is the most common site of damage. Regardless of mechanism, management remains the same.

On evaluation the only findings are visual loss (acuity and/or field) and an afferent pupillary defect (APD). Patterns of visual field loss vary widely, but typically include central depression, which accounts for the decreased acuity. The eye itself, including the optic nerve, should appear normal. Because traumatic optic neuropathies are usually seen with severe trauma, associated injuries—ocular, neurologic, and musculoskeletal—are often found and should be assessed for.

Initial evaluation should involve computed tomography. Fine-cut direct coronal, or reconstructed images through the optic canal, are needed to identify fractures in this area. Fractures of the optic canal and adjacent structures are frequently present but are not necessary to make the diagnosis.

Management of traumatic optic neuropathy is controversial, with many opposing opinions. Consistently proposed management options are largely limited to steroids of various doses and optic canal decompression. Others recommend only observation. Several studies have looked at the natural course, without intervention. Spontaneous improvement has been described in 20% to 50% of cases, with a variable degree of visual acuity recovery.[26,27] Despite these reports, significant recovery to near-normal vision is rare.

Several anecdotal studies showed improvement in visual acuity with corticosteroids.[26,28] The initial rationale was that steroids reduced edema of the nerve within the optic canal, limiting compressive damage to the nerve. More recently it has been suggested that, among other things, corticosteroids inhibit oxygen free radical–induced lipid peroxidation and decrease vasospasm. This finding comes primarily from work on spinal cord injuries. The National Acute Spinal Cord Injury Studies (NASCIS) suggested that methylprednisolone given as a bolus of 30 mg/kg intravenously, followed by 5.4 mg/kg/h for 48 hours, had improved neurologic function after spinal cord injury.[29] Although optic nerve injury was not specifically addressed, advocates for the use of "spinal dose" steroids for the management of indirect traumatic optic neuropathy use this as their basis. Steroid efficacy has recently been called into question, in part because patients in the NASCIS studies were found to have only limited neurologic recovery. More importantly, there was a suggestion that with steroids, there was an increase in life-threatening infections. The CRASH study further elucidated complications of steroid use in head injuries.[30] Available data have shown that the risk to benefit ratio is particularly unfavorable if steroids are not administered within 8 hours of injury. Rarely are patients seen within this 8-hour window, which has greatly reduced the number of patients with traumatic optic neuropathy being treated with high-dose steroids.

Surgical decompression of the optic canal is also advocated by some investigators. The goal of surgical decompression of the optic nerve within the optic canal has been the release of compression by removing bone, possibly improving vascular perfusion. Again, there are anecdotal reports of some success with this approach, but the overall positive effect seems quite low.[31] Also, in the best controlled study assessing optic nerve decompression (International Optic Nerve Trauma Study [IONTS]), no benefit was seen.[27] One exception for which optic canal decompression might be considered is in the rare case where the bony canal is disrupted.

Part of the controversy surrounding the management of traumatic optic neuropathy lies in the lack of solid clinical evidence. Given the rarity of traumatic optic neuropathies combined with the variety among patients, in terms of not only vision but also associated injuries, a proper prospective comparative trial is barely feasible. The best attempt was the IONTS.[27] This trial was a comparative nonrandomized interventional study with concurrent treatment groups that compared the visual outcome in patients with indirect traumatic optic neuropathy treated with corticosteroids, optic canal decompression, or observation alone. After adjustment for baseline vision, there were no significant differences between any of the treatment groups. In fact, although not statistically significant, untreated patients had greater rates of improvement than those treated with steroids or surgery. Although this study was not sufficiently powered to exclude all treatment benefit (the observation group had only 9 subjects), the investigators reasonably concluded that the study was sufficient to exclude a large benefit from steroids or optic canal decompression.

In summary, based the existing literature, neither corticosteroids nor optic canal surgery should be considered the standard of care for patients with traumatic optic neuropathy. It is reasonable for clinicians to use their judgment to decide how to treat an individual patient. If seen acutely (within 8 hours of injury) the use of steroids, following the guidelines outlined by the NASCIS studies, is reasonable.

ORBITAL HEMORRHAGE

Orbital hemorrhage is seen in numerous settings, most commonly in association with orbital fractures or contusion. Hemorrhage is one of the most feared complications of periocular surgery. Its incidence after blepharoplasty with subsequent partial or complete blindness is estimated to be between 6 and 40 per 100,000 (**Fig. 5**).[32] Hemorrhage is also well described in association with retrobulbar or periorbital anesthetic injections.[33] A handful of cases have been described with blood disorders such

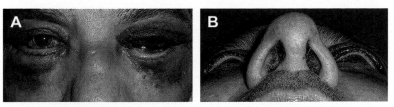

Fig. 5. Bilateral orbital hemorrhage following cosmetic blepharoplasty (*A*). The right eye, in which the blood remained relatively anterior, healed without intervention or consequence. The left eye, with hemorrhage that tracked posterior, evidenced by proptosis (*B*), suffered visual loss to no light perception.

as sickle cell disease, factor VII deficiency, platelet dysfunction, and vitamin C deficiency.[34] Other less common causes, such as extension of subgaleal bleeds, have also been described.[35]

Given the diverse nature of injury, judging the likelihood or degree of visual loss is difficult. The mechanism is presumably due to compressive occlusion of the vasculature supplying the optic nerve or retina. Animal studies have suggested that irreversible damage occurs within 90 to 120 minutes.[36,37] Several investigations have evaluated orbital pressure and associated visual loss. In Graves disease patients with related optic neuropathies, orbital pressures were measured between 17 and 40 mm Hg (mean 28.7 mm Hg).[36] Hargaden and colleagues[38] simulated orbital hemorrhage by inflating balloon catheters within the orbits of 16 nonhuman primates (NHP) for 3 or more hours. When inflated such that intraocular pressure (IOP) was 50 mm Hg or greater, half of the animals suffered irreparable damage. Using a similar technique, Schabdach and colleagues[37] observed permanent injury in only 1 of 9 monkeys. By contrast, Young and colleagues[39] simulated retrobulbar hemorrhage in NHP by autogenous blood injection. In their study all animals regained vision after 120 minutes of ischemia. In NHP, Jordan and colleagues[11] demonstrated that with clamping of the central retinal artery, permanent visual loss occurred after 105 minutes. By contrast, Katz and colleagues[40] described 2 patients with orbital hemorrhage who regained vision following more than 3 hours of no light perception.

Although the details may vary, it is clear that visual loss can occur with elevated orbital pressure (OP), and that this is dependent on the magnitude as well as duration of pressure elevation. Accordingly, treatment has been directed at detecting patients with elevated OP and reducing it. It has been long assumed that OP can be estimated by IOP, which is used as the primary measure in patients with orbit hemorrhage. Experimental evidence has confirmed an extremely close correlation between IOP and OP ($r = 0.97$), with mean IOP remaining on average 11 mm Hg greater than OP.[41]

Management consists largely in estimating OP with IOP and, when elevated, attempting to reduce it, which may ultimately necessitate orbital decompression or exploration with evacuation of any hematoma and ligation or cauterization of problematic vessels. Before an orbitotomy, canthotomy and cantholysis are often employed as an initial attempt at normalizing OP. Canthotomy refers to a horizontal incision, dividing the lateral canthal tendon into its superior crus and inferior crus (**Fig. 6**A). Cantholysis refers to cutting/disinserting the inferior (and less commonly the superior) crus (see **Fig. 6**B). Further decompression can be accomplished by opening the orbital septum bluntly, exposed at the base of the cantholysis incision, with surgical scissors (see **Fig. 6**C). Limited investigative data exist, and impressions of the effectiveness of canthotomy and cantholysis are based largely on anecdotal experiences. Yung and colleagues[42] assessed the effect of canthotomy, cantholysis, and "canthal tendon

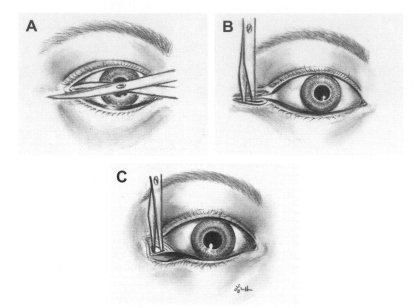

Fig. 6. (*A*) Canthotomy consists of surgically dividing the superior and inferior crura of the lateral canthal tendon. (*B*) Cantholysis refers to lysis of the inferior (and sometimes superior) crus of the lateral canthal tendon. (*C*) Septolysis, opening the orbital septum, can be performed bluntly with a surgical scissors through the incision made during canthotomy and cantholysis. (*Courtesy of* Lynda V McCulley, PharmD.)

disinsertion" on IOP in rabbits following retrobulbar saline injection. These investigators documented a statistically significant decrease in IOP but did not monitor OP.

One additional study has helped to substantiate the effectiveness of canthotomy and cantholysis, with an experimental model in human cadavers using human blood. Significant reductions in OP (58.9% decrease) and IOP (54.9% decrease) were observed after performing a canthotomy, cantholysis, and septolysis (**Fig. 7**).[41] Alarmingly, in the setting of simulated continued bleeding the effect of canthotomy, cantholysis, and septolysis was very short-lived. This observation suggests that this procedure will not have a lasting effect if performed before cessation/control of bleeding (see **Fig. 7**).

One last consideration is evaluation of a bleeding diathesis. A coagulation evaluation is indicated when bleeding occurs spontaneously or with minor trauma. Hemorrhage has been reported to occur in association with numerous blood disorders.[34]

In summary, orbital hemorrhages may be seen in numerous settings. Management consists of monitoring IOP and visual status. If an increase in IOP is seen in association with decreasing vision, attempts should be made to control OP. Canthotomy, cantholysis, and septolysis are effective, but should only be considered temporizing measures in the setting of continued bleeding. Definitive treatment may necessitate orbitotomy with evacuation of a hematoma, control of bleeding and, in the most extreme cases, orbital decompression.

ORBITAL NEOPLASM

One of the most feared diagnoses when evaluating patients with neuro-ophthalmic findings is an orbital tumor. Large portions of textbooks have been written addressing

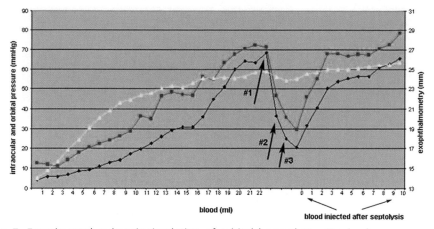

Fig. 7. Experimental cadaveric simulation of orbital hemorrhage. Y-axis gives pressure in mm Hg for orbital and intraocular pressure (*left*) and exophthalmometry measurements in millimeters (*right*). X-axis indicates volume of blood injected in ml. The graph lines illustrate orbital pressure (*blue*), intraocular pressure (*red*), and exophthalmometry measurements (*yellow*). The arrows indicate point when canthotomy (#1), cantholysis (#2), and septolysis (#3) were performed. Note that with injection of just 10 mL of blood following septolysis, orbital pressure returned to the pre-canthotomy level.

orbital oncology.[43,44] Comprehensive coverage is not feasible. This section focuses on commonalities and highlights.

Any cranial nerve (I, II, III, IV, V1, V2, VI) going to or from the eye and extraocular muscles can be affected. Compressive optic neuropathies occur with larger or apical tumors. Intrinsic tumors of the optic nerve include meningiomas and gliomas, and of course can result in visual compromise. Ocular misalignment and diplopia can result from compression of any of the cranial nerves serving the extraocular muscles. More often ocular misalignment results from direct involvement of the muscles.

With virtually any neuro-ophthalmic symptom resulting from orbital neoplasm, many clinical diseases can be mimicked. Often the most useful clue that an orbital neoplasm is responsible is globe malposition. **Fig. 8** illustrates an extreme example. The eye is expected to move opposite to the direction of the tumor. For example, inferomedial displacement of the eye is seen with lacrimal gland tumors (**Fig. 9**). Intraconal tumors usually result in axial proptosis (**Fig. 10**). Most orbital tumors will cause some globe malposition before reaching substantial enough size to cause nerve compression. Therefore, in all patients with a neuropathy of one of the nerves serving they eye, exophthalmometry should be performed. An exception is tumors arising in the confines of the orbital apex. Here a relatively small tumor may compress afferent or efferent nerves before the development of globe malposition.

Ocular findings may include choroidal folds (see **Fig. 9**C), with compression of the posterior globe. Optic nerve edema is seen when optic nerve compression is close to its connection with the eye, usually within 1 cm. With posterior compression, edema is not seen but pallor may be present as atrophy sets in. With extreme proptosis, poor eyelid closure and findings of an exposure keratopathy may develop. With large tumors extending outside the confines of the orbit, facial deformity may be seen.

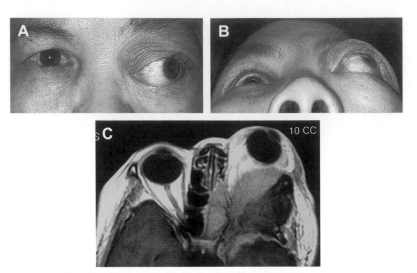

Fig. 8. Globe malposition due to orbital invasion of a sphenoid wing meningioma. From a frontal view (*A*) the eye is seen to be displaced inferiorly (hypoglobus). From below the extreme degree of proptosis is better appreciated (*B*). Magnetic resonance imaging (*C*) confirms the presence of a large orbital mass.

When an intraorbital tumor is suspected, imaging is indicated. Orbital surgeons have traditionally relied on computed tomography, as it was felt to yield superior "spacial resolution." However, with modern imaging techniques, magnetic resonance imaging is likely more sensitive and is the preferred modality in most circumstances. Computed tomography remains the preferred technique when assessment of bone is needed. Numerous clinicians have advocated orbital ultrasound and in rare

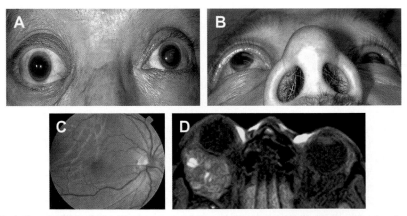

Fig. 9. Inferomedial globe displacement (*A*) and proptosis (*B*) indicate a lacrimal gland tumor. Fundoscopic evaluation reveals choroidal folds (*C*), indicating indentation of the globe. Magnetic resonance imaging (*D*) confirms a large lacrimal gland tumor that proved to be an adenocystic carcinoma.

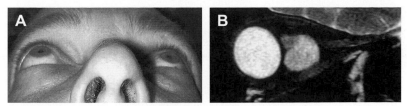

Fig. 10. Cavernous hemangioma: the most common benign orbital tumor of adulthood usually results in axial proptosis (*A*) due to its intraconal location (*B*).

circumstances ultrasound may be adequate. However, it should never be considered a substitute for a formal imaging study.

Individualized treatment and follow-up varies with disease etiology, and often requires a multidisciplinary approach. All malignant tumors warrant evaluation by a skilled oncologist. Tumors with intracranial extension or that involve the adjacent sinuses my require evaluation by a neurosurgeon or an otolaryngologist. Benign tumors are usually amenable to complete excision, whereas malignant tumors often require a more complex approach, including radiation and/or chemotherapy. **Table 2** provides pertinent clinical features of more commonly encountered orbital tumors.

ORBITAL INFLAMMATION

Idiopathic orbital inflammatory syndrome (OIS), formerly called orbital pseudotumor, often presents with ocular motility abnormalities and/or an optic neuropathy. Virtually any neuro-ophthalmic clinical feature can be mimicked by OIS, dependent on the site of inflammation. This section focuses on proper evaluation of a patient with an inflamed orbit, management of idiopathic OIS, and tips on identifying more serious conditions such as infection.

In managing an inflamed orbit the first step is to identify the origin. In some cases the cause cannot be determined, and in these cases the term idiopathic OIS is used. It is important to remember that OIS is a diagnosis of exclusion. Depending on the focus of inflammation, various terminologies may be used. For example, if inflammation is centered primarily within a muscle, the term myositis is used. Myositis is apt to present to the neurologist, as it causes painful diplopia.[45] The pattern of misalignment can be that of paresis, restriction, or both. If it is of the lacrimal gland, the term dacryoadenitis is used. Optic perineuritis refers to inflammation centered around the optic nerve.[46] When the inflammation is of the orbital apex and/or the cavernous sinus, Tolosa-Hunt syndrome is applied.[47] Often there is overlap, with more than one structure being involved.

The first step in evaluating a patient with an inflamed orbit, is obtaining a thorough history. A relatively short duration of hours to days suggests either OIS or an infection. A subacute presentation of days to weeks is more characteristic of Graves disease or a neoplastic process. Any history of rheumatologic disease which might be an associated with soft tissue inflammation should also be noted, as well as a history of thyroid disorder. Pain and tenderness is an important indicator. Nontender swelling is more concerning for neoplasm, some infections, and specific inflammatory syndromes such as Wegener granulomatosis.[48] One should inquire after a history of trauma or insect bites (also indicators of infection) and conditions that might predispose to infections.

Table 2
Neoplasm of the orbit

Category	Specific Neoplasm	Pertinent Details
Vascular tumors	Cavernous hemangioma	Most common benign tumor of adulthood Usually intraconal Slow growing Usually presents with proptosis May be found incidentally
	Capillary hemangioma	Congenital tumor Enlarges first 1–2 years, followed by involution Amblyopia may result from several mechanisms (occlusive, refractive) Intervention is indicated with visual compromise Usually responds well to intralesional or systemic steroids
	Lymphangioma	Benign tumor Composed primarily of lymphatics with variable vascular components Features may overlap with orbital varix Spontaneous hemorrhage may occur (chocolate cyst) May enlarge with upper respiratory or other infections
Neural	Schwannoma	Benign tumor of oligodendrocytes In orbit, most often arises from supraorbital nerve May have intracranial component hindering complete excision
	Meningioma	Most common intrinsic optic nerve tumor of adulthood More common in woman May occasionally be malignant May also reach orbit via intracranial extension May rarely arise from periorbita
	Glioma	Most common intrinsic tumor of childhood Often associated with neurofibromatosis Two distinct growth patterns (intraneural and arachnoid gliomatosis) Most have a benign course and do not require intervention Rarely malignant
	Plexiform neurofibroma	Seen almost exclusively in the setting of neurofibromatosis 1 Often diffusely infiltrative with intracranial involvement
Mesenchymal	Rhabdomyosarcoma	Most common soft tissue malignancy in children May present rapidly resembling a cellulitis Responsive to radiation and chemotherapy

(continued on next page)

Table 2 (continued)		
Category	**Specific Neoplasm**	**Pertinent Details**
Lacrimal gland	Pleomorphic adenoma	Most common benign lacrimal gland neoplasm
		Usually presents with several years history of globe malposition
		Managed with complete excision
		Incisional biopsy may increase risk of malignant transformation
	Adenoid cystic carcinoma	Most common malignant epithelial tumor of the lacrimal gland
		Often presents with pain due to sensory nerve invasion
Cutaneous	Dermoid	Common benign congenital tumor
		Usually detected within first 2 years of life
		May rarely present in adulthood
		Most often located adjacent the frontozygomatic suture
		May have an orbital component "dumbbell lesion"
		May be located entirely within the orbit
		May present as inflammatory lesion if keratin ruptures through cyst wall
	Squamous cell carcinoma (SCC)	May reach orbit due to perineural spread
		Consider in patients with a history of excised periocular SCC
	Basal cell carcinoma (BCC)	Usually from neglected or incompletely excised periocular BCC
Lymphoproliferative	MALT type lymphoma	Most common lymphoproliferative neoplasm of the orbit
		May involve any or multiple orbital structures
		Predilection for lacrimal gland involvement
		May be bilateral
Metastatic disease	Breast cancer	Most common metastasis in woman
	Lung cancer	Most common metastasis in men
	Neuroblastoma	Metastatic tumor of childhood
		May result in characteristic "raccoon eye" hemorrhage
Secondary invasion	Sinus	Mucocele from frontoethmoid sinuses
		Squamous cell and adenocarcinoma carry a poor prognosis
	Intracranial	Most commonly meningioma

Ophthalmic and systemic examinations may help identify an underlying condition. For example, rashes characteristic of systemic lupus erythematosis or polyarteritis nodosa may be identified.[49,50] It is important to note the position of the eyelid; OIS results in blepharoptosis or no change in the eyelid position, whereas Graves disease causes retraction of the eyelid. The age of the patient is also key. Children are more apt to suffer from an infection. The elderly are more apt to have idiopathic OIS.

Following a thorough history and examination, the next step is usually imaging. Most orbital surgeons prefer computed tomography, and in most cases this is adequate.

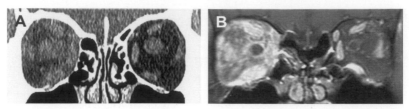

Fig. 11. Imaging of an inflamed orbit. Computed tomography (*A*) shows diffuse enhancement with enlargement of the extraocular muscles. Magnetic resonance imaging (*B*) better delineates areas of involvement. For instance, perineuritis, appreciated on magnetic resonance imaging, is not clearly seen on computed tomography.

However, magnetic resonance imaging provides much more detail (**Fig. 11**). It is reasonable to initiate the evaluation with computed tomography, reserving magnetic resonance imaging for more challenging diagnostic cases. One of the most important things to look for is the presence of sinusitis. Sinusitis is a strong indication of an infection (**Fig. 12**). The lack of sinusitis is suggestive of OIS. Another indication of OIS is focal inflammation within the orbit. Swelling, primarily of one or more structures such as the lacrimal gland, an extraocular muscle, or perineural tissue strongly suggest OIS. Although all of the above may lean toward a diagnosis, unfortunately it is not always possible to definitively distinguish an infection from OIS in a patient with an acutely inflamed orbit.

Management of idiopathic OIS is as follows. A trial of antibiotics can be considered in ambiguous cases. In more clear-cut idiopathic OIS, treatment with steroids usually results in an extremely rapid resolution. The lack of rapid and complete resolution suggests alternative causes. A starting dose of roughly 1 mg/kg, tapered over the course of 1 to 2 months following normalization, is a standard regimen. In recurrent or unresponsive disease a systemic evaluation is appropriate. Laboratory testing for diseases listed in **Table 3** is appropriate; assistance from rheumatology may be helpful. Computed tomography of the chest is also helpful in select cases. Another consideration is orbital biopsy. Opinions vary as to when a biopsy should be considered. In general, an orbital biopsy should be performed with atypical, recurrent, or steroid unresponsive disease.

In recalcitrant disease, if the systemic evaluation identifies a specific cause, treatment is tailored accordingly. If the diagnosis remains idiopathic OIS, the steroid dose can be increased and the duration of the taper lengthened. In cases refractory to steroids, more potent immune suppressive agents such as methotrexate can be considered.[51] There is also recent evidence suggesting rituximab as an alternative

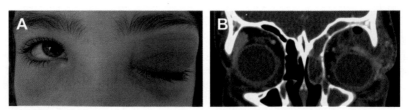

Fig. 12. Orbital cellulitis. A young female with several days of diplopia, blepharoptosis, and painful periocular swelling (*A*). Computed tomography (*B*) clearly demonstrates sinusitis with a superior orbital abscess.

Table 3
Differential diagnosis of an inflamed orbit

Category	Subcategory	Specific Detail
No identifiable cause		Idiopathic orbital inflammatory disease
Inflammatory syndromes	Vasculitis	Wegener granulomatosis
		Systemic lupus erythematosus
		Hepatitis related vasculitis
		Polyarteritis nodosa
		Rheumatoid arthritis
	Miscellaneous	Sarcoidosis
		Graves disease
Infectious	Bacterial	*Staphylococcus aureus*
		Streptococcus pyogenes
	Fungal	Mucormycosis
		Aspergillosis
	Parasitic	Cysticercosis
		Trichinosus
		Microfilaria
		Echinococcus
Neoplastic		Lymphoproliferative
		Ruptured dermoid
		Rhabdomyosarcoma
Vascular		Carotid cavernous fistula
		Lymphangioma

to steroids.[52] Radiation therapy can be used in select cases; however, results are variable and often unsatisfactory.[53]

There are numerous systemic diseases that can be associated with orbital inflammation, and these should be identified. **Fig. 13** illustrates patients with systemic inflammatory syndromes. Sarcoidosis should be suspected and worked up when relatively nontender inflammation of the lacrimal glands is encountered, particularly in African patients. Numerous types of vasculitides can result in orbital inflammation, including systemic lupus erythematosus, rheumatoid arthritis, polyarteritis nodosa, and hepatitis-associated vasculitis, among others.[48–50]

Infectious orbititis can carry grave consequences if misdiagnosed. Bacterial orbital cellulitis is often indistinguishable from OIS. As stated earlier, the presence of sinusitis or an abscess strongly suggests an infectious origin. However, their absence does not exclude it. Often patients' lack of response to antibiotics is needed before more seriously considering the diagnosis of OIS. Two specific entities that should not be missed

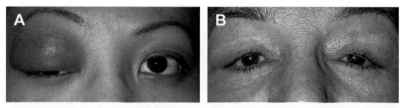

Fig. 13. Two patients who presented with periocular inflammation. Both had relatively little discomfort suggesting diagnosis other than OIS. One proved to have Wegener granulomatosis (*A*) and the other xanthogranuloma (*B*).

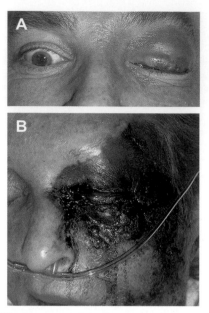

Fig. 14. Necrotizing fasciitis may present in the periocular area. Failure to make a rapid diagnosis results in tissue loss and in extreme cases, death. (*A*) Early necrotizing fasciitis with a relative lack of pain and multiple areas of focal necrosis dotting the supraciliary skin. (*B*) Advanced necrotizing fasciitis, initially misdiagnosed and mistreated, with intracranial spread that resulted in the death of the patient.

are necrotizing fasciitis and mucormycosis. Indications of necrotizing fasciitis are anesthesia of the overlying skin and multiple areas of necrosis (**Fig. 14**).[54] Mucormycosis may be suspected in immune suppressed patients, particularly in those with poorly controlled diabetes (**Fig. 15**).[55]

A relative lack of pain or tenderness is suggestive of malignancy. In children (and rarely adults), rhabdomyosarcoma may present with acute or subacute proptosis and carry with it some inflammation mimicking an OIS. Spontaneous rupture of a dermoid cyst is also a classic cause of acute orbital inflammation. Dermoids are readily detectable with proper imaging. Lastly, lymphoproliferative disease may mimic OIS.

In summary, OIS is a diagnosis of exclusion. Mimickers include infection and neoplasm. A systemic evaluation and biopsy should be considered in atypical,

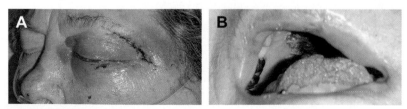

Fig. 15. Advanced mucormycosis initially misdiagnoses and treated as OIS (*A*). Evaluation of the palate reveals characteristic necrosis (*B*).

refractory, or recurrent cases. Most cases of OIS are easily managed with oral prednisone, but occasionally more potent immune suppressive agents are required.

REFERENCES

1. Burnstine MA. Clinical recommendations for repair of isolated orbital floor fractures: an evidence-based analysis. Ophthalmology 2002;109:1207–10.
2. Renzi G, Carboni A, Perugini M, et al. Posttraumatic trigeminal nerve impairment: a prospective analysis of recovery patterns in a series of 103 consecutive facial fractures. J Oral Maxillofac Surg 2004;62:1341–6.
3. Warwar RE, Bullock JD, Ballal DR, et al. Mechanisms of orbital floor fractures: a clinical, experimental, and theoretical study. Ophthal Plast Reconstr Surg 2000;16:188–200.
4. Rhee JS, Kilde J, Yoganadan N, et al. Orbital blowout fractures: experimental evidence for the pure hydraulic theory. Arch Facial Plast Surg 2002;4:98–101.
5. Waterhouse N, Lyne J, Urdang M, et al. An investigation into the mechanism of orbital blowout fractures. Br J Plast Surg 1999;52:607–12.
6. Dal Canto AJ, Linberg JV. Comparison of orbital fracture repair performed within 14 days versus 15 to 29 days after trauma. Ophthal Plast Reconstr Surg 2008; 24:437–43.
7. Westfall CT, Costantino PD, Shore JW. Late orbital reconstruction. Semin Ophthalmol 1994;9:212–7.
8. Putterman AM. Late management of blow-out fractures of the orbital floor. Trans Sect Ophthalmol Am Acad Ophthalmol Otolaryngol 1977;83:650–9.
9. Egbert JE, May K, Kersten RC, et al. Pediatric orbital floor fractures: direct extraocular muscle involvement. Ophthalmology 2000;107:1875–9.
10. Hatton MP, Watkins LM, Rubin PA. Orbital fractures in children. Ophthal Plast Reconstr Surg 2001;17:174–9.
11. Jordan DR, Allen LH, White J, et al. Intervention within days for some orbital floor fractures: the white-eyed blowout. Ophthal Plast Reconstr Surg 1998; 14:379–90.
12. Sires BS, Stanley RB, Levine LM. Oculocardiac reflex caused by orbital floor trapdoor fracture: an indication for urgent repair. Arch Ophthalmol 1998;116:955–6.
13. Bansagi ZC, Meyer DR. Internal orbital fractures in the pediatric age group: characterization and management. Ophthalmology 2000;107:829–36.
14. McCulley TJ, Yip CC, Kersten RC. Medial rectus muscle incarceration in medial orbital wall trapdoor fractures. Eur J Ophthalmol 2004;14:330–3.
15. Cope MR, Moos KF, Speculand B. Does diplopia persist after blow-out fractures of the orbital floor in children? Br J Oral Maxillofac Surg 1999;37:46–51.
16. Kakizaki H, Zako M, Katori N, et al. Adult medial orbital wall trapdoor fracture with missing medial rectus muscle. Orbit 2006;25:61–3.
17. Kum C, McCulley TJ, Yoon MK, et al. Adult orbital trapdoor fracture. Ophthal Plast Reconstr Surg 2009;25:486–7.
18. Parbhu K, Galler K, Li C, et al. Underestimation of soft tissue entrapment by computed tomography in orbital floor fractures in the pediatric population. Ophthalmology 2008;115:1620–5.
19. Millman AL, Della Rocca RC, Spector S, et al. Steroids and orbital blowout fractures—a new systematic concept in medical management and surgical decision-making. Adv Ophthalmic Plast Reconstr Surg 1987;6:291–300.
20. Hawes MJ, Dortzbach RK. Surgery on orbital floor fractures. Influence of time of repair and fracture size. Ophthalmology 1983;90(9):1066–70.

21. Hughes B. Indirect injury of the optic nerves and chiasma. Bull Johns Hopkins Hosp 1962;111:98–126.
22. Turner JWA. Indirect injury of the optic nerves. Brain 1943;66:140–51.
23. Gross CE, DeKock JR, Panje WR, et al. Evidence for orbital deformation that may contribute to monocular blindness following minor frontal head trauma. J Neurosurg 1981;55:963–6.
24. Keane JR. Neurologic eye signs following motorcycle accidents. Arch Neurol 1989;46:761–2.
25. Hwang T, McCulley TJ. Biomechanics of traumatic optic neuropathy. NANOS Annual Meeting, Tucson (AZ), February 26– March 2, 2006.
26. Seiff SR. High dose corticosteroids for treatment of vision loss due to indirect injury to the optic nerve. Ophthalmic Surg 1990;21:389–95.
27. Levin LA, Beck RW, Joseph M, et al. The treatment of traumatic optic neuropathy: the International Optic Nerve Trauma Study. Ophthalmology 1999;106:1268–77.
28. Anderson RL, Panje WR, Gross CE. Optic nerve blindness following blunt forehead trauma. Ophthalmology 1982;80:445–55.
29. Bracken MB, Shepard MJ, Holford TR, et al. Methylprednisolone or tirilazad mesylate administration after acute spinal cord injury: 1 year follow up: results of the Third National Acute Spinal Cord Injury Randomized Controlled Trial. J Neurosurg 1998;89:699–706.
30. Edwards P, Arango M, Balica L, et al. Final results of MR CRASH. Lancet 2005; 365(9475):1957–9.
31. Levin LA, Joseph MP, Rizzo JF III, et al. Optic canal decompression in indirect traumatic optic neuropathy. Ophthalmology 1994;101:566–9.
32. DeMere M, Wood T, Austin W. Eye complications with blepharoplasty or other eyelid surgery. A national survey. Plast Reconstr Surg 1974;53(6):634–7.
33. Davis DB 2nd, Mandel MR. Efficacy and complication rate of 16,224 consecutive peribulbar blocks. A prospective multicenter study. J Cataract Refract Surg 1994; 20:327–37.
34. Oh JY, Khwarg SI. Orbital subperiosteal hemorrhage in a patient with factor VIII and factor XII deficiency. J Pediatr Ophthalmol Strabismus 2004;41:367–8.
35. Yip CC, McCulley TJ, Kersten RC, et al. Proptosis after hair pulling. Ophthal Plast Reconstr Surg 2003;19:154–5.
36. Otto AJ, Koornneef L, Mourits MP, et al. Retrobulbar pressures measured during surgical decompression of the orbit. Br J Ophthalmol 1996;80(12):1042–5.
37. Schabdach DG, Goldberg SH, Breton ME, et al. An animal model of visual loss from orbital hemorrhage. Ophthal Plast Reconstr Surg 1994;10(3):200–5.
38. Hargaden M, Goldberg SH, Cunningham D, et al. Optic neuropathy following simulation of orbital hemorrhage in the nonhuman primate. Ophthal Plast Reconstr Surg 1996;12:264–72.
39. Young VL, Gumucio CA, Lund H, et al. Long-term effect of retrobulbar hematomas on the vision of cynomolgus monkeys. Plast Reconstr Surg 1992; 89(1):70–6.
40. Katz B, Herschler J, Brick DC. Orbital haemorrhage and prolonged blindness: a treatable posterior optic neuropathy. Br J Ophthalmol 1983;67:549–53.
41. Zoumalan CI, Bullock JD, Warwar RR, et al. Evaluation of intraocular and orbital pressure in the management of orbital hemorrhage: an experimental model. Arch Ophthalmol 2008;126:1257–60.
42. Yung CW, Moorthy RS, Lindley D, et al. Efficacy of lateral canthotomy and cantholysis in orbital hemorrhage. Ophthal Plast Reconstr Surg 1994;10(2):137–41.

43. Shields JA, Shields CA. Eyelid, conjunctival, and orbital tumors an atlas and textbook. 2nd edition. Hagerstown (MD): Lippincott Williams & Wilkins; 2007.

44. Rootman J. Diseases of the orbit: a multidisciplinary approach. Hagerstown (MD): Lippincott Williams & Wilkins; 2003.

45. Scott IU, Siatkowski RM. Idiopathic orbital myositis. Curr Opin Rheumatol 1997; 9:504–12.

46. Gordon LK. Diagnostic dilemmas in orbital inflammatory disease. Ocul Immunol Inflamm 2003;11:3–15.

47. Smith JL, Taxdal DS. Painful ophthalmoplegia. The Tolosa-Hunt syndrome. Am J Ophthalmol 1966;61:1466–72.

48. Bhatia A, Yadava U, Goyal JL, et al. Limited Wegener's granulomatosis of the orbit: a case study and review of literature. Eye 2005;19:102–4.

49. Read RW. Clinical mini-review: systemic lupus erythematosus and the eye. Ocul Immunol Inflamm 2004;12:87–99.

50. Akova YA, Jabbur NS, Foster CS. Ocular presentation of polyarteritis nodosa. Clinical course and management with steroid and cytotoxic therapy. Ophthalmology 1993;100(12):1775 81.

51. Shah SS, Lowder CY, Schmitt MA, et al. Low-dose methotrexate therapy for ocular inflammatory disease. Ophthalmology 1992;99:1419–23.

52. Schafranski MD. Idiopathic orbital inflammatory disease successfully treated with rituximab. Clin Rheumatol 2009;28:225–6.

53. Smitt MC, Donaldson SS. Radiation therapy for benign disease of the orbit. Semin Radiat Oncol 1999;9:179–89.

54. Marshall DH, Jordan DR, Gilberg SM, et al. Periocular necrotizing fasciitis: a review of five cases. Ophthalmology 1997;104:1857–62.

55. Warwar RE, Bullock JD. Rhino-orbital-cerebral mucormycosis: a review. Orbit 1998;17:237–45.

Vascular Neuro-Ophthalmology

Cédric Lamirel, MD[a], Nancy J. Newman, MD[a,b],
Valérie Biousse, MD[a,b],*

KEYWORDS

- Stroke • Ischemia • Carotid artery
- Vertebral-basilar circulation • Retinopathy

Vascular neuro-ophthalmology includes visual symptoms and signs found in stroke patients as well as numerous primary vascular disorders involving the eye and the optic nerves. The clinical presentation varies depending on the type of vessel involved (arteries vs veins), the type of stroke (ischemic or hemorrhagic), and the size of the arteries involved (large- vs small-artery disease).

The blood supply to the eye is mostly provided by branches of the ophthalmic artery, which is a branch of the internal carotid artery (ICA) (**Fig. 1**A). For this reason, many patients with cerebral ischemia in the territory of the anterior circulation may present with ipsilateral visual changes. The posterior circulation provides the blood supply to the occipital lobes and posterior fossa; hence, binocular visual loss or abnormal extraocular movements are common with vascular diseases affecting the posterior circulation. In addition, several ocular vascular disorders are associated with specific neurologic manifestations, and numerous systemic inflammatory diseases or hypercoaguable states can affect the eyes and the brain simultaneously.

LARGE-ARTERY DISEASE

Anterior and posterior large-artery circulation ischemia is often associated with visual symptoms and signs that may precede a cerebral infarction.

This work was supported in part by a departmental grant (Department of Ophthalmology) from Research to Prevent Blindness, Inc, New York, New York, and by core grant P30-EY06360 (Department of Ophthalmology) from the National Institute of Health, Bethesda, MD. Dr Newman is a recipient of a Research to Prevent Blindness Lew R. Wasserman Merit Award. Dr Lamirel is supported by research grants from Institut Servier (Paris, France), Fondation Planiol (Varennes, France), and the Philippe Foundation Inc. (New York, USA).
[a] Department of Ophthalmolgy, Emory Eye Center, 1365-B Clifton Road, NE Atlanta, GA 30322, USA
[b] Department of Neurology, Emory University School of Medicine, 1365-B Clifton Road, NE Atlanta, GA 30322, USA
* Corresponding author. Department of Ophthalmolgy, Emory Eye Center, 1365-B Clifton Road, NE Atlanta, GA 30322.
E-mail address: vbiouss@emory.edu

neurologic.theclinics.com

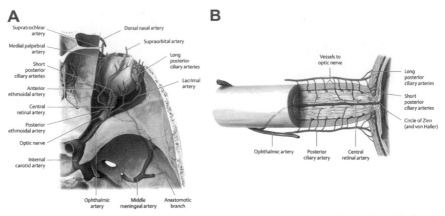

Fig. 1. Blood supply to the eye and optic nerve. (*A*) Superior view of the right orbit showing the ICA, the ophthalmic artery, and its branches in the orbit. (*B*) Lateral view of the optic nerve showing the arterial blood supply of the optic nerve via small branches of the ophthalmic artery (posterior ciliary artery). (*Reprinted from* Biousse V, Newman NJ. Neuro-ophthalmology illustrated. New York: Thieme; 2009. p. 136–7; with permission.)

Anterior Circulation (Carotid Artery Disease)

A variety of transient and permanent visual symptoms and signs may develop in patients with carotid artery disease. The distinguishing feature of most of these disturbances is their monocular nature, ipsilateral to the affected ICA. However, contralateral homonymous visual-field defects, bitemporal visual-field defects, and bilateral simultaneous visual loss may result from diseased carotid arteries and their branches, particularly when the disease is bilateral.

Transient monocular visual loss

Transient monocular visual loss is the most common ophthalmologic symptom of disease of the ICA. The term amaurosis fugax is often used to describe any cause of transient monocular visual loss and should be abandoned.[1] The evaluation and management of patients with transient visual loss are detailed in the article by Foroozan elsewhere in this issue. There are numerous nonvascular causes of transient monocular visual loss that require an emergent detailed ocular examination; an ophthalmic consultation should be obtained before launching an extensive work up for presumed vascular transient monocular visual loss.[2] Multiple episodes of transient visual loss or painful transient visual loss in the elderly should raise the possibility of giant cell arteritis.

Permanent visual loss

Partial or complete monocular loss of vision may occur in patients with carotid artery disease, usually in the ipsilateral eye. This condition most often results from a central retinal artery occlusion (CRAO) or from 1 or multiple branch retinal artery occlusions. In such cases, an embolus may be seen in the affected vessels. Other causes of permanent monocular visual loss in patients with carotid artery disease include venous stasis retinopathy and the ocular ischemic syndrome.[3] Ischemic optic neuropathy, anterior or posterior, results from small-vessel disease (see **Fig. 1**B) and is usually not associated with large-artery disease,[4] explaining why carotid artery evaluation is not usually indicated in patients with classic anterior ischemic optic neuropathy.

The second major visual sign of carotid occlusive disease is a partial or complete contralateral homonymous hemianopic visual-field defect. This condition is most often caused by occlusion of branches of the middle cerebral artery, but it may result from occlusion of the anterior choroidal artery or some of its branches to the optic tract and lateral geniculate body. Rarely, patients with carotid occlusive disease have severe visual deficits caused by a combination of monocular visual loss from ocular circulation insufficiency and contralateral homonymous field loss from damage to the ipsilateral postchiasmal visual sensory pathway.

Central and branch retinal artery occlusion Patients who experience a retinal infarction usually complain of acute loss of visual acuity, visual field, or both. Permanent visual loss may be preceded by episodes of transient monocular visual loss. Patients with a CRAO almost always have extremely poor visual acuity in the affected eye. Acute CRAO is characterized by diffuse pale swelling of the retina, a macular cherry-red spot, and attenuation of the retinal vessels (**Fig. 2**).[5] Within a few weeks, the retinal vessels often recanalize and the retina has an almost normal appearance; however, the optic disc becomes pale (**Fig. 3**).[5] Emboli are seen in up to 40% of CRAOs and in most branch artery occlusions (**Fig. 4**).[5–7] The most common emboli that occlude retinal arterioles are made of cholesterol, fibrin platelets, and calcium fragments (**Table 1**).

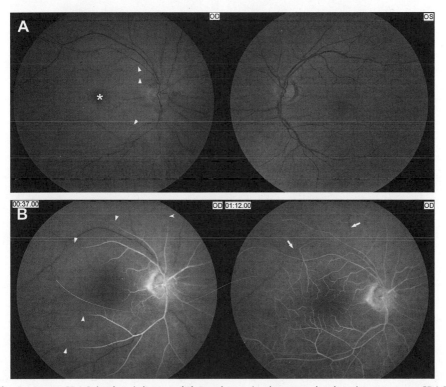

Fig. 2. Acute CRAO in the right eye. (*A*) Funduscopic photographs showing an acute CRAO in the right eye (OD) (*left*). Note the attenuated central retinal artery with segmental arterial narrowing in the right eye (*arrowheads*) compared with the left eye (OS) (*right*). The ischemic retina is edematous and appears whitish compared with the left eye, and there is a cherry-red spot (*asterisk*). (*B*) Fluorescein angiography of the right eye (OD) at 37 seconds after injection of fluorescein dye in an arm vein (*left*), and at more than 1 minute (*right*). There is delayed retinal arterial filling (*arrowheads*). Venous filling (*arrows*) is also delayed at more than 1 minute.

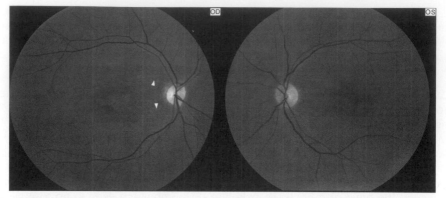

Fig. 3. Right optic atrophy secondary to an old CRAO. Funduscopic photograph showing an old CRAO in the right eye (OD) (*left*). Note the optic disc pallor with narrowing and sheathing of some arterioles in the right eye (*arrowheads*) compared with the left eye (OS) (*right*).

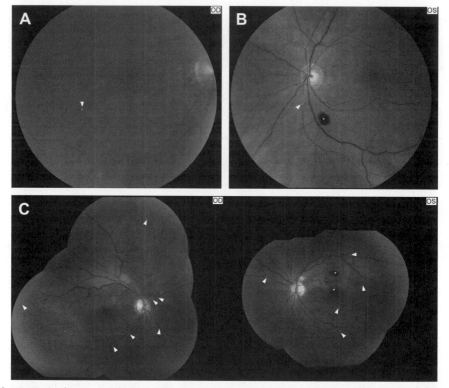

Fig. 4. Retinal artery emboli. Funduscopic photographs showing: (*A*) a refractile cholesterol retinal embolus (Hollenhorst plaque; *arrowhead*) found in the right eye of a patient who had an episode of transient visual loss in the right eye (OD); (*B*) a branch retinal artery embolus in a patient with monocular vision loss in the left eye (OS). The embolus is whitish and disrupts the blood flow within the artery, suggesting a platelet-fibrin embolus (*arrowhead*) from carotid artery atheroma. There is an intraretinal hemorrhage inferiorly related to retinal ischemia (*asterisk*); (*C*) multiple bilateral retinal emboli (*arrowheads*) in the setting of valvular endocarditis (Roth spots) with bilateral branch arterial occlusions and 2 intraretinal hemorrhages (OS; *asterisks*).

Table 1
The most common types of retinal emboli

Type of Retinal Emboli	Source of Emboli	Funduscopic Appearance	Location in the Retina
Cholesterol (Hollenhorst plaque)	Ipsilateral ICA Aortic arch	Yellow, refractile Multiple in 70% of cases Wider than the arteriole	Often at an arteriole bifurcation
Platelet fibrin	Carotid thrombus Aortic arch thrombus Cardiac thrombus Cardiac prosthesis	White-gray, pale, not refractile Often multiple	Within small retinal arterioles
Calcium	Calcified atheromatous plaque or cardiac valve	White and large Usually isolated	In the proximal segment of the central retinal artery or its branches
Infectious	Bacterial endocarditis Candidemia	White spots (Roth spots) Multiple	No specific pattern
Fat	Fat emboli in the setting of leg facture	Whitish spots with hemorrhages and cotton-wool spots Multiple	No specific pattern
Neoplasm	Cardiac myxoma	White, gray Often multiple	No specific pattern
Talc	Intravenous drugs	Yellow, refractile Multiple	No specific pattern

Carotid artery disease is responsible for most retinal infarctions. In patients with embolic retinal infarction who have a normal ICA, the aortic arch or the heart are the most likely sources of emboli.[8] The prognosis of CRAO is poor and treatment is limited. None of the classic treatments offered by ophthalmologists (including ocular massage and anterior chamber paracenthesis) are proven to be useful, and the authors do not recommend them routinely. Selective intra-arterial thrombolysis (directly into the ophthalmic artery) or intravenous thrombolysis are sometimes performed in specialized centers, but will remain debated until a clinical trial shows their efficacy and safety.[9,10]

Ophthalmic artery occlusion Ophthalmic artery occlusion usually results from large emboli in the ophthalmic artery. The visual loss is profound and the prognosis poor. Funduscopic examination shows extensive retinal ischemia which appears white and edematous, often with hemorrhages and with poor or no retinal artery filling, as well as disc edema. Because the choroidal circulation is also compromised, there is no cherry-red spot (**Fig. 5**).

Homonymous visual-field defects Ischemia in the anterior circulation (carotid territory) may be associated with a contralateral homonymous hemianopia when there is a lesion of the optic tract, lateral geniculate body, or anterior optic radiations.

Damage to the optic tract produces a contralateral homonymous hemianopia associated with a relative afferent pupillary defect on the side of the hemianopia, and

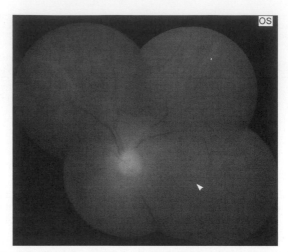

Fig. 5. Left ophthalmic artery occlusion. Funduscopic photograph showing a severe left ophthalmic artery occlusion with massive retinal ischemia and ischemic disc edema. The arteries are barely visible and there is no cherry-red spot (*arrowhead*).

subsequent optic nerve atrophy (because the axons of the optic tract originate in the ganglion cell bodies of the retina).[11] Lesions of the lateral geniculate body may produce a homonymous sectoranopia because of its unique blood supply. Lesions of the anterior optic radiations typically produce a contralateral homonymous hemianopia, usually in association with other neurologic symptoms or signs.[3]

Venous stasis retinopathy and ocular ischemic syndrome Venous stasis retinopathy (also called hypotensive retinopathy) is caused by severe carotid obstructive disease and poor collateral circulation. The retinopathy is characterized by insidious onset, dilated and tortuous retinal veins, peripheral microaneurysms, and dot blot hemorrhages in the midperipheral retina (**Fig. 6**). Patients with this condition complain primarily of generalized blurred vision in the affected eye, or may be asymptomatic. Symptoms of carotid insufficiency, such as transient monocular visual loss, decreased

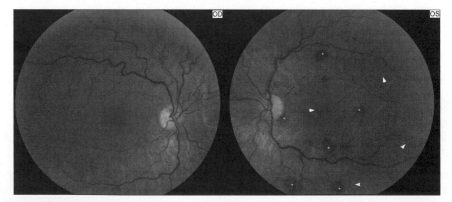

Fig. 6. Left venous stasis retinopathy. Funduscopic photograph showing venous stasis retinopathy in the left eye (OS) (*right*) secondary to a left ICA occlusion. Note the multiple retinal hemorrhages (*asterisks*), with microaneurysms (*arrowheads*).

vision after exposure to bright light, and orbital pain, are common. Venous stasis retinopathy may occur as part of the ocular ischemic syndrome or in isolation. It is found in up to 4% to 18% of patients with carotid occlusive disease, and is often asymptomatic.[12–14] Venous stasis retinopathy usually resolves spontaneously if arterial patency can be restored.[13] However, in many cases there is persistent visual dysfunction from irreversible retinal ischemic changes. If ocular perfusion cannot be improved, the affected eye may develop neovascularization of the iris and optic disc as well as other signs of ocular ischemia. In such cases, ablation of hypoxic retinal tissue by panretinal photocoagulation may prevent progression of the condition and may produce regression of neovascularization.[14,15]

The ocular ischemic syndrome (also called ischemic ocular inflammation or chronic ocular ischemia) is a progressive disorder resulting from chronic hypoperfusion of the eye.[14,16] Patients describe blurry vision that may be transient or persistent. Visual loss is typically insidious and slowly progressive. Some patients describe positive afterimages when exposed to bright light. The affected eye is often red, with episcleral vascular dilation.[15] The ocular fundus shows venous stasis retinopathy, sometimes associated with neovascularization. Some patients will have severe ocular or periorbital pain that is often improved when they lie down.[16] In eyes with persistent hypoperfusion, neovascularization of the iris, retina, optic disc, and anterior chamber angle develop. Other signs of ocular ischemia include corneal edema, uveitis, cataract formation, and a dilated and poorly reactive pupil.[14] The visual prognosis is extremely poor. Although early retinopathy may resolve spontaneously with the development of collateral circulation, severe loss of vision is almost always irreversible once tissue infarction occurs.[14,15]

The treatment of the ocular ischemic syndrome is aimed at preservation and improvement of visual function and treatment of the underlying process.[14,15] The first requires a relative decrease in the oxygen requirements of the eye, thus reducing the drive for neovascularization. This stage is usually accomplished by ablation of retinal tissue by laser panretinal photocoagulation or peripheral retinal cryotherapy. When severe carotid artery stenosis is the underlying condition, endarterectomy or carotid stenting may be used to reestablish flow. The artery is usually occluded, in which case a superficial temporal artery to middle cerebral artery bypass procedure may be beneficial if the external carotid artery is patent. When the internal and external carotid arteries are occluded, some form of revascularization of the external carotid artery may be of benefit. However, revascularization procedures have been associated with ocular complications such as retinal or vitreal hemorrhages and increased intraocular pressure. Moreover, patients with such severe carotid disease and poor collateral circulation often have a high surgical risk. No therapy is clearly effective in reversing the ocular ischemic syndrome.

Horner syndrome
Although it is more common in carotid artery dissections, Horner syndrome may occur in patients with atherosclerotic carotid artery disease (**Fig. 7**).[17] Most such patients have complete occlusion of the ICA, and the Horner syndrome is associated with other neurologic symptoms and signs of carotid artery disease. Horner syndrome occurring in patients with occlusion of the ICA is almost always postganglionic (third order) (see the article by Kawasaki elsewhere in this issue for further exploration of this topic).

Ocular motor nerve paresis
Patients with acute occlusion or severe ICA stenosis may occasionally develop 1 or more ocular motor nerve pareses on the side of the occlusion, in isolation or with signs

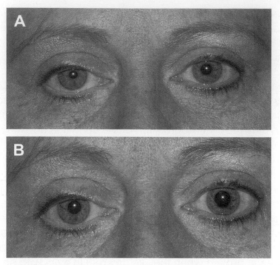

Fig. 7. Right Horner syndrome related to a right ICA occlusion. There is mild right upper lid ptosis and anisocoria with the right pupil being smaller than the left pupil in the light (*A*) and in the dark (*B*). The anisocoria is greater in the dark than in the light, and there was dilation lag of the right pupil in the dark.

of ocular ischemia.[18] In some cases of isolated ocular motor nerve palsy, ischemia of the nerve probably results from reduction of blood flow through mesencephalic branches of the anterior choroidal artery. In other cases, blood supply to the cranial nerves themselves, which originates from branches of the ICA, may be compromised.[3,19]

Referred pain

Isolated ocular pain may be a symptom of carotid occlusive disease, even without other symptoms and signs of vascular disease. It is usually a referred pain resulting from ischemia or compression of the trigeminal branches. It may also be part of the ocular ischemic syndrome.[3]

Posterior Circulation

The vertebrobasilar system supports the neural components of the entire brainstem ocular motor system as well as those of the posterior visual sensory pathways and visual cortex. For this reason, ocular motor and visual symptoms and signs play a major role in the diagnosis of vascular disease in the vertebrobasilar system.

Transient binocular visual loss

Episodes of transient binocular visual loss are common in vertebrobasilar ischemia. The visual loss is always bilateral, with both eyes being affected simultaneously and symmetrically.[3,20–22] The change in vision may be described as a sudden grayout of vision, a sensation of looking through fog or smoke, or the feeling that someone has turned down the lights. Most attacks of blurred vision that result from vertebrobasilar ischemia last less than a minute. Attacks of longer duration may be accompanied by flickering, flashing stars of silvery light in a homonymous or altitudinal field of vision. They may occur alone or in combination with other transient symptoms in the verte-brobasilar territory. The episodes of blurred vision that occur in patients with occipital ischemia must be differentiated from other causes of transient or permanent visual loss. Transient, complete 90° to 180° inversion of the visual image occasionally occurs.

Homonymous visual-field defects

An isolated homonymous visual-field defect of sudden onset is the hallmark of a vascular lesion in the occipital lobe (**Fig. 8**). Such a lesion is usually the result of infarction in the territory supplied by the posterior cerebral artery (PCA) (**Table 2**). The field defect may be complete or incomplete, but, when it is incomplete or scotomatous, it is usually congruous. When there is a complete homonymous hemianopia, macular sparing is common, and the occipital pole is usually spared. Patients with a homonymous visual-field defect caused by ischemia in the PCA territory have normal visual acuity. When both occipital lobes are infarcted, visual acuity is usually severely impaired but the amount of visual loss is symmetric in both eyes (**Fig. 9**). In some cases of occipital lobe infarction, the anterior portion of the lobe is unaffected, resulting in sparing of part or all of the peripheral 30° of the contralateral, monocular

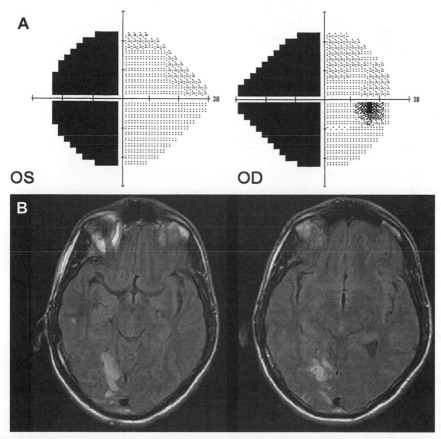

Fig. 8. Left homonymous hemianopia secondary to a right occipital infarction. (*A*) 24-2 Humphrey visual fields showing a complete left homonymous hemianopia. The right eye visual field is on the right and the left eye visual field is on the left. (*B*) Fluid attenuated inversion recovery (FLAIR) axial brain magnetic resonance imaging (MRI) shows a right occipital infarction in the territory of the right posterior cerebral artery.

Table 2
Common causes of cerebral visual loss classified by mechanism

Mechanism	Cause of Vision Loss
Vascular	Vertebrobasilar ischemia (PCA territory) Cerebral anoxia Cerebral venous thrombosis (superior sagittal sinus) Hypertensive encephalopathy (posterior reversible encephalopathy syndrome) Eclampsia
Head trauma	Occipital lobe injury
Occipital mass	Tumor Abscess Vascular (aneurysm, arteriovenous malformation) Hemorrhage
Demyelinating disease	Multiple sclerosis
Infection	Occipital abscess Meningitis Progressive multifocal leucoencephalopathy Creutzfeld-Jacob disease
Toxic	Cyclosporine Tacrolimus
Metabolic	Hypoglycemia Porphyria Hepatic encephalopathy
Migraine	Migrainous visual aura
Seizure	Occipital lobe seizures
Degenerative	Alzheimer disease/posterior cortical atrophy

temporal field (the temporal crescent). Symptoms of PCA occlusion usually occur without warning. The patient may have a slight sensation of dizziness or light-headedness and then become aware of a homonymous visual-field defect. Some patients initially experience complete blindness, with vision returning in the ipsilateral homonymous visual field within minutes. Pain in the ipsilateral eye or over the ipsilateral brow (contralateral to the hemianopia) is an important, although inconstant, symptom in such patients.[23] This pain is referred from the tentorial branches of the trigeminal nerve.

Disorders of higher cortical function

Several syndromes, described by patients as difficulty seeing or difficulty reading, may result from cerebral ischemia.[3,11]

Alexia without agraphia results from infarction of the left occipital lobe and disruption of the left ventral visual association cortex and its outflow tracts to the left angular gyrus, thus interrupting input from the right occipital area to the language verbal-association area. Patients can usually name individual letters or numbers, but they cannot read words or phrases. Although they are able to write, they cannot read it back moments later. Patients in whom there is infarction of the left occipital lobe and the splenium of the corpus callosum have no visual information to send to the language center from the left occipital lobe, and information from the right occipital lobe cannot be transmitted across to the left language center via the corpus callosum.

Gerstmann syndrome results from infarction of the left angular gyrus secondary to an occlusion of the left PCA. Patients have difficulty telling right from left, difficulty in

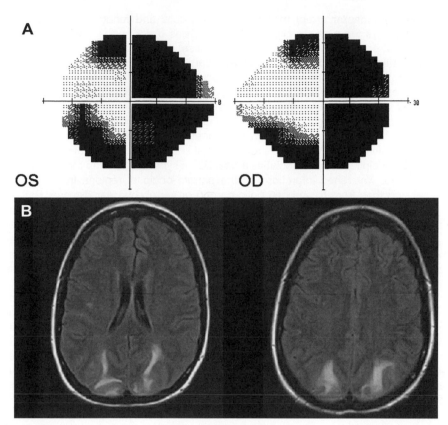

OS   OD

Fig. 9. Bilateral homonymous hemianopia related to posterior reversible encephalopathy syndrome. (*A*) 24-2 Humphrey visual fields showing a complete right homonymous hemianopia and an incomplete congruous left homonymous hemianopia. This patient had malignant hypertension and the FLAIR axial brain MRI (*B*) showed bilateral occipital lesions, suggesting posterior reversible encephalopathy syndrome (PRES). The visual-field defects resolved after treatment of the hypertension, and the brain MRI normalized within 2 weeks.

naming digits on the their own or another's hand, constructional dyspraxia, agraphia, and difficulty calculating.

Associative visual agnosia is present in some patients with a left PCA occlusion. It consists of difficulty understanding the nature and use of objects presented visually. However, they can trace with fingers, and they can copy an object presented in the hand and explored by touch or verbally described by the examiner.

Prosopagnosia results from occlusion of the right PCA. Patients with this condition have difficulty recognizing familiar faces. The patients may also have difficulty revisualizing what a given object or person should look like, and their dreams are often devoid of visual imagery.

Visual neglect is much more common after occlusion of the right PCA with infarction of the right parietal lobe than it is after occlusion of the left PCA.

Cerebral blindness occurs with bilateral PCA occlusions. Patients with this syndrome may have premonitory episodes of bilateral visual blurring or focal brainstem ischemia before they develop acute, bilateral, simultaneous visual loss caused by bilateral simultaneous homonymous hemianopia. Many cases of cortical blindness are caused by basilar artery thrombosis. The pupils and fundus examination are normal. Many of the patients experience photopsias or formed visual hallucinations while they are totally blind. Denial of blindness, known as Anton syndrome, is common. Bilateral occipital lobe infarction can produce decreased central visual acuity in both eyes without any obvious hemianopic defect. The loss of central vision probably results from generalized ischemia of the occipital lobes and is symmetric in both eyes, unless there is an associated unilateral or asymmetric ocular disease.

Balint syndrome can occur in patients who experience bilateral simultaneous or sequential PCA occlusions, although it is most common after bilateral watershed infarctions between the PCA and middle cerebral artery territories, primarily damaging the parieto-occipital visual associative areas. Balint syndrome occurs more frequently after bilateral watershed infarctions of the parieto-occipital regions from systemic hypotension than from thromboembolic carotid or vertebrobasilar disease. Patients with this syndrome present with a triad of psychic paralysis of visual fixation, optic ataxia, and visuospatial disorientation. Patients with Balint syndrome have a variety of abnormalities of fixation and tracking. They have great difficulty locating a stationary object in space, although they can maintain fixation on the object once they locate it. They can track a moving target, but if the target begins to move rapidly, it is lost and cannot be relocated.

Simultagnosia may develop in patients with bilateral superior occipital lobe strokes. Such patients complain of piecemeal perception of the visual environment wherein objects may look fragmented or even appear to vanish from direct view. Simultagnosia is caused by a defect in visual attention that results in an inability to sustain visuospatial processing across simultaneous elements in an array. Simultagnosia, like Balint syndrome and other higher disorders of visual processing and attention, occurs more frequently after systemic hypotension with watershed infarctions than from occlusion of the PCAs. Common causes include cardiac arrest and intraoperative hypotension.

Achromatopsia occurs in association with prosopagnosia when occipital lobe infarction is limited to the lower banks of the calcarine fissures on both sides.

Visual hallucinations

Formed visual hallucinations may be produced by vertebrobasilar ischemia. These hallucinations, which may last 30 minutes or more, may be associated with decreased consciousness, but they usually occur in an otherwise alert patient who is aware that the visual images are not real. The hallucinations are generally restricted to a hemianopic field, and they are often complex. Some of the visual hallucinations that occur in patients with PCA occlusion are palinoptic, with the hallucinations consisting of recently or previously seen images.[3]

Diplopia

Transient binocular horizontal or vertical diplopia is a common manifestation of vertebrobasilar ischemia. The diplopia may result from transient ischemia of the ocular motor nerves or their nuclei (ocular motor nerve paresis), or from transient ischemia to supranuclear or internuclear ocular motor pathways (skew deviation, internuclear ophthalmoplegia, gaze paresis). In most cases, the diplopia is not isolated and the patient has other neurologic symptoms suggesting vertebrobasilar ischemia.[24–29]

Persistent disturbances of eye movements are common in patients with vertebrobasilar ischemia. Ocular motor nerve paresis, internuclear ophthalmoplegia, supranuclear deficits, and nystagmus develop based on the anatomic location of the lesion.

Nystagmus produces oscillopsia, which is often described by the patients as "jumping of vision."

SMALL-ARTERY DISEASE
Arteritis

Infectious and noninfectious inflammation affecting the central nervous system can produce visual symptoms. In some vasculitides with a predilection for large arteries, such as Takayasu arteritis, ocular ischemia is common. Most often, vasculitis produces retinal vasculitis with retinal vascular occlusions and visual loss, often associated with ocular inflammation (uveitis) (**Fig. 10**).[3]

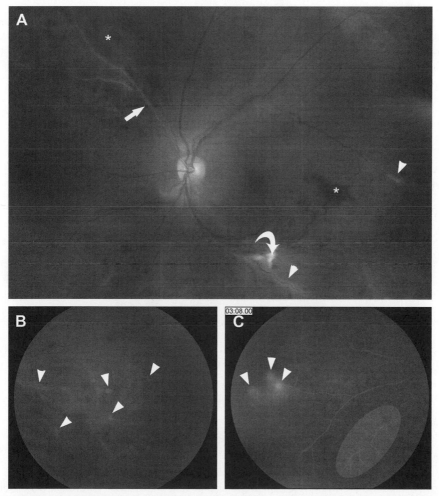

Fig. 10. Retinal vasculitis. (A) Funduscopic photograph of the left eye, showing extensive vasculitis with periarterial sheathing (*arrowheads*), a branch retinal artery occlusion (*arrow*), and retinal ischemia; note the cotton-wool spots (*curved arrow*) and intraretinal hemorrhages (*asterisks*). (B) Magnification of the same photograph showing the periarterial sheathing (*arrowheads*). (C) Fluorescein angiogram (at 3 minutes and 8 seconds) showing arterial leakage (*arrowheads*) and the attenuated arterial vasculature (*white ellipse*).

Giant cell arteritis should be considered in all patients more than 50 years old presenting with acute optic nerve or retinal ischemia.[30] Permanent visual loss is common in giant cell arteritis, and is often preceded by transient monocular visual loss (see the article by Falaradeau elsewhere in this issue for further exploration of this topic).

Susac Syndrome

Susac syndrome describes young patients with multiple bilateral branch retinal arterial occlusions, hearing loss, and neurologic symptoms suggestive of a brain microangiopathy.[31] It classically occurs in young women, but can affect men. Affected patients have recurrent multiple branch retinal occlusions that are most often bilateral, progressive hearing loss, and various neurologic presentations including psychiatric changes and encephalopathy. The disease usually has a chronic relapsing course punctuated by frequent remissions and exacerbations.[31]

Retinal fluorescein angiography classically shows retinal arterial wall hyperfluorescence, which is indicates disease activity (**Fig. 11**) Hearing loss primarily involves low and medium frequencies, and is best identified by audiogram. It is believed to

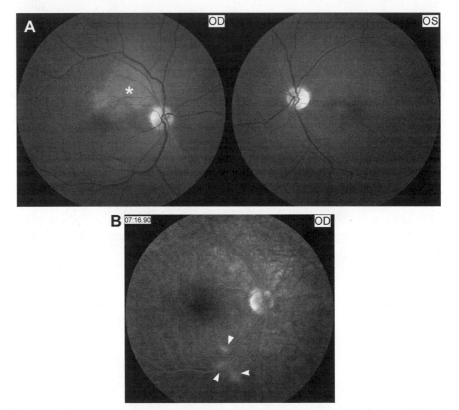

Fig. 11. Funduscopic and fluorescein angiographic findings in Susac syndrome. (*A*) Funduscopic photograph of a young woman with recurrent bilateral branch retinal artery occlusions related to Susac syndrome. There is an area of ischemia superiorly (*asterisk*) in the right eye (OD, *left*). In the left eye (OS, *right*) there is diffuse arterial attenuation and optic disc pallor from prior arterial occlusions. (*B*) Fluorescein angiogram of the right eye showing 3 areas of arterial leakage distant from the ischemic retina (*arrowheads*), highly suggestive of Susac syndrome.

result from cochlear damage caused by occlusions of the cochlear end arterioles. Encephalopathy varies in severity from mild memory loss and personality changes to severe cognitive dysfunction, confusion, psychiatric disorders, seizures, and focal neurologic symptoms and signs. The brain involvement in Susac syndrome is usually the most severe part of the disease and is frequently debilitating.

Electroencephalograms usually show diffuse slowing. Cerebrospinal fluid examination may be normal or show a variable degree of leukocytosis (lymphocytes), with increased protein levels. The neuroimaging modality of choice is brain magnetic resonance imaging (MRI), which typically shows multiple enhancing small lesions in the white and gray matter, with classic involvement of the corpus callosum (an otherwise unusual location for vascular disease).[32] The magnetic resonance angiography is normal, but catheter angiography has shown evidence of vasculopathy in some patients. In a few cases, brain biopsy was performed and showed microinfarcts with some minimal perivascular lymphocytic infiltration, but no true vasculitis.

Because of the spontaneously remitting-relapsing course of Susac syndrome, and the small number of cases reported, it is difficult to assess the efficacy of the various treatments that have been tried. Most patients receive steroids, immunosuppressive agents, and antiplatelet/antithrombotic therapy until the disease becomes clinically inactive.[31,33]

Hereditary Retinopathies

Several rare hereditary retinopathies are associated with central nervous system abnormalities. Recent genetic characterization of 3 of these syndromes has shown that there is an overlap among these entities (**Table 3**).[34]

Miscellaneous Angiopathies of the Central Nervous System with Ocular Manifestations

A variety of other systemic disorders producing strokes may be associated with ocular abnormalities (**Table 4**). Most are inherited disorders, and ophthalmic manifestations may reveal the angiopathy.[3,11]

Table 3
Characteristics of the 3 autosomal dominant cerebro-ocular vasculopathies mapped to chromosome 3

Name	Ocular Findings	Neurologic Findings	Other Findings
Hereditary vascular retinopathy (HVR)	Microangiopathy Retinal periphery and posterior pole	Multiple small lesions in GM and WM Headaches	Raynaud phenomenon
Cerebro-retinal vasculopathy (CRV)	Microangiopathy Posterior pole	Cerebral pseudotumors Extensive WM lesions Dementia Headaches Death <55 years	
Hereditary endotheliopathy, retinopathy, nephropathy, and stroke (HERNS)	Microangiopathy Posterior pole	Cerebral pseudotumors Extensive WM lesions Dementia Headaches Stroke Death <55 years	Renal involvement

Abbreviations: WM, white matter, GM, gray matter.

Table 4
Miscellaneous angiopathies of the central nervous system with ocular manifestations

Disease	Ocular Manifestations	Mechanism of Angiopathy	Transmission
Neurofibromatosis I	Neurofibromas, iris Lish nodules, optic nerve gliomas, retinal hamartomas	Arterial dissections, aneurysms, fistulae ganglioneuromas, neurofibromas	Autosomal dominant
von Hippel-Lindau syndrome	Retinal angiomas	Cerebellar, brainstem, and spinal cord hemangioblastoma	Autosomal dominant
Tuberous sclerosis (Bourneville disease)	Retinal hamartomas	Intracranial aneurysms, moyamoya syndrome	Autosomal dominant
Rendu-Osler-Weber syndrome (hereditary hemorrhagic telangiectasia)	Retinal telangiectasia	Arteriovenous malformations, venous angiomas, aneurysms, meningeal telangiectasia	Autosomal dominant
Sturge-Weber syndrome (encephalofacial angiomatosis)	Skin, conjunctiva, episclera, uveal angiomas; glaucoma	Leptomeningeal venous angioma, arteriovenous malformations, venous and dural sinus abnormalities	Possibly autosomal dominant Mostly sporadic
Wyburn-Mason syndrome (Racemose angioma)	Retinal arteriovenous malformations	Cerebral arteriovenous malformations (usually brainstem)	Sporadic
Ataxia-telangiectasia (Louis-Bar syndrome)	Oculocutaneous telangiectasia	Telangiectasia	Autosomal recessive
Marfan syndrome	Lens subluxation, retinal detachment	Aneurysms, aortic dissection	Autosomal dominant
Fibromuscular dysplasia	Retinal emboli	Arterial stenosis, arterial dissections aneurysms, carotid cavernous fistula	Possibly autosomal dominant. Mostly sporadic

Disease	Ocular findings	Vascular/pathologic features	Inheritance
Ehler-Danlos syndrome (type IV)	Ocular ischemia, angioid streaks	Aneurysms, carotid cavernous fistula carotid or vertebral artery dissection	Heterogeneous
Pseudoxanthoma elasticum (Gronblad-Strandberg syndrome)	Angioid streaks, peau d'orange fundus	Premature atherosclerosis, aneurysms, carotid cavernous fistula	Heterogenous
Moyamoya syndrome	Morning glory disc, ocular ischemia	Noninflammatory occlusive intracranial vasculopathy	May be associated with other hereditary disorders
Menkes syndrome (kinky hair disease)	Ocular ischemia	Tortuosity, elongation, and occlusion of cerebral arteries	X-linked recessive
Fabry disease (angiokeratoma corporis diffusum)	Whorl-like corneal opacification, tortuosity of vessels	Glycosphingolipid deposit in endothelial cells, cerebral aneurysms	X-linked recessive
Homocystinuria and homocysteinemia	Retinal ischemia, lens subluxation	Premature atherosclerotic occlusion of carotid arteries and large cerebral arteries	Autosomal recessive
Cerebral autosomal dominant arteriopathy with subcortical infarcts and leukoencephalopathy (CADASIL)	Valcular retinopathy	Nonatherosclerotic, nonamyloidotic angiopathy of leptomeningeal and small penetrating arteries	Autosomal dominant
MELAS (mitochondrial myopathy, encephalopathy, lactic acidosis, strokelike episodes)	Optic atrophy, chronic progressive external ophthalmoplegia, pigmentary retinopathy	Proliferation of mitochondria in smooth muscle cells of cerebral vessels	Maternally inherited (point mutation in mitochondrial DNA)

Hypertensive Encephalopathy

Patients with systemic hypertension may develop a severe encephalopathy often associated with reversible visual loss (also called posterior reversible encephalopathy syndrome) (see **Fig. 9**).[35,36] Hypertensive retinopathy may also be present bilaterally and does not always correlate with the severity of the hypertensive encephalopathy. There may be associated optic nerve head edema that may mimic that of increased intracranial pressure (**Fig. 12**).

Ischemic Optic Neuropathies

Most vascular diseases involving the optic nerve are in the category of anterior and posterior ischemic optic neuropathies believed to be small-vessel diseases.[4] (See the article by Bonelli and Arnold elsewhere in this issue for further exploration of this topic.)

Retinopathy and Retinal Vascular Caliber and the Risk of Stroke and Coronary Artery Disease

Several studies have shown that retinal microvascular changes are related to clinical stroke, stroke mortality, coronary artery disease, cognitive changes, cerebral white matter changes detected by MRI, and cerebral atrophy.[37–40] In these studies, retinal vascular changes (generalized and focal narrowing of the retinal arterioles, arteriovenous nicking, microaneurysms) and retinopathy (cotton-wool spots, retinal hemorrhages) were evaluated on fundus photographs.[37–40]

ANEURYSMS, FISTULAS, AND VASCULAR MALFORMATIONS
Aneurysms

The most common neuro-ophthalmic manifestations of intracranial aneurysms are secondary to a local mass effect on adjacent cranial nerves. The pulsatile process of the aneurysm may be as important as the direct mass effect.[41] Manifestations of the aneurysm depend on its location and its size. Aneurysms arising from the ophthalmic artery, the cavernous carotid artery, the anterior communicating artery, or the ICA can result in unilateral optic neuropathy or chiasmal visual-field defects.[42]

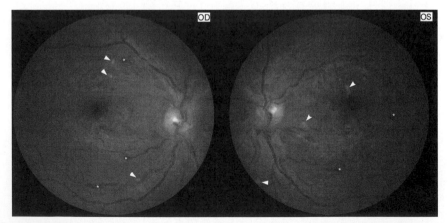

Fig. 12. Hypertensive retinopathy stage IV. Funduscopic photographs showing severe bilateral retinal changes with disc edema, suggesting hypertensive retinopathy stage IV. Note the bilateral optic nerve head edema, cotton-wool spots (*arrowheads*) and superficial retinal hemorrhages (*asterisks*). Blood pressure was 200/130 mm Hg.

Rarely, a homonymous hemianopia can result from compression of the optic tract. Multiple ocular nerve palsies can result from an aneurysm involving the cavernous carotid artery. Posterior communicating artery aneurysms classically produce an isolated third nerve palsy, whereas isolated trochlear or abducens nerve palsies only rarely result from aneurysmal compression (see the article by Volpe and Prasad elsewhere in this issue for further exploration of this topic).[43]

Aneurysmal rupture producing a subarachnoid hemorrhage may be associated with retinal, subhyaloid, and vitreal hemorrhages in 1 or both eyes (Terson syndrome) (**Fig. 13**). The presumed mechanism is that of acute increased intracranial pressure with sudden increase of ocular central-venous pressure. Vision loss is variable but is not associated with a relative afferent pupillary defect unless the retina is detached. The diagnosis is often delayed in intensive care unit (ICU) patients who may not be aware of visual loss. Unless there is an associated retinal detachment, treatment is usually deferred, and a vitrectomy is performed only if the hemorrhage does not resolve spontaneously.[42,43]

When an aneurysm arises from the cavernous carotid artery or from its branches in the cavernous sinus, rupture results in carotid cavernous fistula, not subarachnoid hemorrhage.

Carotid Cavernous Sinus Fistula

Direct carotid cavernous fistula results from direct communication of the cavernous carotid artery and the cavernous sinus with resultant high velocity of blood flow.[44] Direct carotid cavernous fistulas can result from trauma or from rupture of a preexisting aneurysm of the cavernous carotid artery. Ocular manifestations are usually obvious and include proptosis, periorbital swelling, chemosis, dilation of the episcleral vessels, orbital bruit, ophthalmoplegia, increased intraocular pressure, dilation or occlusion of the retinal veins, and optic disc edema.[45]

Dural carotid cavernous sinus fistulas result from indirect communications between branches of the internal and external carotid arteries and the cavernous sinus. They are more common in middle-aged and elderly women. Neuro-ophthalmic

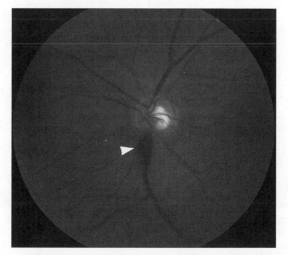

Fig. 13. Left Terson syndrome. Funduscopic photograph showing a preretinal hemorrhage inferior to the optic nerve (*arrowhead*) in a patient with subarachnoid hemorrhage, consistent with Terson syndrome.

manifestations depend on the blood-flow velocity and vary from the full classic appearance of direct fistulas to isolated bruit, cranial nerve palsies, or simply a red eye (**Fig. 14**). Their diagnosis is therefore more difficult and is often delayed.

Orbital imaging with computerized tomography (CT) or MRI classically shows dilatation of the superior ophthalmic veins, enlargement of the extraocular muscles, or enlargement of the cavernous sinus (see **Fig. 14**). Catheter angiography is the best way to confirm a carotid cavernous fistula, which can often be treated with an endovascular approach at the same time.

Arteriovenous Malformations

Intracranial arteriovenous malformations may result in intraparenchymal hemorrhage, subarachnoid hemorrhage, seizures, or mass effect.[46,47] Occipital arteriovenous malformations can cause episodic visual symptoms mimicking the visual aura of migraine. Homonymous hemianopia is common in occipital lesions, most often as the result of bleeding or as a complication of treatment (**Fig. 15**). Posterior fossa arteriovenous

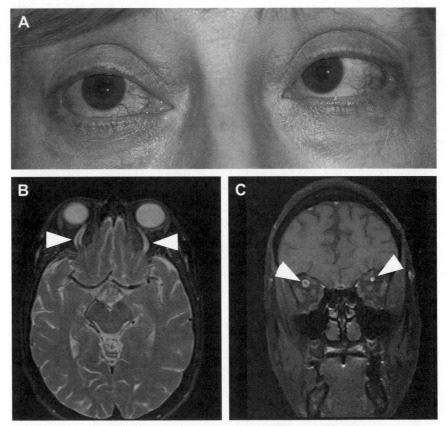

Fig. 14. Indirect dural carotid cavernous fistula with bilateral sixth nerve palsies. (*A*) A 55-year-old woman with bilateral sixth nerve palsies with esotropia, and dilation of the episcleral vessels in both eyes. T2-axial brain MRI through the upper part of the orbits (*B*) and T1-coronal orbital MRI with contrast and fat suppression showing dilation of both superior ophthalmic veins (*arrowheads*). A catheter angiogram showed a complex indirect dural carotid cavernous fistula draining mostly posteriorly.

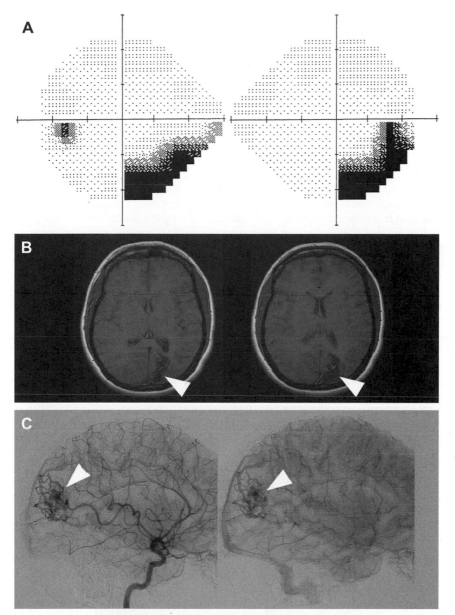

Fig. 15. Right homonymous hemianopia related to a left occipital arteriovenous malforma-tion. (*A*) 24-2 Humphrey visual fields showing an incomplete congruous right homonymous hemianopia. (*B*) Brain MRI showed a heterogeneous and irregular hyposignal in the left occipital lobe on the axial-T1–weighted image. (*C*) Catheter cerebral angiogram confirmed a left occipital arteriovenous malformation.

malformations usually cause intermittent or permanent diplopia, often associated with other neurologic signs. Orbital arteriovenous malformations produce an acute or subacute orbital syndrome, including proptosis, chemosis, ophthalmoplegia, visual loss, and increase of the intraocular pressure.

Retinal arteriovenous malformations are rare. They are sometimes isolated or are associated with intracranial or facial arteriovenous malformations.[48]

Cavernous Hemangioma

Cavernous hemangiomas are most common in the posterior fossa and usually produce diplopia when they bleed.[46] Familial cavernous hemangiomas are often multiple and may be associated with grapelike small retinal hemangiomas that are usually asymptomatic (**Fig. 16**).

VENOUS DISEASE
Central and Branch Retinal Vein Occlusion

Central retinal vein occlusion (CRVO) is a common ocular disorder in elderly patients, often associated with atheromatous vascular risk factors.[49] Occlusion of the central retinal vein is presumed to result from compression by the central retinal artery within the optic nerve. CRVO is also the most common ocular vascular occlusion associated with hypercoaguable states, whereas CRAO and ischemic optic neuropathy are rarely associated with hypercoaguable states. Patients with CRVO complain of blurry vision, the severity of which depends on the severity of the CRVO and associated retinal ischemia. Funduscopic examination reveals diffusely spread retinal superficial hemorrhages, retinal and macular edema, dilated and tortuous veins, and optic disc edema (**Fig. 17**). Cotton-wool spots suggest associated retinal ischemia, indicating a worse visual prognosis. Neovascularization of the retina, optic disc, and iris predisposes the patient to intravitreous hemorrhage, traction retinal detachment, and neovascular glaucoma. This disorder is primarily managed by the ophthalmologist, and the goals of the treatment are to treat macular edema and to prevent or treat neovascularization and its complications.[50]

Branch retinal vein occlusions (BRVO) result from direct compression from a retinal branch artery sharing a common sheath at an arteriovenous crossing (**Fig. 18**). The signs of vein occlusion are limited to the retinal area drained by the occluded

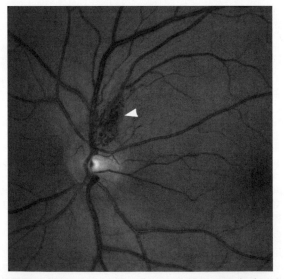

Fig. 16. Retinal cavernous hemangioma. Funduscopic photograph showing a small retinal cavernous hemangioma superior to the optic nerve in the left eye (*arrowhead*).

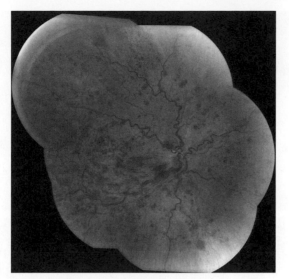

Fig. 17. Right CRVO. Funduscopic photograph showing a right CRVO with dilation and tortuosity of the veins, multiple retinal hemorrhages, and disc edema.

branch vein. Vision loss depends on the localization of the occluded vein branch and the involvement or sparing of the macula; prognosis is usually better than for CRVO.[51]

Cerebral Venous Thrombosis

Cerebral infarction related to cerebral venous thrombosis may present with acute focal neurologic signs, including homonymous hemianopia or cranial nerve palsies, usually in the setting of headaches or altered mental status.[52,53] However, most neuro-

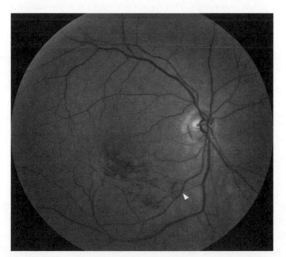

Fig. 18. BRVO. Funduscopic photograph showing an inferior temporal BRVO in the right eye. The vein is occluded by the artery at an arteriovenous crossing (*arrowhead*). The area of superficial retinal hemorrhages is limited to the territory drained by the occluded vein.

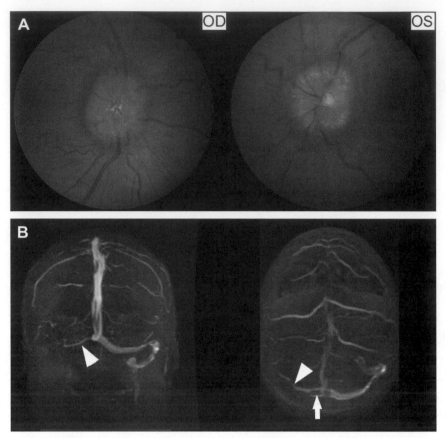

Fig. 19. Cerebral venous thrombosis. (*A*) Fundus photographs showing bilateral prominent papilledema from increased intracranial pressure. (*B*) Brain magnetic resonance venogram (*left*, coronal; *right*, axial) showing occlusion of the right transverse sinus and right sigmoid sinus (*arrowheads*).

ophthalmic manifestations of cerebral venous thrombosis are related to increased intracranial pressure,[54] and include papilledema and diplopia from uni- or bilateral sixth-nerve palsies (**Fig. 19**). Diagnosis and management of cerebral venous thrombosis are detailed in the article by Wall elsewhere in this issue.

Cavernous sinus thrombosis is extremely rare and produces acute painful proptosis with chemosis, ophthalmoplegia, venous stasis retinopathy, and visual loss.[55]

SUMMARY

Cerebrovascular diseases are commonly associated with neuro-ophthalmologic symptoms or signs, which mostly depend on the type, size, and location of the vessels involved, and the mechanism of the vascular lesion. Funduscopic examination allows direct visualization of the retinal circulation, which shares many common characteristics with the cerebral microcirculation, and can be used as a marker of vascular disease.

REFERENCES

1. Fisher CM. 'Transient monocular blindness' versus 'amaurosis fugax'. Neurology 1989;39(12):1622–4.
2. Biousse V, Trobe JD. Transient monocular visual loss. Am J Ophthalmol 2005; 140(4):717–21.
3. Biousse V. Cerebrovascular diseases. In: Miller N, Newman N, Biousse B, et al, editors. Walsh & Hoyt's clinical neuro-ophthalmology. 6th edition. Philadelphia: Williams & Wilkins; 2005. p. 1967–2168.
4. Luneau K, Newman NJ, Biousse V. Ischemic optic neuropathies. Neurologist 2008;14(6):341–54.
5. Hayreh SS, Zimmerman MB. Fundus changes in central retinal artery occlusion. Retina 2007;27(3):276–89.
6. Ros MA, Magargal LE, Uram M. Branch retinal-artery obstruction: a review of 201 eyes. Ann Ophthalmol 1989;21(3):103–7.
7. Hayreh SS, Podhajsky PA, Zimmerman MB. Branch retinal artery occlusion: natural history of visual outcome. Ophthalmology 2009;116(6):1188–94, e1–4.
8. Hayreh SS, Podhajsky PA, Zimmerman MB. Retinal artery occlusion: associated systemic and ophthalmic abnormalities. Ophthalmology 2009;116(10):1928–36.
9. Biousse V, Calvetti O, Bruce BB, et al. Thrombolysis for central retinal artery occlusion. J Neuroophthalmol 2007;27(3):215–30.
10. Biousse V. Thrombolysis for acute central retinal artery occlusion: is it time? Am J Ophthalmol 2008;146(5):631–4.
11. Biousse V, Newman N. Neuro-ophthalmology illustrated. New York: Thieme; 2009.
12. Russell RW, Page NG. Critical perfusion of brain and retina. Brain 1983;106(Pt 2): 419–34.
13. Klijn CJ, Kappelle LJ, van Schooneveld MJ, et al. Venous stasis retinopathy in symptomatic carotid artery occlusion: prevalence, cause, and outcome. Stroke 2002;33(3):695–701.
14. Mendrinos E, Machinis TG, Pournaras CJ. Ocular ischemic syndrome. Surv Ophthalmol 2010;55(1):2–34.
15. Mizener JB, Podhajsky P, Hayreh SS. Ocular ischemic syndrome. Ophthalmology 1997;104(5):859–64.
16. Hazin R, Daoud YJ, Khan F. Ocular ischemic syndrome: recent trends in medical management. Curr Opin Ophthalmol 2009;20(6):430–3.
17. Biousse V, Touboul PJ, D'Anglejan-Chatillon J, et al. Ophthalmologic manifestations of internal carotid artery dissection. Am J Ophthalmol 1998;126(4): 565–77.
18. Schievink WI, Mokri B, Garrity JA, et al. Ocular motor nerve palsies in spontaneous dissections of the cervical internal carotid artery. Neurology 1993;43(10): 1938–41.
19. Lapresle J, Lasjaunias P. Cranial nerve ischaemic arterial syndromes. A review. Brain 1986;109(Pt 1):207–16.
20. Hoyt WF. Some neuro-ophthalmological considerations in cerebral vascular insufficiency; carotid and vertebral artery insufficiency. AMA Arch Ophthalmol 1959; 62(2):260–72.
21. Caplan L. Posterior circulation ischemia: then, now, and tomorrow. The Thomas Willis Lecture-2000. Stroke 2000;31(8):2011–23.
22. Devuyst G, Bogousslavsky J, Meuli R, et al. Stroke or transient ischemic attacks with basilar artery stenosis or occlusion: clinical patterns and outcome. Arch Neurol 2002;59(4):567–73.

23. Knox DL, Cogan DG. Eye pain and homonymous hemianopia. Am J Ophthalmol 1962;54:1091–3.
24. Amarenco P. The spectrum of cerebellar infarctions. Neurology 1991;41(7): 973–9.
25. Bassetti C, Bogousslavsky J, Barth A, et al. Isolated infarcts of the pons. Neurology 1996;46(1):165–75.
26. Bogousslavsky J, Maeder P, Regli F, et al. Pure midbrain infarction: clinical syndromes, MRI, and etiologic patterns. Neurology 1994;44(11):2032–40.
27. Hommel M, Bogousslavsky J. The spectrum of vertical gaze palsy following unilateral brainstem stroke. Neurology 1991;41(8):1229–34.
28. Moncayo J, Bogousslavsky J. Vertebro-basilar syndromes causing oculo-motor disorders. Curr Opin Neurol 2003;16(1):45–50.
29. Vuilleumier P, Bogousslavsky J, Regli F. Infarction of the lower brainstem. Clinical, aetiological and MRI-topographical correlations. Brain 1995;118(Pt 4):1013–25.
30. Melson MR, Weyand CM, Newman NJ, et al. The diagnosis of giant cell arteritis. Rev Neurol Dis 2007;4(3):128–42.
31. Susac JO. Susac's syndrome: the triad of microangiopathy of the brain and retina with hearing loss in young women. Neurology 1994;44(4):591–3.
32. Susac JO, Murtagh FR, Egan RA, et al. MRI findings in Susac's syndrome. Neurology 2003;61(12):1783–7.
33. Rennebohm RM, Susac JO. Treatment of Susac's syndrome. J Neurol Sci 2007; 257(1–2):215–20.
34. Ophoff RA, DeYoung J, Service SK, et al. Hereditary vascular retinopathy, cerebroretinal vasculopathy, and hereditary endotheliopathy with retinopathy, nephropathy, and stroke map to a single locus on chromosome 3p21.1-p21.3. Am J Hum Genet 2001;69(2):447–53.
35. Bartynski WS. Posterior reversible encephalopathy syndrome, part 2: controversies surrounding pathophysiology of vasogenic edema. AJNR Am J Neuroradiol 2008;29(6):1043–9.
36. Bartynski WS. Posterior reversible encephalopathy syndrome, part 1: fundamental imaging and clinical features. AJNR Am J Neuroradiol 2008;29(6): 1036–42.
37. Wong TY, Klein R, Couper DJ, et al. Retinal microvascular abnormalities and incident stroke: the Atherosclerosis Risk in Communities Study. Lancet 2001; 358(9288):1134–40.
38. Wong TY, Klein R, Sharrett AR, et al. The prevalence and risk factors of retinal microvascular abnormalities in older persons: the Cardiovascular Health Study. Ophthalmology 2003;110(4):658–66.
39. Wang JJ, Mitchell P, Leung H, et al. Hypertensive retinal vessel wall signs in a general older population: the Blue Mountains Eye Study. Hypertension 2003; 42(4):534–41.
40. Sun C, Wang JJ, Mackey DA, et al. Retinal vascular caliber: systemic, environmental, and genetic associations. Surv Ophthalmol 2009;54(1):74–95.
41. Rodriguez-Catarino M, Frisen L, Wikholm G, et al. Internal carotid artery aneurysms, cranial nerve dysfunction and headache: the role of deformation and pulsation. Neuroradiology 2003;45(4):236–40.
42. Biousse V, Newman NJ. Aneurysms and subarachnoid hemorrhage. Neurosurg Clin N Am 1999;10(4):631–51.
43. Newman SA. Aneurysm. In: Miller N, Newman N, Biousse B, et al, editors. Walsh & Hoyt's clinical neuro-ophthalmology. 6th edition. Philadelphia: Williams & Wilkins; 2005. p. 2169–262.

44. Miller N. Carotid-cavernous sinus fistulas. In: Miller N, Newman N, Biousse B, et al, editors. Walsh & Hoyt's clinical neuro-ophthalmology. 6th edition. Philadelphia: Williams & Wilkins; 2005. p. 2263–96.

45. Kupersmith MJ, Berenstein A, Flamm E, et al. Neuroophthalmologic abnormalities and intravascular therapy of traumatic carotid cavernous fistulas. Ophthalmology 1986;93(7):906–12.

46. Biousse V, Newman NJ. Intracranial vascular abnormalities. Ophthalmol Clin North Am 2001;14(1):243–64.

47. Qureshi AI, Tuhrim S, Broderick JP, et al. Spontaneous intracerebral hemorrhage. N Engl J Med 2001;344(19):1450–60.

48. Singh AD, Rundle PA, Rennie I. Retinal vascular tumors. Ophthalmol Clin North Am 2005;18(1):167–76.

49. Hayreh SS, Zimmerman MB, Podhajsky P. Incidence of various types of retinal vein occlusion and their recurrence and demographic characteristics. Am J Ophthalmol 1994;117(4):429–41.

50. Mohamed Q, McIntosh RL, Saw SM, et al. Interventions for central retinal vein occlusion: an evidence based systematic review. Ophthalmology 2007;114(3): 507–19, 524.

51. McIntosh RL, Mohamed Q, Saw SM, et al. Interventions for branch retinal vein occlusion: an evidence-based systematic review. Ophthalmology 2007;114(5): 835–54.

52. Ameri A, Bousser MG. Cerebral venous thrombosis. Neurol Clin 1992;10(1): 87–111.

53. Ferro JM, Canhao P, Stam J, et al. Prognosis of cerebral vein and dural sinus thrombosis: results of the International Study on Cerebral Vein and Dural Sinus Thrombosis (ISCVT). Stroke 2004;35(3):664–70.

54. Biousse V, Ameri A, Bousser MG. Isolated intracranial hypertension as the only sign of cerebral venous thrombosis. Neurology 1999;53(7):1537–42.

55. DiNubile MJ. Septic thrombosis of the cavernous sinuses. Arch Neurol 1988; 45(5):567–72.

Thyroid Eye Disease

Kimberly P. Cockerham, MD*, Stephanie S. Chan, OD

KEYWORDS
- Graves disease • Thyroid eye disease
- Thyroid-associated ophthalmopathy
- Compressive optic neuropathy

Thyroid eye disease (TED) causes visual disability, discomfort, and facial disfigurement. These symptoms and signs are caused by immune-mediated, inflammatory events that may result in irreversible tissue alterations. Considerable controversy exists as to whether treatment is better than observation during the active phase of disease. Even those who favor treatment disagree on which patients should be treated, which antiinflammatory treatment to use, and how to measure treatment outcome. In the chronic phase, surgical options provide relief for decreased vision, diplopia, and eyelid malpositions. However, even with appropriate interventions at each stage of the disorder, TED patients often suffer a dramatic reduction in their quality of life.

BACKGROUND

TED is the most common cause of orbital inflammation and proptosis in adults. TED should always be a consideration in patients with unexplained diplopia, pain, or optic nerve dysfunction. TED can mimic a partial third nerve palsy, a sixth or fourth nerve palsy, or develop in a patient with known myasthenia gravis.

At least 80% of TED is associated with Graves disease (GD), but it can occur in patients with hypothyroidism, subacute thyroiditis, and even thyroid cancer. In patients with thyroid cancer, the association may be incidental or due to a dysregulation that stems from the neoplasia. At least 50% of patients with GD develop clinically evident symptomatic TED.[1,2] The most confusing patients for doctors of all subspecialties are the patients with eye symptoms and signs that precede serum evidence of a thyroid imbalance. TED is a clinical diagnosis with no ancillary test support in 20% of patients.

GD and TED affect more than 20 million previously healthy and productive adults in the United States alone. The peak incidence is in the fourth and fifth decades.[3] However, TED also presents in children and the elderly.

There is a classic curve to the activity (deterioration, plateau, improvement, and burnt-out stabilization) of TED. The classic teaching 2 decades ago was to provide only supportive care (such as preservative-free artificial tears) as patients move

Department of Ophthalmology, Stanford University, Stanford, CA, USA
* Corresponding author. 762 Altos Oaks Drive, Suite 2, Los Altos, CA 94024.
E-mail address: dr@cockerhammd.com

Neurol Clin 28 (2010) 729–755
doi:10.1016/j.ncl.2010.03.010
0733-8619/10/$ – see front matter © 2010 Elsevier Inc. All rights reserved.

through these phases.[4] However, this philosophy ignores the significant visual disability that can occur at home and at work.[5–7] Excessive tearing, foreign-body sensation, bulging of the eyes, swelling of the eyelids, retro-orbital pain, blurred vision, inability to focus, and double vision characterize early active TED. In 5% to 10% of TED patients, visual loss occurs as a result of corneal decompensation or optic nerve compression.[4,8,9]

During the active phase, the symptoms and signs of TED might fluctuate from hour to hour or day to day. As the TED progresses to the inactive, chronic, and stable phase, the redness, swelling, and retro-orbital pain resolve. Stabilization typically occurs in the second or third year but may be delayed in men, older patients, smokers, and those with prolonged hypothyroidism. Anecdotally, with the advent of the recent recession, the role of stress, especially at work, has become a particular concern for patients' disease stabilization. Once stable and inactive, symptoms and disfiguring signs are often present because of restriction of eye movement and fibrotic proptosis. Visual blurring, doubling, distortion, and tearing cause difficulties with driving, reading, and computer use. Bulging eyes, retracted lids, and misaligned eyes from enlarged, restricted muscles disfigure patients.

Many TED patients become depressed, withdraw socially, lose self-esteem, and suffer job dislocation, divorce, and emotional devastation. The economic effect of this disease is great because it affects women and, less commonly, men in their peak years of productivity, affecting their families, communities, and workplaces.[5,6] The most frustrated patients are those with normal thyroid function tests who often elude diagnosis for months or even years.

Disease management varies widely by practitioner, institution, state, and country.[2,10–15] The first step is a comprehensive evaluation; the second step is a frank discussion with the patient about clinical and surgical options depending on the patients' needs, desires, and expectations.

If patients have active TED that is disrupting their visual function, job, and life, there are several therapeutic options to consider. The most common medical interventions (corticosteroids or external beam radiation) are typically reserved for patients with pain, severe diplopia, excessive inflammation, vision-threatening active-phase orbitopathy, or rapidly progressive orbitopathy. This article details potential first-step therapeutics to improve patient's comfort and functionality.

Unless the patient is going blind from corneal breakdown or an optic neuropathy, or is in pain from a congestive orbitopathy, surgery is delayed until the patient recedes from active disease to a more stable chronic picture. Surgery can dramatically improve the patients' quality of life by decreasing disfigurement and allowing the patient to see a single image when looking straight ahead, down, and in most needed gazes. However, the tissue alterations are irreversible so there is often no way to restore normal eye-muscle movement or predisease appearance. Thus, many of the manifestations of TED are permanent, which can be frustrating for patients who are models, flight attendants, pilots, and engineers. We tell patients that 80% restoration is our realistic goal.

IMMUNOLOGY

GD is a systemic autoimmune disease associated with overactivity and dysregulation of the thyroid gland. This condition is typically accompanied by extensive remodeling of orbital and, less commonly, pretibial dermal connective tissues. The pathogenic relationship between the thyroid dysfunction and inflammation of the orbital tissues is an enigma. The immune response in TED is humoral and cell mediated. Monocytes, lymphocytes, and mast cells are known to participate but the mechanism for the activation and trafficking of these cells is unknown.[16–21]

The acute phase is driven by mononuclear cells (primarily lymphocytes and mast cells) that infiltrate the extraocular muscles (EOMs), orbital fat, and periorbital tissues such as the orbicularis and Mueller muscle. The site-specific response is explained in part by the unique phenotype of resident fibroblasts that respond to proinflammatory cytokines at a 100-fold greater rate than abdominal fibroblasts. In TED, orbital fibroblasts orchestrate the recruitment of immunocompetent cells and initiate tissue remodeling. Activated fibroblasts drive the disease process through expression of molecular mediators including cytokines and chemoattractants that promote ongoing inflammation and immune recruitment.[22–28]

Inflammation-mediated production and accumulation of orbital glycosaminoglycans (GAGs) are characteristic of active TED.[29–36] The highly charged, hydrophilic, hyaluronan molecules attract water, and thereby contribute to orbital tissue expansion and orbital congestion. The combination of muscle and fat expansion results in proptosis, restricted eye-muscle movement and, in some patients, optic neuropathy. Irreversible changes occur when fibroblast activity induces fibrosis at the level of the fibrovascular matrix of the orbital soft tissue.[37–40]

CLINICAL PRESENTATION
Eyelid Retraction

Upper eyelid retraction with a stare (**Fig. 1**) is a common presenting feature in patients with GD and TED. The increased circulating thyroid hormones initially induce eyelid retraction but, with time, the Mueller muscle becomes infiltrated with mast cells, lymphocytes, and fibroblasts, resulting in hypertrophy and scarring that is permanent. Eyelid retraction refers to the eyelid position when the patient is looking straight ahead (**Fig. 2**A), lid lag refers to a slowed downward vertical saccade of the eyelid, and lagophthalmos is the failure to close the eyelid in passive downward closure (see **Fig. 2**B). Bilateral upper and lower lid retraction often results in the classic lid stare appearance of TED (**Fig. 3**).

If ptosis is present intermittently or at the end of the day, the patient may suffer from TED and myasthenia gravis (**Fig. 4**). Look for difficulties with sustained upgaze, a Cogan lid twitch, and other systemic evidence of myasthenia gravis (proximal muscle weakness, difficulty swallowing or breathing) (**Fig. 5**).

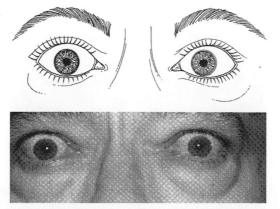

Fig. 1. Bilateral upper eyelid retraction is a common presenting sign of TED.

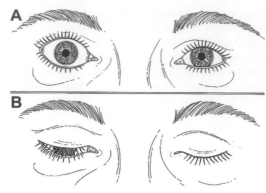

Fig. 2. (*A*) Unilateral lid retraction often leads to (*B*) lagophthalmos, or failure of the eyelid to close fully in passive closure.

Double Vision

TED dysmotility often presents as intermittent diplopia that is initially more symptomatic in the morning because of edema that results from sleeping in a supine position. The saccadic speed and accuracy is normal in TED. In contrast, a patient with a cranial nerve palsy will have slowed saccades. Myasthenia gravis patients can exhibit rapid saccades or intrasaccadic delay. Esotropia is more common than hypotropia, but any pattern of deviation can occur. TED can occasionally mimic a partial third, fourth or sixth nerve palsy. In the example in **Fig. 6**, there is a right hypertropia that is worse on right head tilt and left gaze, due to restriction of the left inferior rectus instead of a right fourth nerve deficit. Saccadic velocity and accuracy should be intact in a patient with TED dysmotility. The intraocular pressure can be measured in upgaze to confirm restriction of the inferior rectus (**Fig. 7**).

Optic Neuropathy

TED optic neuropathy is slowly progressive and begins with loss of color perception, (reds start to look orange or brown,) and progresses to decreased vision due to compression of macular fibers (as manifested as a central scotoma on visual field testing) (**Fig. 8**). However, any optic nerve pattern of visual field alteration is possible (eg, arcuate defect, nasal step, peripheral constriction that respects the horizontal meridian) (**Fig. 9**). This pattern is in contrast to visual field defects from the chiasm

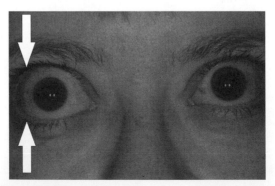

Fig. 3. Upper and lower eyelid retraction that is most pronounced laterally (*arrow*).

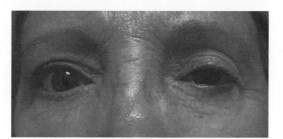

Fig. 4. Unilateral ptosis combined with lid retraction in the other eye; the patient may suffer from TED and myasthenia gravis.

posteriorly, which respect the vertical meridian (eg, bitemporal or homonomous field defects) (**Fig. 10**).

The optic nerve is often normal until late in the process, so the vision loss is often reversible even after months of compression. Nerve fiber analysis with optical coherence tomography (OCT) can be helpful in identifying occult nerve fiber layer loss and in predicting postsurgical visual function in TED and other compressive optic neuropathies from parasellar processes, such as pituitary tumors.

Eyelid and Orbital Inflammation

Most patients with TED experience an active phase of the disease in which symptoms and signs of inflammation are present. Erythema and edema of the eyelids are often prominent in the morning. The conjunctival vessels are engorged and fluid accumulates between the white of the eye (sclera) and the thin overlying layer (conjunctiva); this is called chemosis. The caruncle can be particularly hyperemic and edematous (**Fig. 11**). A vague ache that increases with eye movement can be present. The degree of pain appreciated by the patient can occasionally confuse the clinical diagnosis.

CLINICAL MEASURES TO ASSESS TED ACTIVITY AND SEVERITY

The duration (months to years) and severity of active TED are unpredictable in individual cases. Male gender, older age, degree of initial thyroid imbalance, prolonged hypothyroidism, and cigarette smoking are risk factors for longer duration and severity of the initial active phase.[41–52]

The most widely used disease activity classification system is NOSPECS, which documents the presence of specific symptoms and signs, of which only some are characteristic of active disease.[53] A higher score (clinical worsening) may not represent increased inflammatory activity, but progressive fibrosis associated with resolving inflammation.[54–59]

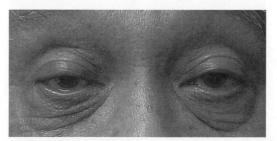

Fig. 5. Bilateral symmetric ptosis is more typical of a patient with myasthenia gravis.

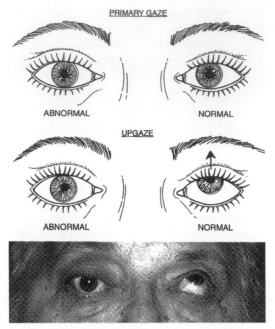

Fig. 6. (*Top*) Patient looking straight ahead (primary gaze). (*Middle, bottom*) Patient looking up; the right eye is unable to supraduct at all due to the restrictive thyroid process.

More recently, the modified clinical activity score (CAS) for TED has been used. The CAS assigns a point to each symptom or sign (retrobulbar pain, eyelid erythema, conjunctival injection, chemosis, swelling of the caruncle, and eyelid edema or fullness) and is a simple summation that does not provide information regarding overall progression or severity of TED. In practice, the identification of active TED remains

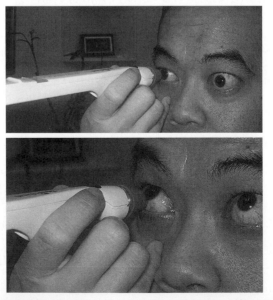

Fig. 7. Tono-pen intraocular pressure measurement in primary and upgaze.

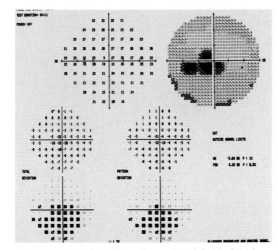

Fig. 8. Central scotoma on automated Humphrey visual fields (HVF).

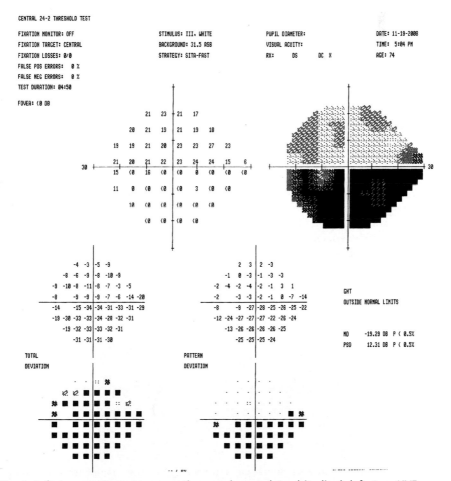

Fig. 9. Inferior arcuate scotoma creating nearly complete altitudinal defect on HVF.

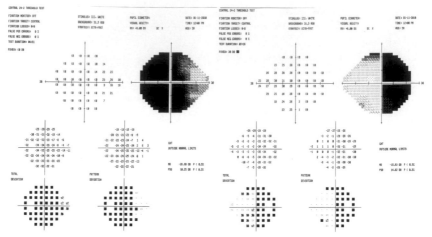

Fig. 10. Junctional defect that respects the vertical meridian unilaterally.

an imperfect combination of the patient's impression and the clinician's interpretation of the physical symptoms and signs.

CAS

- Pain: pain on eye movement, or pain or oppressive feeling on or behind the globe, in last 4 weeks
- Redness: conjunctival or eyelid injection
- Swelling: chemosis, eyelid or caruncular edema, increasing proptosis of more than 2 mm in last 1 to 3 months
- Impaired function: decrease in eye movement or visual acuity in last 1 to 3 months.

OBJECTIVE DISEASE ASSESSMENT TOOLS

Potential candidates for objective assessment of TED disease activity currently include (1) eye muscle reflectivity on A-mode ultrasound of 40% or less;[60] (2) increased urine or plasma GAGs;[61–64] (3) high orbital uptake on Octreoscan;[65,66] (4) increased thyroid-stimulating immunoglobulin (TSI);[67–83] (5) detection of EOM edema by magnetic resonance imaging (MRI).[84–99]

EYE MUSCLE REFLECTIVITY ON A-MODE ULTRASOUND

B-mode ultrasound has been used for decades to identify the gross size and shape of the EOMs. More recently, A-mode ultrasound has been used in TED patients to detect

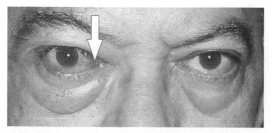

Fig. 11. Active TED with edema, erythema, and chemosis of the conjunctiva and caruncle (*arrow*).

edema (low eye-muscle reflectivity as measured as a percent of the initial sclera spike). The reflectivity can be reliably measured; low reflectivity correlates with active TED and accurately predicts response to immunosuppressive treatment.[100] However, it has a poor negative predictive value and therefore cannot be used in isolation.[60]

Urine and Plasma GAGs

GAGs are hydrophilic and participate in the expansion of intraconal fat and EOMs in TED. GAGs can be isolated from plasma and urine specimens by protein elimination, dialysis, and precipitation techniques. TED patients had higher plasma GAGs than controls, whereas previous corticosteroid therapy in a TED patient normalized the GAG content. Using highly specific high-pressure liquid chromatography (HPLC), the urinary concentration of GAGs, hyaluronic acid, and chondroitin sulfate A were increased in untreated TED patients. GAGs play a role in the pathogenesis of TED and may be a useful marker for active disease and a conformational marker for successfully treated TED with immunosuppressives.[61–63]

Octreoscan

Pentetreotide, a synthetic derivative of ^{111}In-labeled somatostatin, is combined with a γ camera to detect tumors that have somatostatin surface receptors. ^{111}In-DTPA-D-Phe octreotide scintigraphy (Octreoscan) can identify active TED. If the peak activity in the orbit at hour 5 after injection is 100%, a decrease in the orbit of 40%, compared with an expected plasma decrease of 15% at 24 hours, confirms the presence of activated lymphocytes with somatostatin receptors. Issues include cost, lack of availability, radiation exposure, and the possibility that the binding is to myoblasts, fibroblasts, or endothelial cells.[101,102] Orbital MRI T2 relaxation times correlate with octreotide uptake and are statistically significant in discerning active from inactive TED.[65]

SERUM IMMUNOLOGY MEASURES

Laboratory tests to detect thyroid dysfunction, including thyroid-stimulating hormone, thyrotropin, and serum-free T3 and T4 levels, do not correlate with TED disease activity.[67,72,82,83] In contrast, TSI have been found in more than 90% of patients with active GD and in 50% to 90% of euthyroid TED patients.

TSI levels and TED

- Significantly higher in GD patients with TED
- Correlate with the presence of active TED signs such as eyelid edema
- Higher when EOM and orbital fat expansion are present on orbital computerized tomography (CT).[67–83]

TED is also associated with antibodies that recognize and activate the receptor for insulin growth factor 1 (IGF-1). Virtually all individuals with early GD and TED exhibit antibodies that bind to the IGF-1 receptor (IGF-1R) and activate this protein. There is a specific relationship between these antibodies and receptor activation in orbital fibroblasts from patients with severe TED.[103–110]

TSI is considered to be increased if more than 125; active TED patients often have levels in the 300 to 500 range. TSI levels decline as TED becomes inactive. In contrast, anti–IGF-1R is not detectable in patients without an active autoimmune disease such as TED, so the test result is positive or negative in TED and not a continuous variable.

In summary, patients with GD and TED have higher levels of TSI than patients with GD alone. Increase in TSI seems to be a prerequisite for the development of active TED. IGF-1 is increased in early, active TED and GD. In contrast, other antibody levels (thyroid stimulating hormone binding inhibitory immunoglobulin [TBII], antithyroid peroxidase, and antithyroglobulin) are often found to be significantly lower in GD/TED patients compared with patients who have GD alone.

MRI

In an effort to identify a noninvasive objective tool to detect active TED, several small studies have explored the usefulness of MRI as a tool to identify EOM enlargement and to quantify EOM edema. The magnetic resonance image acquisition is predicated on the differential behavior of soft tissues in a magnetic field, which is based primarily on the water content of the tissues. The increased water content caused by active inflammation is characterized by prolonged T2 relaxation times (a continuous variable), and by decreased gadolinium contrast enhancement of fat-saturation T1 imaging (a subjective interpretation).[84–99]

MRI results were compared with subjective, nonvalidated clinical, and often inadequate, measures of disease severity or disease activity.[85–96] However, MRI seems to be predictive of response to therapeutic interventions such as intravenous pulse corticosteroids, orbital radiotherapy, and cyclosporine.[97–99] In one study, MRI T2 relaxation had a 64% positive predictive value and a 92% negative predictive value for the response to orbital radiotherapy as subjectively reported by the patient and managing physician.[10] Response to treatment included improvement in diplopia, proptosis, and soft-tissue swelling.

The role of gadolinium enhancement of EOMs in fat-suppressed T1-weighted images is more controversial. The literature depicts mixed results with increased and decreased enhancement described in active and posttreatment TED.[88,90,95,98,99] These studies are also limited in size and differ regarding TED disease activity. Systematic evaluation of EOM enhancement and multiple measures of disease activity are needed to determine the usefulness of this measure in TED.

The use of prolongation of T2 relaxation times to identify EOM edema is the technique that has been the most widely studied, seems likely to be the most specific, and has the fewest technical difficulties (**Fig. 12**).

PRACTICAL CLINICAL EVALUATION OF THE NEW TED PATIENT

When a patient presents with double vision or decreased vision that may be due to TED, a comprehensive ophthalmic workup is indicated.

To assess afferent function, best corrected visual acuity, color testing with pseudoisochromatic plates, color and light desaturation, pupillary function looking for an relative afferent pupillary defect, and examination of the optic nerve are performed. Ancillary testing includes formal visual field testing (eg, Humphrey visual field [HVF] 24-2).

To assess efferent function, saccades and pursuits are tested, and versions and ductions are documented. Intraocular pressure testing in upgaze is helpful if there is restriction of upgaze. External gaze photographs are helpful to follow dysmotility (**Fig. 13**). TED patients should have normal saccadic velocity and accuracy accompanied by positive forced ductions (Tono-pen is used in opposite gaze to demonstrate the same principle).

Eyelid position should be examined and eyelid retraction documented. If there is ptosis, it should be considered that the patient may have TED and myasthenia gravis. Look for difficulty with sustained upgaze and look for a Cogan lid twitch. Look at the dynamic movement of the eyelid when the patient is asked to perform vertical saccades to ascertain whether the eyelid descends more slowly than the globe; this

A   **B**

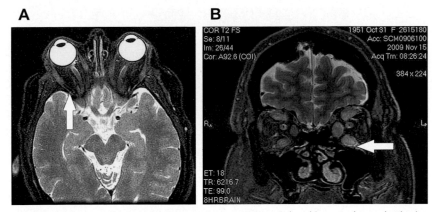

Fig. 12. (*A*) Axial MRI of the orbits shows edema on T2-weighted images (*arrow*). The lateral rectus is bright in areas of fluid accumulation and dark where edema is absent. (*B*) Coronal MRI shows edema in the inferior rectus (*arrow*).

is called lid lag. failure of the eyelid to close completely with passive eyelid closure (ie, not squeezing the eyelids shut) is called lagophthalmos (**Fig. 14**).

Evidence of active disease should be sought. The history is important: do the symptoms vary from day to day and over the course of the day (eg, diplopia and swelling are worse in the morning)? On examination, do the eyelids, conjunctiva, and caruncle appear red (injected) and retain fluid (periorbital edema and chemosis) (**Fig. 15**)?

Bulging of the eye forward is called exophthalmos or proptosis and can be quantified with a Hertel exophthalmometer (**Fig. 16**).

A dilated fundus examination should be performed. Despite prolonged compression or stretch, the optic nerve appearance is often grossly normal. Fundus photography is useful but OCT may also be helpful to detect preclinical optic nerve fiber loss (**Fig. 17**).

Depending on the clinical situation, CT scan of the orbits with no contrast (**Fig. 18**) or MRI of the orbits with gadolinium (**Fig. 19**), thyroid-function tests, or TSI could be obtained.

MANAGEMENT OPTIONS
Conservative Therapy

A variety of noninvasive patient recommendations can be provided to TED patients. These include using only artificial tears without preservatives to avoid toxicity, and

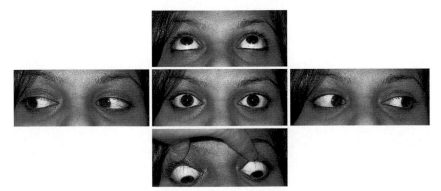

Fig. 13. A young woman with inactive TED showing mild proptosis, eyelid retraction, and excellent motility.

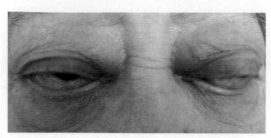

Fig. 14. Inability to close the eyes with passive closure (lagophthalmos) is accompanied by conjunctival injection, eyelid erythema and edema, and proptosis.

adding measures to keep the ocular surface moist at night even if the eyes open slightly (lagophthalmos). A bland topical eye ointment can be applied followed by Saran wrap and an eye mask. Details of an eye mask for patients with dry eyes or lagophthalmos from TED, seventh nerve dysfunction, or postsurgical conditions can be found at www.EyeEco.com. To improve ocular comfort, smoking should be discontinued.

Things to avoid or minimize in patients with TED

- Stress
- Tobacco, including secondhand smoke
- Salt and monosodium glutamate (MSG) in foods
- Fluorescent lighting
- Dry heat.

Ocular Therapeutics

In addition to artificial tears without preservatives, mast cell inhibitors (eg, Pataday) or topical T-cell modulators (cyclosporine formulated as Restasis or higher

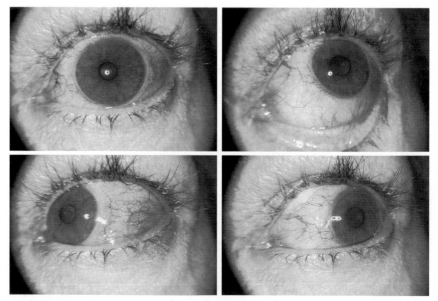

Fig. 15. Although the conjunctival injection associated with TED is classically most significant overlying the recti muscles, diffuse injection is common, as shown here.

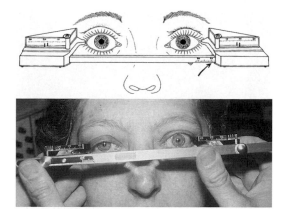

Fig. 16. Quantification of eye bulging (proptosis) with a Hertel exophthalmometer.

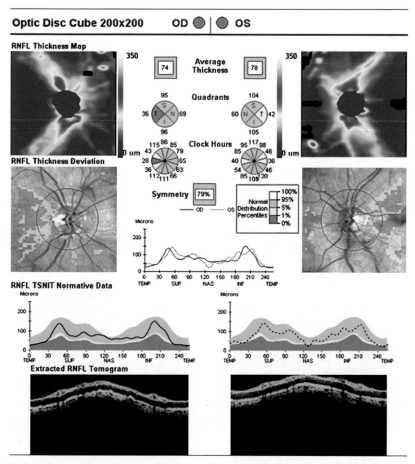

Fig. 17. OCT shows bilateral nerve fiber layer loss; green is normal for age, yellow is borderline, and red is abnormal.

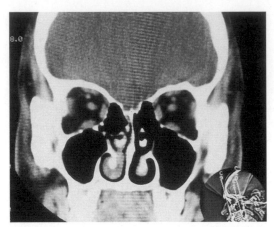

Fig. 18. Coronal CT of the orbits without contrast shows expanded intraconal fat with mildly enlarged EOM that are symmetric. This combination is most commonly misread as normal CT by radiology personnel.

concentrations by a compounding pharmacy) can be extremely helpful in controlling eye symptoms of itching, tearing, and irritation. Topical corticosteroids and nonsteroidal antiinflammatory drops have been remarkably disappointing in controlling the activity of disease or improving comfort.

Intranasal Therapeutics

The orbit is adjacent to the nasal cavity. The anterior and posterior ethmoidal foramen allow for egress, and the ethmoid thins and cracks in response to expansion of the

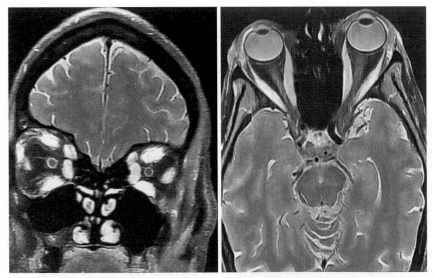

Fig. 19. Coronal and axial MRI shows the more classic enlargement of the EOMs with sparing of the tendons. The optic nerve is on stretch and the orbital apex crowded. This patient should be evaluated closely for optic neuropathy; OCT would be particularly helpful to identify occult optic nerve damage.

medial rectus and the intraorbital space. Nasonex (mometasone furoate monohydrate) is particularly hydrophilic, allowing entrance into the orbit. The side-effect profile is excellent; mild nasal bleeding or a sore throat may occur. Bone loss, gastrointestinal irritation, cholesterol, and glucose alterations are avoided. Retrobulbar injections of corticosteroids have also been used with success.

Corticosteroids

Options include topical, intranasal, retrobulbar, oral, and intravenous routes of administration. Topical steroids have not been found to be particularly helpful because the preservatives in the products are toxic and can exacerbate the disease.

Oral corticosteroids in an actively inflamed TED patient can result in a decrease in soft-tissue swelling, optic neuropathy, and EOM size in up to 65% of cases.[2,10,14] The effect is often short-term, with recurrence of symptoms and signs with taper. However, a short course of high-dose prednisone (60 mg each morning for 1 week) can be a useful test to predict the efficacy of external beam irradiation or other immunomodulation therapy.

The clinical response to intravenous corticosteroids is as high as 85%, with fewer side effects than oral prednisone. One meta-analysis of the literature suggests an overall corticosteroid-mediated treatment response of 69% in TED patients, which is similar to previously reported rates.[15,111–132] However, such statistical analyses are limited by a suboptimal definition of active disease, inconsistent inclusion criteria and outcome measures, dissimilar treatment protocols, and failure to assess long-term efficacy. Therefore, there is no evidence-based guidance or uniform opinion regarding therapeutic intervention with corticosteroids in TED.[2,4,14,133]

External-beam Radiation

Orbital irradiation remains an effective tool in the management of select TED patients in the active phase of the disease. Side effects include induction of a temporary dry eye state, mild erythema, and, rarely, eyelash or eyebrow hair loss. Visually significant radiation optic neuropathy and retinopathy occur infrequently in nondiabetic patients. Microaneurysm formation in retinal vessels has been reported but seems to have no clinical importance.

The use of orbital radiation varies widely and reflects the personal or regional experience of clinical groups. A well-controlled prospective clinical trial has not been performed. Prior studies failed to control for placebo effect of noncontrolled trials, had inadequate clinical assessment tools, and failed to control for variability of disease course. Recent prospective controlled trials reached conflicting conclusions that have generated confusion about the role of orbital irradiation in the treatment of thyroid-associated orbitopathy.[8,134–137] At least 7 investigators have called for further study or randomized controlled trials in peer-reviewed journals since the publication of the frequently cited study by Gorman and colleagues.[136–145]

Data addressing the efficacy of orbital irradiation, alone or in combination with other treatment modalities (corticosteroids, steroid sparing agents, surgery), are conflicting. A meta-analysis of 36 studies, with at least 20 subjects, suggests a 71% response rate of TED to orbital irradiation in 2048 irradiated patients.[138–166,157,167–174] This efficacy is similar to reported overall improvement rates of 60% to 65% in less inclusive meta-analyses in the literature.[142] Any future trial of radiation therapy must be a prospective, double-masked, placebo-controlled study, must include a direct comparison with corticosteroid treatment, and must recognize the potential for the 2 treatment methods to be additive or synergistic.

Other Immunomodulators

A variety of other therapies have been used with mixed success and significant side effects, including methotrexate, CellCept (mycophenolate mofetil), and cyclosporin. Somatostatin analogs that initially looked promising in retrospective case reports have not shown efficacy in subsequent systematic meta-analysis.[175]

Rituximab (RTX) has recently been used in severe, corticosteroid-resistant, or orbital decompression TED. RTX promotes antibody- and complement-dependent cellular toxicity and has been used to treat non-Hodgkin B-cell lymphomas. In a retrospective case series (n = 6), vision improved and inflammatory signs responded to a combination of oral or intravenous corticosteroids in combination with RTX infusion without relapse after discontinuation of therapy. Two infusions of 1 g of RTX were administered 2 weeks apart (the protocol used for rheumatoid arthritis).[176] Previous studies found clinical improvement and reduction of TSI levels in response to RTX, so a prospective clinical study is warranted.[177,178]

Surgical Rehabilitation

If optic nerve dysfunction is present as a result of compression or being on stretch, and the patient is also proptotic, orbital decompression is performed. If the globe position is normal, then external beam radiation is a potential stand-alone treatment or adjunct to surgical decompression.

In patients without visual compromise, reconstructive surgery is typically delayed until the TED patient is in the chronic phase of disease. Surgery can help restore the function and appearance that are crucial to their self-esteem and functioning. Surgical options include strabismus surgery to maximize visual function in primary gaze and down gaze. This surgery is typically performed after decompression surgery if it is needed. Eyelid and orbital reconstruction is performed to restore facial appearance (**Fig. 20**). However, no combination of therapies will completely restore eye movement or facial appearance, so communication with these challenging patients is crucial at each step of the rehabilitation.

Surgical options

- Eyelid retraction repair. Goal: eyelid closure, corneal protection, comfort
- Eye muscle surgery (strabismus surgery). Goal: single vision
- Orbital decompression. Goal: reduction of bulging, relief of pain, reduction of intraocular pressure, restoration of physical appearance.

QUALITY-OF-LIFE TOOLS

The TEDQOL (Thyroid Eye Disease Quality of Life) questionnaire was designed and used as a supplement to the 25-item National Eye Institute Visual Function Questionnaire (VFQ-25).[179,180] The TEDQOL supplement uses a combination of questions from other quality-of-life questionnaires to address double vision, difficulty focusing on or

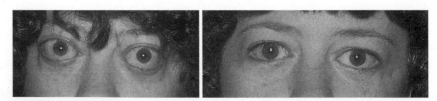

Fig. 20. Pre- and postoperative appearance after eyelid retraction repair of upper lids.

following moving objects, difficulty with vision when the eyes are tired (from the 10-item Neuro-ophthalmic Supplement [10-NOS]),[181–183] and self-esteem, self-confidence, and social interactions (from the European Graves Ophthalmopathy Quality-of-life Questionnaire [GO-QoL]).[184–189] The higher the TEDQOL score, the poorer the TED subjects' quality of life from a standpoint of visual disability and physical disfigurement. A prospective study of chronic TED patients found that 72% reported limitations in daily activities due to visual dysfunction, and 63% complained of the psychosocial consequences of disfigurement years after resolution of the active TED phase.[190]

SUMMARY

TED is a common disease that affects women more than men in the fourth and fifth decades of life. The inflammatory process is more severe in smokers, men, and the elderly. Myasthenia gravis may complicate the management of some TED patients. Visual dysfunction and facial alterations result in severely diminished quality of life for these patients.

TED patients may present to a neurologist's office with complaints of decreased vision, pain, or double vision. TED can mimic a partial third, sixth, or fourth nerve palsy or develop in a known myasthenia gravis patient.

TED suggestions for your practice

- Look for the stare; the look of TED
- Do not worry if the thyroid function tests are normal; TED is a clinical diagnosis
- Consider TED in all case of double vision
- Ptosis plus eyelid retraction should prompt myasthenia gravis evaluation
- TED can cause unexplained eye pain and headache.

Management of TED may include immunosuppressive medications, radiation, or surgery. A team approach is ideal, with the endocrinologist working closely with an ophthalmologist who has interest and subspecialty training in this disorder (ie, has completed a plastics, orbit, or neuro-ophthalmic fellowship; ophthalmology does not have subspecialty boards like those of neurology).

Although the prognosis for optic nerve function is excellent, the restrictive dysmotility can only be partially treated with strabismus surgery. There is no way to restore full pursuits. Orbit and eyelid reconstruction are the final steps in minimizing facial alterations and enhancing the patient's daily functioning.

ADDENDUM

The International Thyroid Eye Disease Study (ITEDS) group has developed VISA (Vision-Inflammation-Soft tissue-Activity). The score is detailed and requires significant time to prepare, making it most useful for prospective research purposes.

REFERENCES

1. Char DH. Thyroid eye disease. Br J Ophthalmol 1996;80:922–6.
2. Bartalena L, Pinchera A, Marcocci C. Management of Graves' ophthalmopathy: reality and perspectives. Endocr Rev 2000;21:168–99.
3. Wiersinga WM, Bartalena L. Epidemiology and prevention of Graves' ophthalmology. Thyroid 2002;12:855–60.

4. Kennerdell JS, Cockerham KP, Maroon JP, et al. Dysthyroid orbitopathy. In: Kennerdell JS, Cockerham KP, editors. Practical diagnosis and management of orbital disease. Boston: Butterworth/Heinemann Press; 2001. p. 53–75.
5. Kahaly GJ, Hardt J, Petrak F, et al. Psychosocial factors in subjects with thyroid-associated ophthalmopathy. Thyroid 2002;12(3):237–9.
6. Wiersinga WM, Prummel MF, Terwee CB. Effects of Graves' ophthalmopathy on quality of life. J Endocrinol Invest 2004;27(3):259–64.
7. Bahn RS. Pathophysiology of Graves' ophthalmology: the cycle of disease. J Clin Endocrinol Metab 2003;88:1939–46.
8. Kahaly GJ, Gorman CA, Kal HB. Radiotherapy for Graves' ophthalmopathy. In: Lightman S, McCluskey P, editors. Recent developments in Graves' ophthalmopathy. Boston: Kluwer Academic Publishers; 2000. p. 115–31.
9. Bartley GB, Fatourechi V, Kadrmas EF, et al. Clinical features of Graves' ophthalmopathy in an incidence cohort. Am J Ophthalmol 1996;121:284–90.
10. Clauser L, Galie M, Sarti E, et al. Rationale of treatment in Graves' ophthalmopathy. Plast Reconstr Surg 2001;108(7):1880–94.
11. Denniston A, Dodson P, Reuser T. Diagnosis and management of thyroid eye disease. Hosp Med 2002;63(3):153–6.
12. Krassas GE, Heufelder AE. Immunosuppressive therapy in patients with thyroid eye disease: an overview of current concepts. Eur J Endocrinol 2001;144:311–8.
13. Marcocci C, Bartalena L, Marino M, et al. Current medical management of Graves' ophthalmopathy. Ophthal Plast Reconstr Surg 2002;18(2):402–8.
14. Weetman AP, Wiersinga WM. Current management of thyroid associated ophthalmopathy in Europe. Results of an International Survey. Clin Endocrinol 1998;49:21–8.
15. Prummel MF, Bakker A, Wiersinga WM, et al. Multi-center study on the characteristics and treatment strategies of patients with Graves' orbitopathy: the first European Group on Graves' orbitopathy experience. Eur J Endocrinol 2003; 148(5):491–5.
16. De Carli M, D'Elios MM, Mariotti S, et al. Cytolytic T cells with Th1-like cytokine profile predominate in retroorbital lymphocytic infiltrates of Graves' ophthalmopathy. J Clin Endocrinol Metab 1994;77:1120–4.
17. Pritchard J, Han R, Horst N, et al. Immunoglobulin activation of T cell chemoattractant expression in fibroblasts from patients with Graves' disease is mediated through the insulin-like growth factor I receptor pathway. J Immunol 2003;170: 6348–54.
18. Makinen T, Wagar G, Apter L, et al. Evidence that the TSH receptor acts as a mitogenic antigen in Graves' disease. Nature 1978;275:314–5.
19. Heufelder AE, Dutton CM, Sarkar G, et al. Detection of TSH receptor RNA in cultured fibroblasts from patients with Graves' ophthalmopathy and pretibial dermopathy. Thyroid 1993;3:297–300.
20. Bell A, Gagnon A, Grunder L, et al. Functional TSH receptor in human abdominal preadipocytes and orbital fibroblasts. Am J Physiol Cell Physiol 2000;279.
21. Crisp M, Lane C, Hallwell M, et al. Thyrotropin receptor transcripts in human adipose tissue. J Clin Endocrinol Metab 1997;82:2003–5.
22. Smith TJ, Koumas L, Gagnon A, et al. Orbital fibroblast heterogeneity may determine the clinical presentation of thyroid-associated ophthalmopathy. J Clin Endocrinol Metab 2002;87:385–92.
23. Smith TJ. Orbital fibroblasts exhibit a novel pattern of responses to proinflammatory cytokines: potential basis for the pathogenesis of thyroid-associated ophthalmopathy. Thyroid 2002;12:197–203.

24. Bahn RS, Gorman CA, Woloschak GE, et al. Human retroocular fibroblasts in vitro: a model for the study of Graves' ophthalmopathy. J Clin Endocrinol Metab 1987;65:665–70.
25. Bahn RS, Heufelder AE. Retroocular fibroblasts: important effector cells in Graves' ophthalmopathy. Thyroid 1992;2:89–94.
26. Pritchard J, Horst N, Cruikshank W, et al. Immunoglobulins from patients with Graves' disease induce the expression of T cell chemoattractants in their fibroblasts. J Immunol 2002;168:942–50.
27. Bahn RS. The fibroblast is the target cell in the connective tissue manifestations of Graves' disease. Int Arch Allergy Immunol 1995;106:213–8 [Review] [44 refs].
28. Hufnagel TJ, Hickey WF, Cobbs WH, et al. Immunohistochemical and ultrastructural studies on the exenterated orbital tissues of a patient with Graves' disease. Ophthalmology 1984;91:1411–9.
29. Wang HS, Cao HJ, Winn VD, et al. Leukoregulin induction of prostaglandin-endoperoxide H synthase-2 in human orbital fibroblasts. J Biol Chem 1996; 271:22718–28.
30. Smith TJ, Bahn RS, Gorman CA, et al. Stimulation of glycosaminoglycan accumulation by interferon gamma in cultured human retroocular fibroblasts. J Clin Endocrinol Metab 1991;72:1169–71.
31. Spicer AP, Kaback LA, Smith TJ, et al. Molecular cloning and characterization of the human and mouse UDP-glucose dehydrogenase genes. J Biol Chem 1998; 273:25117–24.
32. Smith TJ, Wang HS, Evans C. Leukoregulin is a potent inducer of hyaluronan synthesis in cultured human orbital fibroblasts. Am J Physiol 1995;268: C382–8.
33. Cao HJ, Smith TJ. Leukoregulin up regulation of prostaglandin endoperoxide H synthase-2 expression in human orbital fibroblasts. Am J Physiol 1999;277 (6 Pt 1):C1075–85.
34. Muhlberg T, Heberling HJ, Joba W, et al. Detection and modulation of interleukin-1 receptor antagonist messenger ribonucleic acid and immunoreactivity in Graves' orbital fibroblasts. Invest Ophthalmol Vis Sci 1997;38:1018–28.
35. Sempowski GD, Rozenblit J, Smith TJ, et al. Human orbital fibroblasts are activated through CD40 to induce proinflammatory cytokine production. Am J Physiol 1998;274(3 Pt 1):C707–14.
36. Cao HJ, Wang HS, Zhang Y, et al. Activation of human orbital fibroblasts through CD40 engagement results in a dramatic induction of hyaluronan synthesis and prostaglandin endoperoxide H synthase-2 expression. Insights into potential pathogenic mechanisms of thyroid-associated ophthalmopathy. J Biol Chem 1998;273:29615–25.
37. Stassi G, Di Liberto D, Todaro M, et al. Control of target cell survival in thyroid autoimmunity by T helper cytokines via regulation of apoptotic proteins [see comment]. Nat Immunol 2000;1:483–8.
38. Yang D, Hiromatsu Y, Hoshino T, et al. Dominant infiltration of T (H) 1-type CD4+ T cells at the retrobulbar space of patients with thyroid-associated ophthalmopathy. Thyroid 1999;9:305–10.
39. Aniszewski JP, Valyasevi RW, Bahn RS. Relationship between disease duration and predominant orbital T cell subset in Graves' ophthalmopathy. J Clin Endocrinol Metab 2000;85:776–80.
40. Smith TJ, Wang HS, Hogg MG, et al. Prostaglandin E2 elicits a morphological change in cultured orbital fibroblasts from patients with Graves ophthalmopathy. Proc Natl Acad Sci U S A 1994;91:5094–8.

41. Tallstedt L, Lundell G, Torring O, et al. Occurrence of ophthalmopathy after treatment for Graves' hyperthyroidism. N Engl J Med 1992;326:1733–8.
42. Kung AEC, Yau CC, Cheng A. The incidence of ophthalmopathy after radioiodine therapy for Graves' disease: prognostic factors and the role of methimazole. J Clin Endocrinol Metab 1994;79:542–6.
43. Noury AMS, Stanford MR, Graham EM. Radioiodine and Graves' ophthalmopathy reconsidered. Nucl Med Commun 2001;22:1167–9.
44. Bartalena L. Radioiodine therapy and Graves' ophthalmopathy. Nucl Med Commun 2002;23:1143–5.
45. Rasmussen AK, Nygaard B, Feldt-Rasmussen U. I131 and thyroid-associated ophthalmopathy. Eur J Endocrinol 2000;143:155–60.
46. Bartalena L, Marcocci C, Bogazzi F, et al. Relation between therapy for hyperthyroidism and the course of Graves' ophthalmopathy. N Engl J Med 1998;338:73–8.
47. Bartalena L, Marococci C, Pinchera A. Graves' ophthalmology: a preventable disease? Eur J Endocrinol 2002;146:457–61.
48. Tallstedt L, Lundell G, Taube A. Graves' ophthalmopathy and tobacco smoking. Acta Endocrinologica 1993;129:147–50.
49. Prummel MF, Wiersinga WM. Smoking and risk of Graves' disease. JAMA 1993;260:479–82.
50. Pfelschifter J, Ziegler R. Smoking and endocrine ophthalmopathy: impact of smoking severity and current vs. lifetime cigarette consumption. Clin Endocrinol 1996;45:477–81.
51. Vestergaard P. Smoking and thyroid disorders – a meta-analysis. Eur J Endocrinol 2002;146:153–61.
52. Eckstein A, Quadbeck B, Mueller G, et al. Impact of smoking on the response to treatment of thyroid associated ophthalmopathy. Br J Ophthalmol 2003;87(6):773–6.
53. Werner SC. Modification of the classification of the eye changes of Graves' disease: recommendations of the Ad Hoc Committee of the American Thyroid Association. J Clin Endocrinol Metab 1977;44:203–4.
54. Mourits MP, Koornneef L, Wiersinga WM, et al. Clinical criteria for the assessment of disease activity in Graves' ophthalmopathy: a novel approach. Br J Ophthalmol 1989;73:639–44.
55. Wiersinga WM, Prummel MF, Mourits MP, et al. Classification of the eye changes of Graves' disease. Thyroid 1991;1(4):357–60.
56. Gorman CA. The measurement of change in Graves' ophthalmopathy. Thyroid 1998;8:539–43.
57. Dickinson AJ, Perros P. Controversies in the clinical evaluation of active thyroid-associated orbitopathy: use of a detailed protocol with comparative photographs for objective assessment. Clin Endocrinol (Oxf) 2001;55:283–303.
58. Bartley GB, Gorman CA. Diagnostic criteria for Graves' ophthalmopathy. Am J Ophthalmol 1995;119:792–5.
59. Mourits MP, Prummel MF, Wiersinga WM, et al. Clinical activity score as a guide in the management of patients with Graves' ophthalmopathy. Clin Endocrinol (Oxf) 1997;47:9–14.
60. Gerding MN, Prummel MF, Wiersinga WM. Assessment of disease activity in Graves' ophthalmopathy by orbital ultrasonography and clinical parameters. Clin Endocrinol (Oxf) 2000;52:641–6.
61. Kahaly G, Schuler M, Sewell AC, et al. Urinary glycosaminoglycans in Graves' ophthalmopathy. Clin Endocrinol (Oxf) 1990;33:35–44.

62. Kahaly G, Hansen C, Beyer J, et al. Plasma glycosaminoglycans in endocrine ophthalmopathy. J Endocrinol Invest 1994;17:45–50.
63. Kahaly G, Forster G. Hansen glycosaminoglycans in thyroid eye disease. Thyroid 1998;8:429–32.
64. Martins JR, Furlanetto RP, Oliveira LM, et al. Comparison of practical methods for urinary glycosaminoglycans and serum hyaluronan with clinical activity scores in patients with Graves' ophthalmopathy. Clin Endocrinol (Oxf) 2004;60:726–33.
65. Kahaly G, Diaz M, Just M, et al. Role of Octreoscan and correlation with MR imaging in Graves' ophthalmopathy. Thyroid 1995;5:107–11.
66. Postema PT, Krenning EP, Wijngaarde R, et al. van der Loos T [111In-DTPA-D-Phe1] octreotide scintigraphy in thyroid and orbital Graves' disease: a parameter for disease activity? J Clin Endocrinol Metab 1994;79:1845–51.
67. Morris JC 3rd, Hay ID, Nelson RE, et al. Clinical utility of thyrotropin-receptor antibody assays: comparison of radioreceptor and bioassay methods. Mayo Clin Proc 1988;63:707–17.
68. Jiang NS, Fairbanks VF, Hay ID. Assay for thyroid stimulating immunoglobulin. Mayo Clin Proc 1986;61:753–5.
69. Gerding MN, van der Meer JW, Broenink M, et al. Association of thyrotropin receptor antibodies with the clinical features of Graves' ophthalmology. Clin Endocrinol (Oxf) 2000;52:267–71.
70. Noh JY, Hamada N, Inoue Y, et al. Thyroid-stimulating antibody is related to Graves' ophthalmopathy, but thyrotropin-binding inhibitor immunoglobulin is related to hyperthyroidism in patients with Graves' disease. Thyroid 2000;10:809–13.
71. Khoo DH, Ho SC, Seah LL, et al. The combination of absent thyroid peroxidase antibodies and high thyroid-stimulating immunoglobulin levels in Graves' disease identifies a group at markedly increased risk of ophthalmopathy. Thyroid 1999;9:1175–80.
72. Khoo DH, Eng PH, Ho SC, et al. Graves' ophthalmopathy in the absence of elevated free thyroxine and triiodothyronine levels: prevalence, natural history, and thyrotropin receptor antibody levels. Thyroid 2000;10:1093–100.
73. Goh SY, Ho SC, Seah LL, et al. Thyroid autoantibody profiles in ophthalmic dominant and thyroid dominant Graves' disease differ and suggest ophthalmopathy is a multiantigenic disease. Clin Endocrinol (Oxf) 2004;60:600–7.
74. De Bellis A, Bizzarro A, Conte M, et al. Relationship between longitudinal behaviour of some markers of eye autoimmunity and changes in ocular findings in patients with Graves' ophthalmopathy receiving corticosteroid therapy. Clin Endocrinol (Oxf) 2003;59:388–95.
75. Rapoport B, Greenspan FS, Filetti S, et al. Clinical experience with a human thyroid cell bioassay for thyroid-stimulating immunoglobulin. J Clin Endocrinol Metab 1984;58:332–8.
76. Kazuo K, Fujikado T, Ohmi G, et al. Value of thyroid stimulating antibody in the diagnosis of thyroid associated ophthalmopathy of euthyroid patients. Br J Ophthalmol 1997;81:1080–3.
77. Strakosch CR, Wenzel BE, Row VV, et al. Immunology of autoimmune thyroid diseases. N Engl J Med 1982;307:1499–507.
78. Kashiwai T, Tada H, Asahi K, et al. Significance of thyroid stimulating antibody and long term follow up in patients with euthyroid Graves' disease. Endocr J 1995;42:405–12.
79. Teng CS, Smith BR, Clayton B, et al. Thyroid-stimulating immunoglobulins in ophthalmic Graves' disease. Clin Endocrinol (Oxf) 1977;6:207–11.

80. Fenzi G, Hashizume K, Roudebush CP, et al. Changes in thyroid-stimulating immunoglobulins during antithyroid therapy. J Clin Endocrinol Metab 1979;48: 572–6.
81. Salvi M, Zhang ZG, Haegert D, et al. Patients with endocrine ophthalmopathy not associated with overt thyroid disease have multiple thyroid immunological abnormalities. J Clin Endocrinol Metab 1990;70:89–94.
82. Rapoport B, Chazenbalk GD, Jaume JC, et al. The thyrotropin receptor: interaction with thyrotropin and autoantibodies. Endocr Rev 1998;19:673–716.
83. Wu YJ, Clarke SEM, Shepherd P. Prevalence and significance of antibodies reactive with eye muscle membrane antigens in sera from patients with Graves' ophthalmopathy and other thyroid and non-thyroid diseases. Thyroid 1998;8:167.
84. Villadolid MC, Yokoyama N, Izumi M, et al. Untreated Graves' disease patients without clinical ophthalmopathy demonstrate a high frequency of extraocular muscle (EOM) enlargement by magnetic resonance. J Clin Endocrinol Metab 1995;80:2830–3.
85. Hosten N, Schorner W, Lietz A, et al. [The course of the disease in endocrine orbitopathy. Magnetic resonance tomographic documentation]. Rofo 1992; 157:210–4 [in German].
86. Yokoyama N, Nagataki S, Uetani M, et al. Role of magnetic resonance imaging in the assessment of disease activity in thyroid-associated ophthalmopathy. Thyroid 2002;12:223–7.
87. Prummel MF, Gerding MN, Zonneveld FW, et al. The usefulness of quantitative orbital magnetic resonance imaging in Graves' ophthalmopathy. Clin Endocrinol (Oxf) 2001;54:205–9.
88. Weber AL, Dallow RL, Sabates NR. Graves' disease of the orbit. Neuroimaging Clin N Am 1996;6:61–72.
89. Nishida Y, Tian S, Isberg B, et al. MRI measurements of orbital tissues in dysthyroid ophthalmopathy. Graefes Arch Clin Exp Ophthalmol 2001;239:824–31.
90. Cakirer S, Cakirer D, Basak M, et al. Evaluation of extraocular muscles in the edematous phase of Graves ophthalmopathy on contrast-enhanced fat-suppressed magnetic resonance imaging. J Comput Assist Tomogr 2004;28:80–6.
91. Hoh HB, Laitt RD, Wakeley C, et al. The STIR sequence MRI in the assessment of extraocular muscles in thyroid eye disease. Eye 1994;8(Pt 5):506–10.
92. Sillaire I, Ravel A, Dalens H, et al. Graves' ophthalmopathy: usefulness of T2 weighted muscle signal intensity. J Radiol 2003;84:139–42.
93. Laitt RD, Hoh B, Wakeley C, et al. The value of the short tau inversion recovery sequence in magnetic resonance imaging of thyroid eye disease. Br J Radiol 1994;67:244–7.
94. Mayer E, Herdman G, Burnett C, et al. Serial STIR magnetic resonance imaging correlates with clinical score of activity in thyroid disease. Eye 2001;15:313–8.
95. Utech CI, Khatibnia U, Winter PF, et al. MR T2 relaxation time for the assessment of retrobulbar inflammation in Graves' ophthalmopathy. Thyroid 1995;5:185–93.
96. Ohnishi T, Noguchi S, Murakami N, et al. Extraocular muscles in Graves ophthalmopathy: usefulness of T2 relaxation time measurements. Radiology 1994; 190:857–62.
97. Ott M, Breiter N, Albrecht CF, et al. Can contrast enhanced MRI predict the response of Graves' ophthalmopathy to orbital radiotherapy? Br J Radiol 2002;75:514–7.
98. Sato M, Hiromatsu Y, Tanaka K, et al. [Prediction for effectiveness of steroid pulse therapy by MRI in Graves' ophthalmopathy]. Nippon Naibunpi Gakkai Zasshi 1992;68:143–53 [in Japanese].

99. Hiromatsu Y, Kojima K, Ishisaka N, et al. Role of magnetic resonance imaging in thyroid-associated ophthalmopathy: its predictive value for therapeutic outcome of immunosuppressive therapy. Thyroid 1992;2:299–305.

100. Prummel MF, Suttorp-Schulten MSA, Wiersinga WM, et al. A new ultrasonographic method to detect disease activity and predict response to immunosuppressive treatment in Graves' ophthalmopathy. Ophthalmology 1993;100:556–61.

101. Krassas GE, Kahly GJ. The role of Octreoscan in thyroid eye disease. Eur J Endocrinol 1999;140(5):373–5.

102. Krassas GE. Octreoscan in thyroid associated ophthalmopathy. Thyroid 2002; 12(3):229–33.

103. Rosenfeld RG, Doll LA. Characterization of the somatomedin C/insulin like growth factor I (SM-C/IGF-I) receptor on cultured human fibroblast monolayers. Regulation of receptor concentrations by SM-C/IGF-I and insulin. J Clin Endocrinol Metab 1982;55:434–40.

104. Jacobs S. Somatomedin-C stimulates the phosphorylation of the beta-subunit of its own receptor. J Biol Chem 1983;258:9581–4.

105. Prisco M, Hongo A, Rizzo MG, et al. The insulin like growth factor I receptor as a physiologically relevant target of p53 in apoptosis caused by interleukin 3 withdrawal. Mol Cell Biol 1997;17:1084–92.

106. Mashikian MV, Ryan TC, Seman A, et al. Reciprocal desensitization fo CCR5 and CD4 is mediated by IL-16 and macrophage-inflammatory protein-1 beta, respectively. J Immunol 1999;163(6):3123–30.

107. Adams TE, Epa VC, Garrett TP, et al. Structure and function of the type 1 insulin-like growth factor receptor. Cell Mol Life Sci 2000;57:1050–93.

108. Grimberg A, Cohen P. Role of insulin-like growth factors and their binding proteins in growth control and carcinogenesis. J Cell Physiol 2000;183:1–9.

109. De Meyts P, Palsgaard J, Sajid W, et al. Structural biology of insulin and IGF-1 receptors. Novartis Found Symp 2004;262:160–71 [discussion: 171–6, 265–8].

110. Smith TJ, Hoa N. Immunoglobulins from patients with Graves' disease induce hyaluronan synthesis in their orbital fibroblasts through the self-antigen, insulin-like growth factor-I receptor. J Clin Endocrinol Metab 2004; 89:5076–80.

111. Bartalena L, Marcocci C, Chiovato L, et al. Orbital cobalt irradiation combined with systemic corticosteroids for Graves' ophthalmopathy: comparison with systemic corticosteroids alone. J Clin Endocrinol Metab 1983;56(6):1139–44.

112. Bartalena L, Marcocci C, Bogazzi F, et al. Use of corticosteroids to prevent progression of Graves' ophthalmopathy after radioiodine therapy for hyperthyroidism. N Engl J Med 1989;321:1349–52.

113. Baschieri L, Antonelli A, Nardi S, et al. Intravenous immunoglobulin vs. corticosteroids in treatment of Graves' ophthalmopathy. Thyroid 1997;7:579–85.

114. Chang T-C, Kao SC, Hsiao YL, et al. Therapeutic responses to corticosteroids in Graves' ophthalmopathy. J Formos Med Assoc 1996;95(11):833–8.

115. Chang TC, Huang KM, Hsiao YL, et al. Relationships of orbital computed tomography and activity scores to the prognosis of corticosteroid therapy in patients with Graves' ophthalmopathy. Acta Ophthalmol Scand 1997;75(3):301–4.

116. Dandona P, Havard CW, Mier A. Methylprednisolone and Graves' ophthalmopathy. BMJ 1989;298(6676):830.

117. Ebner R, Devoto MH, Weil D, et al. Treatment of thyroid associated ophthalmopathy with periocular injections of triamcinolone. Br J Ophthalmol 2004;88(11):1380–6.

118. Guy JR, Fagien S, Donovan JP, et al. Methylprednisolone pulse therapy in severe dysthyroid optic neuropathy. Ophthalmology 1989;96:1048–53.

119. Hiromatsu Y, Tanaka K, Sato M, et al. Intravenous methylprednisolone pulse therapy for Graves' ophthalmopathy. Endocr J 1993;40:63–72.
120. Kauppinen-Makelin R, Karma A, Leinonen E, et al. High dose intravenous methylprednisolone pulse therapy versus oral prednisone for thyroid-associated ophthalmopathy. Acta ophthalmol Scand 2002;80(3):316–21.
121. Kazim M, Trokel S, Moore S. Treatment of acute Graves' orbitopathy. Ophthalmology 1991;98(9):1443–8.
122. Kendall-Taylor P, Crombie AL, Stephenson AM, et al. Intravenous methylprednisolone in the treatment of Graves' ophthalmopathy. Br Med J 1988;297:1574–8.
123. Koshiyama H, Koh T, Fujiwara K, et al. Therapy of Graves' ophthalmopathy with intravenous high-dose steroid followed by orbital irradiation. Thyroid 1994;4:409–13.
124. Matejka G, Verges B, Vaillant G, et al. Intravenous methylprednisolone pulse therapy in the treatment of Graves' ophthalmopathy. Horm Metab Res 1998; 30(2):93–8.
125. Noth D, Gebauer M, Muller B, et al. Graves' ophthalmopathy: natural history and treatment outcomes. Swiss Med Wkly 2001;131(41–42):603–9.
126. Nagayama Y, Izumi M, Kiriyama T, et al. Treatment of Graves' ophthalmopathy with high-dose intravenous methylprednisolone pulse therapy. Acta Endocrinol 1987;116:513–8.
127. Nakahara H, Noguchi S, Murakami N, et al. Graves ophthalmopathy: MR evaluation of 10-Gy versus 24-Gy irradiation combined with systemic corticosteroids. Radiology 1995;196(3):857–62.
128. Ohtsuka K, Sato A, Kawaguchi S, et al. Effect of steroid pulse therapy with and without orbital radiotherapy on Graves' ophthalmopathy. Am J Ophthalmol 2003; 135(3):285–90.
129. Staar S, Muller RP, Hammer M, et al. Results and prognostic factors in retrobulbar radiotherapy combined with systemic corticosteroids for endocrine orbitopathy (Graves' disease). Front Radiat Ther Oncol 1997;30:206–17.
130. Prummel MF, Mourits MP, Berghout A, et al. Prednisolone and cyclosporine in the treatment of severe Graves' ophthalmopathy. N Engl J Med 1989;321:1353–9.
131. Scott IU, Siatrkowski M. Thyroid eye disease. Semin Ophthalmol 1999;14(2):52–61.
132. Tagami T, Tanaka K, Sugawa H, et al. High-dose intravenous steroid pulse therapy in thyroid-associated ophthalmopathy. Endocr J 1996;43(6):689–99.
133. Zoumalan CI, Cockerham KP, Turbin RE. Efficacy of corticosteroids and external beam radiation in the management of moderate to severe thyroid eye disease. J Neuroophthalmol 2007;27:205–14.
134. Bartley GB, Gorman CA. Perspective–Part I: the Mayo Orbital Radiotherapy for Graves Ophthalmopathy (ORGO) study: lessons learned. Ophthal Plast Reconstr Surg 2002;18(3):170–2.
135. Mourits MP, van Kempen-Harteveld ML, Garcia MB, et al. Radiotherapy for Graves' orbitopathy: randomized placebo-controlled study. Lancet 2000;355:1505–9.
136. Gorman CA, Garrity JA, Fatourechi V, et al. A prospective, randomized, double blind, placebo-controlled study of orbital radiotherapy for Graves' ophthalmopathy. Ophthalmology 2001;108:1523–34.
137. Prummel MF, Terwee CB, Gerding MN, et al. A randomized controlled trial of orbital radiotherapy versus sham irradiation in patients with mild Graves' ophthalmopathy. J Clin Endocrinol Metab 2004;89(1):15–20.
138. Perros P, Krassas GE. Orbital irradiation for thyroid-associated orbitopathy: conventional dose, low dose or no dose? Clin Endocrinol 2002;56(6):689–91.
139. Cockerham KP, Kennerdell JS. Does radiotherapy have a role in the management of thyroid orbitopathy? Br J Ophthalmol 2002;86(1):102–4.

140. McNab AA. Does radiotherapy have a role in the management of thyroid orbitopathy? Comment. Br J Ophthalmol 2002;86(1):106–7.
141. Feldon SE. Radiation therapy for Graves' ophthalmopathy: trick or treat? Ophthalmology 2001;108(9):1521–2.
142. Bartalena L. Orbital radiation therapy for Graves' ophthalmopathy. Ophthalmology 2003;110(3):452–3.
143. Meyer DR. Orbital radiation therapy for Graves' ophthalmology. (letter). Ophthalmology 2003;110(3):450–1.
144. Ainbinder DJ, Halligan JB. Orbital radiation therapy for Graves' ophthalmology. (letter). Ophthalmology 2003;110:449.
145. Beckendorf V, Maalouf T, George JL, et al. Place of radiotherapy in the treatment of Graves' orbitopathy. Int J Radiat Oncol Biol Phys 1999;43(4):805–15.
146. Claridge KG, Ghabrial R, Davis G, et al. Combined radiotherapy and medical immunosuppression in the management of thyroid eye disease. Eye 1997; 11(Pt 5):717–22.
147. Donaldson SS, Bagshaw MA, Kriss JP. Supervoltage orbital radiotherapy for Graves' ophthalmopathy. J Clin Endocrinol Metab 1973;37(2):276–85.
148. Erickson BA, Harris GJ, Lewandowski MF, et al. Echographic monitoring of response of extraocular muscles to irradiation in Graves' ophthalmopathy. Int J Radiat Oncol Biol Phys 1995;31(3):651–60.
149. Ferris JD, Dawson EL, Plowman N, et al. Radiotherapy in thyroid eye disease: the effect on the field of binocular single vision. J AAPOS 2002;6(2):71–6.
150. Friedrich A, Kamprad F, Goldmann A. Clinical importance of radiotherapy in the treatment of Graves' disease. Front Radiat Ther Oncol 1997;30:195–205.
151. Jing J, Kommerell G, Henne K, et al. Retrobulbar irradiation for thyroid-associated orbitopathy: double-blind comparison between 2.4 and 16 Gy. Int J Radiat Oncol Biol Phys 2003;55(1):182–9.
152. Gorman CA, Garrity JA, Fatourechi V, et al. The aftermath of orbital radiotherapy for Graves' ophthalmopathy. Ophthalmology 2002;109(11):2100–7.
153. Gorman CA. Radiotherapy for Graves' ophthalmopathy: results at one year. Thyroid 2002;12:251–5.
154. Heyd R, Strassmann G, Herkstroter M, et al. Hypofractionated radiotherapy for Graves' orbitopathy. Rontgenpraxis 2001;54(3):94–100.
155. Hurbli T, Char DH, Harris J, et al. Radiation therapy for thyroid eye diseases. Am J Ophthalmol 1985;99(6):633–7.
156. Just M, Kahaly G, Higer HP, et al. Graves's ophthalmopathy: role of MR imaging in radiation therapy. Radiology 1991;179(1):187–90.
157. Kahaly GJ, Rosler HP, Pitz S, et al. Low- versus high-dose radiotherapy for Graves' ophthalmopathy: a randomized, single blind trial. J Clin Endocrinol Metab 2000;85(1):102–8.
158. Kao SC, Kendler DL, Nugent RA, et al. Radiotherapy in the management of thyroid orbitopathy. Computed tomography and clinical outcomes. Arch Ophthalmol 1993;111(6):819–23.
159. Lloyd WC 3rd, Leone CR Jr. Supervoltage orbital radiotherapy in 36 cases of Graves' disease. Am J Ophthalmol 1992;113(4):374–80.
160. Marcocci C, Bartalena L, Panicucci M, et al. Orbital cobalt irradiation combined with retrobulbar or systemic corticosteroids for Graves' ophthalmopathy: a comparative study. Clin Endocrinol 1987;27(1):33–42.
161. Marquez SD, Lum BL, McDougall IR, et al. Long-term results of irradiation for patients with progressive Graves' ophthalmopathy. Int J Radiat Oncol Biol Phys 2001;51(3):766–74.

162. Olivotto IA, Ludgate CM, Allen LH, et al. Supervoltage radiotherapy for Graves' ophthalmopathy: CCABC technique and results. Int J Radiat Oncol Biol Phys 1985;11(12):2085–90.

163. Palmer D, Greenberg P, Cornell P, et al. Radiation therapy for Graves' ophthalmopathy: a retrospective analysis. Int J Radiat Oncol Biol Phys 1987;13(12): 1815–20.

164. Petersen IA, Kriss JP, McDougall IR, et al. Prognostic factors in the radiotherapy of Graves' ophthalmopathy. Int J Radiat Oncol Biol Phys 1990;19(2):259–64.

165. Pigeon P, Orgiazzi J, Berthezene F, et al. High voltage orbital radiotherapy and surgical orbital decompression in the management of Graves' ophthalmopathy. Horm Res 1987;26:172–6.

166. Prummel MF, Mourits MP, Blank L, et al. Randomized double-blind trial of prednisone versus radiotherapy in Graves' ophthalmopathy. Lancet 1993;342(8877): 949–54.

167. Sakata K, Hareyama M, Oouchi A, et al. Radiotherapy in the management of Graves' ophthalmopathy. Jpn J Clin Oncol 1998;28(6):364–7.

168. Sandler HM, Rubenstein JH, Fowble BL, et al. Results of radiotherapy for thyroid ophthalmopathy. Int J Radiat Oncol Biol Phys 1989;17(4):823–7.

169. Seegenschmiedt MH, Keilholz L, Becker W, et al. Radiotherapy for severe, progressive thyroid-associated ophthalmopathy: long-term results with comparison of scoring systems. Front Radiat Ther Oncol 1997;30:218–28.

170. Steinsapir KD, Goldberg RA. Orbital radiation therapy for Graves' ophthalmology. (letter). Ophthalmology 2003;110:451–2.

171. Teng CS, Crombie AL, Hall R, et al. An evaluation of supervoltage orbital irradiation for Graves' ophthalmopathy. Clin Endocrinol 1980;13:545.

172. van Ouwerkerk BM, Wijngaarde R, Hennemann G, et al. Radiotherapy of severe ophthalmic Graves' disease. J Endocrinol Invest 1985;8(3):241–7.

173. Wiersinga WM, Smit T, Schuster-Uittenhoeve AL, et al. Therapeutic outcome of prednisone medication and of orbital irradiation in patients with Graves' ophthalmopathy. Ophthalmologica 1988;197(2):75–84.

174. Wilson WB, Prochoda M. Radiotherapy for thyroid orbitopathy. Effects on extraocular muscle balance. Arch Ophthalmol 1995;113(11):1420–5.

175. Stiebel-Kalish H, Robenshtok E, Hasanreisoglu M, et al. Treatment modalities for Graves' ophthalmopathy: systemic review and metaanalysis. J Clin Endocrinol Metab 2009;94(8):2708–16.

176. Khanna D, Chong K, Nikoo A, et al. Rituximab Treatment of patients with severe, corticosteroid resistant thyroid associated ophthalmopathy. Ophthalmology 2010;117:133–9.

177. El Fassi D, Nielsonen CH, Hasselbalch HC, et al. The rationale for B lymphocyte depletion in Graves' disease: monoclonal anti-CD20 antibody therapy as a novel treatment option. Eur J Endocrinol 2006;154:623–32.

178. El Fassi D, Banga JP, Gilbert JA, et al. Treatment of Graves' disease with Rituximab specifically reduces the production of thyroid stimulating autoantibodies. Clin Immunol 2009;130:252–8.

179. Mangione CM, Berry S, Spritzer K, et al. Identifying the content area for the 51-item National Eye Institute Visual Function Questionnaire: results from focus groups with visually impaired persons. Arch Ophthalmol 1998;116:227–33.

180. Mangione CM, Lee PP, Gutierrez PR, , et alNational Eye Institute Visual Function Questionnaire Field Test Investigators. Development of the 25-Item National Eye Institute Visual Function Questionnaire (VFQ-25). Arch Ophthalmol 2001;119: 1050–8.

181. Mangione CM, Lee PP, Pitts J, , et alNEI-VFQ Field Test Investigators. Psycho-metric properties of the National Eye Institute Visual Function Questionnaire (NEI-VFQ). Arch Ophthalmol 1998;116:1496–504.

182. Ma SL, Shea JA, Galetta SL, et al. Self-reported visual dysfunction in multiple sclerosis: new data from the VFQ-25 and development of an MS-specific vision questionnaire. Am J Ophthalmol 2002;133:686–92.

183. Raphael BA, Galetta K, Nano-Schiavi ML, et al. Validation of a 10-Item Neuro-Ophthalmic Supplement to the VFQ-25. Neurology 2005;64(Suppl 1):A37.

184. Terwee CB, Gerding MD, Dekker FW, et al. Test-retest reliability of the GO-QOL: a disease-specific quality of life questionnaire for patients with Graves' oph-thalmopathy. J Clin Epidemiol 1999;52(9):875–84.

185. Terwee C, Wakelkamp I, Tan S, et al. Long-term effects of Graves' ophthalmop-athy on health-related quality of life. Eur J Endocrinol 2002;146:751–7.

186. Terwee CB, Gerding MD, Dekker FW, et al. Development of a disease specific quality of life questionnaire for patients with Graves' ophthalmopathy: the GO-QOL. Br J Ophthalmol 1998;82:773–9.

187. Tehrain M, Krummenauer F, Mann WJ, et al. Disease-specific assessment of quality of life after decompression surgery for Graves' ophthalmopathy. Eur J Ophthalmol 2004;14(3):193–9.

188. Park JJ, Sullivan TJ, Mortimer RH, et al. Assessing quality of life in Australian patients with Graves' ophthalmopathy. Br J Ophthalmol 2004;99:75–8.

189. Terwee CB, Dekker FW, Mourits MP, et al. Interpretation and validity of changes in scores on the Graves' ophthalmopathy quality of life questionnaire (GO-QOL) after different treatments. Clin Endocrinol 2001;54:391–8.

190. Eberling TV, Ramussen AK, Feldt-Ramussen U, et al. Impaired health-related quality of life in Graves' disease. A prospective study. Euro J of Endocrinol 2004;151:549–55.

Neuroimaging in Neuro-Ophthalmology

Fiona E. Costello, MD, FRCP[a,b,*], Mayank Goyal, MD, FRCP[a,c,d]

KEYWORDS

- Magnetic resonance imaging • Computed tomography
- Ultrasound • Angiography • Clinical-anatomic localization

The modern imaging era has introduced a variety of techniques that aid in the evaluation of complex neurologic problems. To optimize the yield of neuroimaging the clinician must, first and foremost determine the nature of the neuro-ophthlamic disorder; and then localize the lesion. Once the localization of the neuro-ophthalmic problem is understood, the optimal imaging modality can be directed toward the anatomic region of interest. In this article the approach to neuroimaging is discussed, with emphasis on the anatomic localization of lesions affecting afferent and efferent visual function.

REVIEWING THE OPTIONS: THE ADVANTAGES AND DISADVANTAGES OF COMMON NEUROIMAGING TECHNIQUES
Magnetic Resonance Imaging

Magnetic resonance imaging (MRI) is based on the principle that atoms consist of charged particles (protons and electrons), which rotate about their axes. Atoms with an odd number of atomic particles, such as hydrogen (a single proton nucleus), possess a larger magnetic moment than those with an even number of particles.[1] Because hydrogen is abundant in human tissue, it is an ideal element to measure with MRI. Protons in tissues normally spin to produce tiny magnetic fields that are randomly aligned.[2] When placed in a magnetic field, the magnetic axes align along that field. Once a radiofrequency pulse is applied, the proton axes of hydrogen atoms momentarily align against the field in a high-energy state.[2] After the magnetic pulse,

[a] Department of Clinical Neurosciences, Foothills Medical Centre, University of Calgary, Room AC164, 1403–29 Street North West, Calgary, Alberta T2N 2T9, Canada
[b] Department of Surgery, Foothills Medical Centre, University of Calgary, Room AC164, 1403–29 Street North West, Calgary, Alberta T2N 2T9, Canada
[c] Department of Radiology, Foothills Medical Centre, University of Calgary, 1403–29 Street North West, Calgary, Alberta T2N 2T9, Canada
[d] High Field Program, Seaman Family MR Research Centre, Foothills Medical Centre, University of Calgary, 1403–29 Street North West, Calgary, Alberta T2N 2T9, Canada
* Corresponding author. Department of Clinical Neurosciences, Foothills Medical Centre, University of Calgary, Room AC164, 1403–29 Street North West, Calgary, Alberta T2N 2T9, Canada.
E-mail address: Fiona.Costello@albertahealthservices.ca

Neurol Clin 28 (2010) 757–787
doi:10.1016/j.ncl.2010.03.011
0733-8619/10/$ – see front matter © 2010 Elsevier Inc. All rights reserved.

neurologic.theclinics.com

Table 1
Neuro-ophthalmic indications and recommended imaging study

Clinical Indication	Preferred Imaging Study	Contrast Material	Comment
Optic nerve drusen	CT scan of the orbit may show calcification	Not necessary	Orbital ultrasound is less costly and more sensitive than a CT scan for optic disc head drusen
Bilateral optic disc swelling	MRI head (with MRV) CT scan might be first-line study in emergent setting	Yes	Consider concomitant contrast MRV to exclude venous sinus thrombosis, especially in atypical cases of pseudotumor cerebri who are thin, male, or elderly
Transient monocular visual loss (amaurosis fugax) due to ischemia	MRA or CTA of neck for carotid stenosis or dissection	Depends on clinical situation	Carotid Doppler study might be first line and may still require follow-up catheter angiography
Demyelinating optic neuritis	MRI head and orbit	Yes (enhancing lesions suggest acute disease)	FLAIR to look for demyelinating white matter lesions. MRI has prognostic significance for development of multiple sclerosis
Inflammatory, infiltrative, or compressive optic neuropathy	MRI head and orbit	Yes	Fat suppression to exclude intraorbital optic nerve enhancement. CT is superior in traumatic optic neuropathy for canal fractures
Junctional scotoma (ie, optic neuropathy in one eye and superotemporal field loss in fellow eye)	MRI head (attention to sella)	Yes	Junctional lesions are typically mass lesions
Bitemporal hemianopsia	MRI head (attention to chiasm and sella)	Yes	Consider CT of sella if an emergent scan is needed (eg, pituitary or chiasmal apoplexy) or if imaging for calcification (eg, meningioma or craniopharyngioma or aneurysm)

Indication	Imaging study	Contrast	Comments
Homonymous hemianopsia	MRI head	Yes	Retrochiasmal pathway. DWI may be useful if acute ischemic infarct or PRES. If structural imaging negative and organic loss consider functional imaging like PET
Cortical visual loss or visual association cortex (eg, cerebral achromatopsia, alexia, prosopagnosia, simultagnosia, optic ataxia, Balint syndrome)	MRI head	Yes	Retrochiasmal pathway. Consider DWI in ischemic infarct. If structural imaging negative and organic loss consider functional imaging (eg, PET, SPECT, or MRS)
Third, fourth, sixth nerve palsy or cavernous sinus syndrome	MRI head with attention to the skull base. Isolated vasculopathic cranial neuropathies may not require initial imaging	Yes	Rim calcification in aneurysm, calcification in tumors, and hyperostosis may be better seen on CT
Internuclear ophthalmoplegia (INO), supranuclear or nuclear gaze palsies, dorsal midbrain syndrome, skew deviation	MRI head (brainstem)	Yes	Rule out demyelinating or other brainstem lesion. Include a FLAIR sequence
Nystagmus	MRI brainstem	Yes	Localize nystagmus
Hemifacial spasm	MRI brainstem (with or without MRA)	Yes	Facial nerve compression at root exit zone
Horner syndrome: preganglionic	MRI head and neck to second thoracic vertebra (T2) in chest with neck MRA[a]	Yes	Rule out lateral medullary infarct, brachial plexus injury, apical lung neoplasm, carotid dissection, and so forth
Horner syndrome: postganglionic	MRI head and neck to level of superior cervical ganglion (C4 level) with MRA neck[b]	Yes	Rule out carotid dissection. Isolated postganglionic lesions are often benign
Thyroid eye disease	CT or MRI of orbit	Iodinated contrast may interfere with evaluation and treatment of systemic thyroid disease	Bone anatomy is better seen on a CT scan especially if orbital decompression is being considered

(continued on next page)

Table 1
(continued)

Clinical Indication	Preferred Imaging Study	Contrast Material	Comment
Orbital cellulitis and orbital disease secondary to sinus disease	CT orbit and sinuses	Depends on clinical situation	MRI and/or CT with CTA may be useful adjunct to a CT alone; especially if possible concomitant cavernous sinus thrombosis is present
Idiopathic orbital inflammation	CT or MRI of orbit (with fat suppression)	Yes	Beware fat suppression artifact
Orbital tumor (eg, proptosis or enophthalmos, gaze-evoked visual loss)	CT or MRI of orbit	Yes	Include head imaging if lesion could extend intracranially. MRI with contrast is superior at determining intracranial extent of primary optic nerve tumors (eg, optic nerve glioma or sheath meningioma). CT scan may be superior if looking for hyperostosis or calcification
Orbital trauma (eg, fracture, subperiosteal hematoma, orbital foreign body, orbital emphysema)	CT scan of orbit with direct coronal	Not generally necessary	CT is superior to MRI for bone fractures
Traumatic optic neuropathy	CT of optic canal (thin sections)	Not generally necessary	CT is superior for visualizing fracture or bone fragment
Carotid-cavernous sinus or dural fistula (eg, orbital bruit, arterialization of conjunctival and episcleral vessels, glaucoma)	CT or MRI of head and orbit (with contrast enhanced MRA)	Yes	CT or MRI may show enlarged superior ophthalmic vein. May require catheter angiogram for final diagnosis and therapy. Color flow Doppler studies may be useful for detecting reversal of orbital venous flow

Abbreviations: CT, computed tomography; CTA, computed tomographic angiography; DWI, diffusion-weighted imaging; FLAIR, fluid attenuation inversion recovery; MRA, magnetic resonance angiography; MRI, magnetic resonance imaging; MRS, magnetic resonance spectroscopy; MRV, magnetic resonance venography; PET, positron emission tomography; PRES, posterior reversible encephalopathy syndrome; SPECT, single-photon emission computed tomography.
[a] When the presumed lesion is in the lung, mediastinum, or anterior aspect of the neck, contrast-enhanced axial CT may be sufficient for localization.
[b] Imaging the entire pathway (MRI head and neck down to T2 with MRA neck) may be necessary if further localization cannot be performed due to difficulties with hydroxyamphetamine availability.
Modified from Lee AG, Brazis PW, Garrity J, et al. Imaging in orbital and neuro-ophthalmic disease. Am J Ophthalmol 2004;138:852–62; with permission.

protons release energy over a short period of time according to 2 relaxation constants known as T1 and T2.[1–3] By controlling the radiofrequency pulse and gradient wave-forms, computer programs are used to produce specific pulse sequences that determine how various tissues appear.[2] Fatty tissue appears bright (high signal intensity or hyperintense) on T1-weighted (T1W) MRI, and relatively dark (low signal intensity or hypointense) on T2-weighted (T2W) images. Water and fluids appear relatively dark on T1W scans, relative to T2W images, in which they appear bright.[1] T1W studies demonstrate normal soft tissue anatomy and fat, whereas T2 studies show fluid changes arising from tumors and inflammation.[2] Rapid blood flow is decreased on T1W and T2W scans, because the velocity of blood is high enough that it passes through a tissue volume without being exposed to both pulses. This decreased signal intensity on both scan types is referred to as the "flow void" phenomenon.[1] Gadolinium is a paramagnetic contrast material that can be used in concert with T1W to better delineate lesions in the brain and spinal cord. As a contrast agent, gadolinium is quite safe to use, with the only relative contraindication being in hemolytic or sickle cell anemia. Other adverse side effects of gadolinium include allergic reactions, headache, hypotension, and transient increase in iron and serum bilirubin.[3] In patients with renal impairment, nephrogenic systemic fibrosis, a rare but life-threatening condition, can occur.[2] In addition to T1W and T2W imaging, other commonly used MR techniques include the following.

1. *Gradient echo imaging (GRE)*: Pulse sequences can be used for fast imaging of moving blood and cerebrospinal fluid (CSF). Because this technique is fast it can reduce motion artifacts and increase sensitivity in detecting early hemorrhagic changes.[2,3]
2. *Diffusion-weighted imaging (DWI)*: Signal intensities are related to diffusion of water molecules in tissue.[1–3] Water molecules in tissue are in continuous Brownian motion, termed diffusion, which is quantified as apparent diffusion coefficient (ADC).[3] Neuronal ischemia leads to a failure of the membrane-bound ATP-dependent ionic channels responsible for both neuron resting membrane potentials and the generation of action potentials. This metabolic aberration results in accumulation of intracellular ions, creating an intracellular gradient responsible for intracellular accumulation of water (cytotoxic edema).[3] Approximately 3 to 4 hours after the onset of cerebral ischemia, the integrity of the blood-brain barrier becomes compromised, and plasma proteins pass into the extracellular space. The intravascular water follows when reperfusion occurs (vasogenic edema).[3] This process begins 6 hours after the onset of stroke and reaches a maximum 2 to 4 days after the onset of stroke.[3] Diffusion tensor imaging (DTI) can reliably distinguish cytotoxic from vasogenic edema, such that vasogenic edema is characterized by elevated diffusion due to a relative increase in the water in the extracellular compartment, where water is more mobile, whereas cytotoxic edema causes restricted diffusion.[4] DWI is very sensitive and relatively specific in detecting acute ischemic stroke, and has been shown to reveal diffusion abnormalities in almost 50% of patients with clinically defined transient ischemic attacks.[3] In addition to being sensitive to detecting early cerebral ischemia and infarction, DWI can also help differentiate cysts from solid masses.[2]
3. *Fluid attenuated inversion recovery (FLAIR)*: Sequences show a heavily weighted T2W sequence, without a bright CSF signal. FLAIR can be used to demonstrate regions of the brain where there is a partial volume effect from CSF, such as the periventricular regions. This technique is especially useful in studying tumors, ischemic lesions, and demyelination in the brain and spinal cord.[1]

Table 2
Imaging characteristics of orbital lesions

Orbital Lesion	Imaging Features
Dermoid cyst	Orbital US of superficial lesions shows medium to high internal reflectivity, whereas deep lesions show low internal reflectivity. CT shows a well-defined lesion with rim enhancement and calcification, which may be associated with a bony defect.[6] Most dermoid tumors have signal intensity characteristics similar to fat, and are hyperintense on T1W images and hypointense on T2W images. Fat-suppression techniques may be helpful in confirming the presence of fat in the lesion[7]
Cavernous hemangioma	B-scan US shows high internal reflectivity with prominent anterior and posterior spikes.[6] MRI may show lesions that are isointense to hypointense on T1W imaging, and hyperintense on T2W imaging[8]
Orbital lymphoma	B-scan US shows low internal reflectivity.[6] CT and MRI show a well-defined intraconal mass that is hypointense on T1W and hyperintense on T2W images.[6] There is molding to surrounding tissues. Bony erosion or infiltration is not seen, except with high-grade lesions[6]
Lacrimal gland pleomorphic adenoma	US shows well-defined surface spikes with medium to high reflectivity.[6] CT shows a well-circumscribed lesion with remodeling of bone, which may appear cystic and show calcification.[6] On MRI, small lesions appear as relatively homogeneous lesions with low signal intensities on T1W imaging, and appear as high signal intensities on T2W images. Large tumors with hemorrhage or necrosis exhibit heterogeneous signal intensities on T1W and T2W images[9]
Lacrimal gland adenoid cystic carcinoma	CT and MRI show an irregular lesion, with bony destruction.[6] MRI may show an isointense signal on T1W images, a hyperintense signal on T2W images, and moderate contrast enhancement[10]
Fibrous histiocytoma	Orbital imaging with CT or MRI shows a well-circumscribed lesion in benign cases, whereas malignant lesions show local infiltration[6]
Rhabdomyosarcoma	CT shows bony destruction. MRI shows an irregular mass that enhances with contrast.[6] On T1W images the lesion may be isointense with muscle, whereas T2W imaging shows hyperintense signal[11]
Metastatic lesions: breast, lung, prostate, leukemia, lymphoma	CT and MRI scan may show mass or infiltrate with IV contrast enhancement involving the optic nerve, extraocular muscles, and soft tissue structures in the orbit (Fig. 22). Brain CT and MRI may show parenchymal lesions and dural enhancement. CT can show bone erosion or infiltrate
Carotid-cavernous sinus fistula	Orbital signs evolve due to venous congestion. US, CT, and MRI show a dilated superior ophthalmic vein and enlargement of the extraocular muscles.[6] US can show arterialized blood flow through the superior ophthalmic vein. Angiography shows a direct communication between the cavernous internal carotid artery and the neighboring cavernous sinus[6]

Cellulitis	CT with/without contrast in axial and coronal planes localizes the process to the orbit, and determines whether the sinuses are involved and whether there is bone and intracranial extension.[12] On MRI, orbital cellulitis appears hypointense on T1W images and hyperintense on T2W images.[13] MRI with fat-suppressed gadolinium-enhanced views may show the extent of orbital and intracranial involvement.[12] There may be opacification of the paranasal sinuses.[12] In preseptal cellulitis the orbital compartments are spared infiltration.[12] A subperiosteal abscess appears as a homogeneous collection adjacent to an orbital wall, surrounded by an enhancing layer on contrast enhanced CT or MRI. The mass may displace orbital structures and be associated with enhancing orbital fat. Increased radiodensity with intervening lucencies may indicate gas-forming organisms[12]
Fungal infections: zygomycetes, ascomycetes, histoplasmosis, blastomycosis, sporotrichosis	CT and MRI (fat-suppressed, enhanced views) show opacification of the sinuses with adjacent orbital mass, with or without bone erosion.[12] Orbital soft tissues, including the optic nerve, may be enlarged.[12] A normal enhancement pattern may not be seen with fungal infections, because fungal invasion of vessels erodes the vascular pathways required for contrast enhancement to be visualized.[12] MRI findings in orbital fungal infections include hypo- to isointense signals on T1W images, and hypointense changes on T2W images, enhancement on post-gadolinium T1W images[14,15]
Parasitic infections: echinococcus, cysticercus, trichinosis, onchocerca, ascaris, schistosoma, entamoeba	CT and MRI (fat-suppressed, gadolinium-enhanced) of the orbits and head (axial and coronal planes) show intraorbital cysts with centers of water density.[12] There may be associated tissue enhancement consistent with inflammation. Calcification can be seen with trichinosis, and cysts may be seen in the extraocular muscles with trichinosis and cysticercosis.[12] US can also identify intraorbital cysts.[12] Orbital neurocysticercosis: T1W MRI noncontrast studies appear; on T2W imaging the lesion appears hypointense[15]
Orbital vasculitis: Wegener granulomatosis (WG), polyarteritis nodosa (PAN), giant cell arteritis (GCA)	WG: MRI may show an enhancing optic nerve lesion. MRI and CT may demonstrate infiltration and inflammation of the orbits and frequently involve the mastoid regions. Orbital masses with infiltration and obliteration of the orbital fat planes is seen, and midline involvement can include bone erosion. MRI shows a marked decrease in the T2W signal, which is a characteristic feature of this entity. The unenhanced, nonfat-suppressed T1-weighted sequence is the preferred method for lesion detection and for definition of the pattern of anatomic involvement.[12,16] PAN: CT scan of head and orbits with axial and coronal views can show orbital, sinus, parasellar, and intracranial involvement. GCA: MRI brain and orbits with axial and coronal views may show an enhancing lesion within the optic nerve. Enhancement of the orbit and intracranial vasculitis may also be seen with MRI[12]
Granulomatous inflammation: sarcoidosis, Erdheim Chester disease (ECD), adult orbital xanthogranuloma, necrobiotic xanthogranuloma (NXG) Sjögren syndrome	Sarcoidosis: CT and MRI may show enlargement of the lacrimal gland, occasionally beyond the orbital rim. Orbital involvement is seen as diffuse enhancement within the orbital fat, optic nerve, and extraocular muscles.[12] ECD: CT and MRI views of the orbits, parasellar structures, and pituitary can be used to define the extent of involvement.[12] NXG: CT and fat-suppressed MRI can show opacification and enlargement of the eyelids and anterior orbital structures. Sjögren: CT and fat-suppressed MRI scans of the orbit can show nonspecific enlargement of the lacrimal glands; however, significant enlargement or bony erosion should prompt consideration of other diagnoses[12]

(continued on next page)

Table 2
(continued)

Orbital Lesion	Imaging Features
Graves orbitopathy	CT and MRI reveal enlarged extraocular muscles, with sparing of the tendinous insertions.[17,18] The inferior and medial recti are often involved. Isolated lateral rectus muscle enlargement without other evidence of muscle enlargement is uncommon, and suggests another disease process, such as orbital myositis.[18] Apical crowding of the optic nerve is well visualized on MRI, which is more sensitive for showing optic nerve compression. CT may be used to delineate the bony architecture of the orbit before decompression. CT and MRI may show straightening of the optic nerve, increased orbital fat, lacrimal gland enlargement, and eyelid edema[18]
Idiopathic orbital inflammatory pseudotumor	CT shows involvement of adjacent bone or paranasal sinuses. MRI shows the extent of soft tissue involvement in the orbit, and demonstrates extension into the cavernous sinus.[12] CT with contrast shows diffuse orbital involvement that in anterior cases is ragged on the edges and conforms to the curvature of the globe. There can be thickening and enhancing of the sclera. Bony remodeling and hyperostosis can also be shown with CT.[12] In posterior cases there is also involvement of the perineural fat or posterior portions of the extraocular muscles.[12] US (A- and B-mode) can show evidence of scleritis with effusion at Tenson's capsule that can create a T sign[12]
Idiopathic sclerosing inflammation of the orbit (ISIO)	CT allows visualization of bone and paranasal sinuses. Fat-suppressed orbit and brain MRI views can show involvement of the cavernous sinuses and soft tissues within the orbits.[12] Orbital studies show homogeneously enhanced areas of opacification with ragged margins.[12] There may also be opacification of the extraocular muscles and/or the lacrimal gland.[12] In severe cases, there may be wall-to-wall opacification of all the orbital structures except the globe.[12] MRI shows low signal intensities on T1W and T2W images[19]
Orbital myositis	CT/MRI shows diffuse enlargement of affected extraocular muscles including the tendinous insertion, which differentiates myositis from thyroid orbitopathy.[12,17,18] Orbital tissue adjacent to the muscle may be locally infiltrated, showing a ragged enhancement on contrast CT adjacent to the muscle substance.[12] MRI features include focal enlarged muscular lesions showing increased T2W and decreased T1W signals with contrast enhancement[20]
Nonspecific inflammatory dacryoadenitis	CT generally shows oblong enlargement of the lacrimal gland, which molds to the curvature of the globe as it extends posteriorly.[12] Primary epithelial tumors of the lacrimal gland show a more rounded appearance. If erosion of the bony orbit is seen, a neoplasm should be suspected.[12] US (A- and B-mode) can be used to differentiate lacrimal gland lesions. The lacrimal gland shows enlargement with internal reflectivity. Echolucency is apparent anteriorly near the sclera if the lateral rectus involvement occurs.[12] MRI may show isointense signal changes on T1W images, a hypointense signal on T2W images, and moderate contrast enhancement

Data from Refs.[6,12,17,18,49]

Axial   Coronal

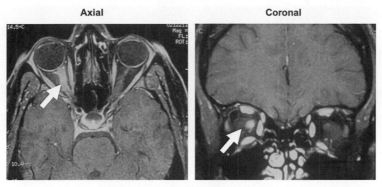

Fig. 1. A 30-year old woman with optic neuritis presented with vision loss in the right eye and pain with eye movements. Visual acuity was 20/200 in the right eye and 20/20 in the left eye. There was a right relative afferent pupil defect. The fundus examination was normal in both eyes. T1-weighted (T1W), fat-suppressed, gadolinium-enhanced MRI (axial and coronal views) studies showed a thickening and enhancement of the right optic nerve (*arrows*).

4. *Fat suppression and short-time inversion recovery (STIR) techniques*: These methods reduce the fat signal and improve tissue contrast. Fat suppression increases the detection of many orbital lesions, eliminates chemical shift artifacts, and decreases motion-related ghost artifacts.[1]

Generally speaking, MRI is superior to computed tomography (CT) in the evaluation of most neuro-ophthalmic lesions, with the exception of acute hemorrhage and bony abnormalities. When compared with CT, MRI provides superior contrast between normal and abnormal tissue; shows better sensitivity in detecting demyelinating pathology; and allows for direct, multiplanar imaging without patient repositioning. Because of the effects of beam-hardening artifact in CT imaging, MRI provides better

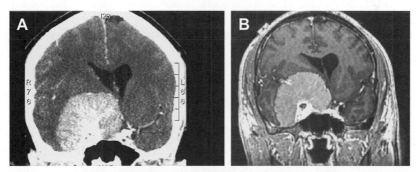

Fig. 2. A 34-year-old man presented with painless vision loss in the right eye and associated personality change. He had count-fingers vision, a relative afferent pupil defect, and optic atrophy in the right eye. Although he denied any vision loss in the left eye, formal perimetry showed a superior temporal visual field defect on the left and a dense central scotoma in the right eye. (*A*) Contrast-enhanced CT (coronal view) and (*B*) MRI (T1W with gadolinium) showed a large, extra-axial homogeneously enhancing mass, centered at the right sphenoid wing and extending into the sellar, parasellar, and right posterior frontal regions. The location, shape, and enhancement patterns were consistent with a meningioma, and this diagnosis was confirmed with surgical pathology.

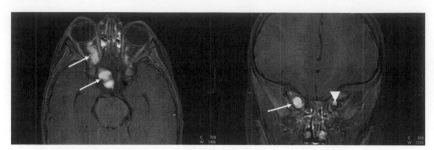

Fig. 3. Axial MRI scans showing optic glioma.

resolution of posterior fossa structures. MRI has some disadvantages relative to CT, including its higher cost and the increased time required to obtain images. Furthermore, motion-related artifacts can degrade image quality in MRI studies. Claustrophobia may prevent some patients from being able to tolerate MRI, and a proportion of patients may require some sedation to complete the procedure for this reason.[1,2] Obesity is another patient-related contraindication for MRI, as some patients cannot fit into the core of the magnet or may exceed the weight limitations of the scanning table.[1] MRI is relatively contraindicated in patients with implanted materials that can be affected by powerful magnetic fields including metallic substances, magnetically activated or electronically controlled devices (cardiac pacemakers, cochlear implants), and nonferromagnetic metal, electronically conductive wires or materials.[2] Because ferromagnetic material may be moved by the magnetic field of the MRI, all patients suspected of having a ferromagnetic foreign body should be initially evaluated with CT.[1,2]

Computed Tomography

As an x-ray beam is transmitted through tissue, the beam energy is attenuated as a function of the tissue's electron density.[1] Using mathematical algorithms, the attenuation in each volume of a particular plane (voxel) can be reconstructed.[1] Images are reconstructed into 2-dimensional (2D) image (tomograms) or detailed 3-dimensional (3D) images.[2] Gray scales are used to display the value of each

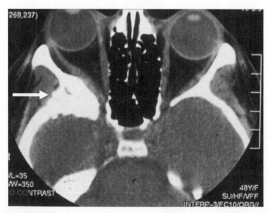

Fig. 4. A CT scan of the orbital (axial view) showing hyperostosis of bone (*arrow*) in a patient with sphenoid wing meningioma.

data point on film, and reflect the range of attenuation coefficients.[1] CT imaging provides more spatial detail and can better differentiate between soft tissue densities as compared with conventional x-ray imaging.[2] Unenhanced CT is used to detect acute hemorrhage in the brain and to characterize bone lesions. Intravenous iodinated contrast shows enhancement in areas of increased vascular supply and in regions of blood-brain barrier breakdown.[1,2] CT generally provides good visualization of most anterior orbital pathologic processes, but lesions at or beyond the orbital apex tend to be better visualized with MRI. Relative to MRI, advantages of CT include faster scanning times, decreased motion artifact, and reconstruction algorithms that enable reformations in any plane.[1] Disadvantages of CT include ionizing radiation, and beam hardening artifacts from bone, metallic clips, and fillings. The iodinated contrast used to enhance CT scans may also cause nephrotoxicity and allergic reactions in some patients.[1,2]

Ultrasonography

Ultrasonography (US) uses reflection of ultrasound waves at acoustic interfaces to provide real-time display of tissues.[1,2] US creates sound waves, which are reflected back (echoes) and converted into electrical signals. This imaging technique is useful in visualizing the globe, and can differentiate papilledema from pseudo-papilledema secondary to optic disc drusen.[1] A computer analyzes the signals and displays information in different ways:[2]

1. *A-mode US*: Shows signals, which are recorded as spikes on a graph. The vertical (Y) axis of the display shows the echo amplitude and the horizontal (X) axis shows depth or distance into the patient.[2] This US technique is often used in ophthalmic scanning.
2. *B-mode (gray-scale) US*: displays signals as 2D anatomic images. B-mode US is fast enough to allow real-time motion to be detected (including pulsating blood vessels), and can be used to provide anatomic and functional information.[2]

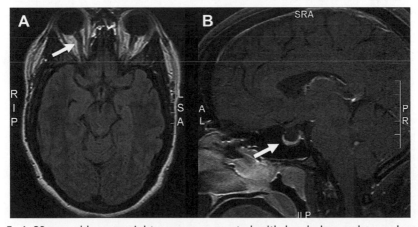

Fig. 5. A 39-year-old, overweight woman presented with headaches, pulse synchronous tinnitus, and transient visual obscurations. The examination showed a visual acuity of 20/20 in both eyes and bilateral optic disc edema. The cranial CT scan was normal. Lumbar puncture revealed an elevated opening pressure of 40 cm of water and normal CSF constituents. (A) An MRI (axial) showed some subtle mild flattening of the posterior sclera with distension of the optic nerve sheaths (*arrow*), and (B) a partially empty sella (sagittal MRI scan) (*arrow*).

Table 3
Imaging features of optic nerve lesions

Optic Nerve Lesion	Imaging Features
Idiopathic optic neuritis	Gadolinium-enhanced, fat-suppressed MRI views of the orbit can show increased signal change in the optic nerve (see Fig. 1)
Inflammatory optic neuropathies: sarcoidosis, tuberculosis (TB), syphilis, Wegener's granulomatosis, Lyme disease, Autoimmune optic neuropathy	In sarcoidosis, TB, syphilis, and Lyme disease, there may be enhancement of the meninges at the base of the skull anterior to the chiasm. TB can also show MRI features of hydrocephalus, cerebral edema, and tuberculomas (see Fig. 6). In syphilis, stroke like lesions from vasculitic involvement of the brain can occur. Syphilitic gummas have increased signal on T2W MRI and may or may not enhance. In Lyme disease cranial nerve enhancement may be seen.[22] If there is cerebral vasculitis, cerebral angiography may show stenotic lesions in the posterior circulation and irregularities of small vessel walls.[22] Patients with autoimmune optic neuropathy may have clinically silent brain white matter lesions on MRI[22]
Compressive optic neuropathies: pituitary macroadenoma, cranopharyngioma, aneurysm, optic nerve sheath meningioma, optic nerve glioma, metastases	Optic nerve gliomas have a distinctive "kinking" sign within the orbit, and a double-intensity tubular thickening of the nerve best seen on MRI (see Fig. 3). This is called the pseudo-cerebrospinal fluid sign because the increased in T2W signal surrounding the nerve may be misinterpreted as CSF.[23] Fat-suppressed, gadolinium MRI views will show demarcation of the optic nerve sheath meningiomas.[23] For metastatic lesions, MRI can show intraparenchymal lesions, generalized or focal dural enhancement, or both
Optic disc drusen	CT shows calcified optic disc drusen in cases of pseudo-papilledema. US can show elevation of the optic disc, and when gain is increased noncalcified ocular tissue loses brightness; whereas drusen, if calcified, remain bright. B-scan US shows calcified drusen to have high reflectivity.[26,27]
Traumatic optic neuropathy	CT is the study of choice for patients with suspected orbital and facial fractures, foreign bodies, and orbital and optic nerve sheath hemorrhage.[28] MRI is inferior to CT in evaluating fractures, but can detect nonmetallic substances including wood.[28] MRI is superior for evaluating the intracanalicular and intracranial sections of the optic nerve and may show orbital, subperiosteal, or intradural hemorrhage.[28] MRI is contraindicated if a ferromagnetic foreign body is suspected. B-scan US can be used to assess ocular and optic nerve head and for following progressive enlargement of the optic nerve sheath

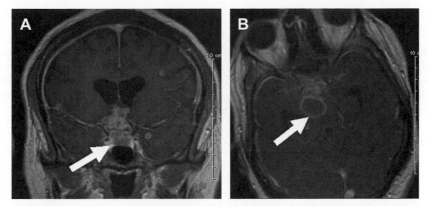

Fig. 6. A 19-year-old man presented with fever, headache, and vision loss. CSF cultures were positive for tuberculosis. The examination showed a visual acuity of count-fingers vision in the right eye and 20/25 in the left eye. There was a large right relative afferent pupil defect. Visual field testing showed a dense central scotoma in the right eye and a temporal hemifield defect in the left eye. There was bilateral optic atrophy, and a third nerve palsy in the right eye with aberrant regeneration. T1W gadolinium-enhanced MRI studies [(*A*) coronal and (*B*) axial views] showed an enhancing suprasellar cystic lesion, consistent with tuberculoma.

3. *Doppler US*: uses the Doppler effect (alteration of sound frequency by reflection off a moving object) to examine blood flow, such that the moving objects are red blood cells.[2] Changes in the frequency of the reflected sound waves are converted into images showing blood flow and velocity.[2] For Doppler US, color is superimposed on a gray-scale anatomic image to indicate the direction of blood flow. By convention, the color red indicates flow toward the transducer, and blue represents flow away from the transducer.[2] In neuro-ophthalmology, Doppler US is used to look

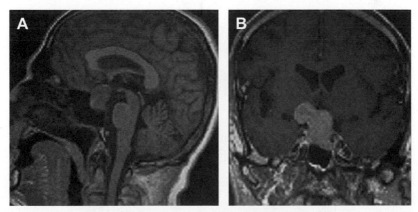

Fig. 7. A 48-year-old man presented with painless, progressive vision loss in the right eye. Examination revealed a visual acuity of 20/50 in the right eye and 20/20 in the left eye. There was a right relative afferent pupil defect. Fundus examination was normal. MRI [(*A*) sagittal and (*B*) coronal] studies showed a large sellar mass that was isointense with brain on T1W images and enhanced with gadolinium. Postsurgical pathologic pathology confirmed that the lesion was a nonsecreting pituitary macroadenoma.

for carotid artery abnormalities in patients with amaurosis fugax or central retinal artery occlusion.[1]

The advantage of US is that it is widely available, noninvasive, involves no ionizing radiation, and provides real-time information regarding vascular anatomy and blood flow.[1,2] The major disadvantage of US is that the quality of the results is highly operator dependent. Furthermore, US cannot be used to image through bone or gas. Finally, obtaining clear US images of target structures can be technically difficult in overweight patients.[2]

Catheter Angiography

Catheter angiography is considered the gold standard for evaluating cerebrovascular lesions including aneurysms, vascular stenoses, vessel occlusions, and dissections.[1] Digital subtraction angiography (DSA) refers to a process in which images of the arteries are taken before and after contrast injection. A computer subtracts one image from another, which enables better visualization of arteries.[2] The disadvantages of this "conventional" angiography include the invasive nature of the study, radiation exposure, and possible adverse reactions to the contrast agent. In addition, injection sites can become painful and hematomas can occur. Rare complications of angiography include shock, seizures, renal failure, and stroke.[2] Recent advances in CT and MRI have allowed for noninvasive angiographic methods to study the head and neck vasculature.[1] Computer reconstruction and maximum intensity techniques generate 3D angiographic images that can be viewed in multiple projections. Strategies have evolved to optimize signal differences between flowing blood and stationary tissue. Spiral CT scanning allows for continuous data acquisition and advanced cross-sectional imaging of vascular structures. CT angiography (CTA) requires multidetector scanners so that very thin slices can be obtained in a short period of time. The data are the used to create 3D maps of the vascular anatomy.[1] MR angiography (MRA) implements time of flight (TOF) and dynamic 3D contrast-enhanced techniques, which may be performed in concert with conventional MRI to detect diffusion-perfusion mismatch in acute stroke, vulnerable plaque, and evolving blood products.[1,4,5] MRA is complemented by fat saturation sequences that aid in detection and characterization

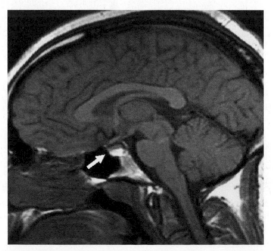

Fig. 8. A sagittal T1W MRI scan showed hyperintense signal change in the region of the pituitary (*arrow*) in a patient with pituitary apoplexy.

of dissecting hematomas and pseudoaneurysms in arterial structures. In general, MRA has a sensitivity and specificity similar to CTA for detection of aneurysms that are 5 mm or larger in diameter, but may have lower sensitivity for detection of lesions smaller than 5 mm.[1] MRA may exaggerate the appearance of vascular stenoses, causing vessels to appear smaller than with catheter angiography because slower blood flow at the site of the vessel wall causes signal loss.[1] The clinical setting in which MRA is superior to CTA is in the assessment of aneurysms previously treated with endovascular coils.

OPTIMIZING THE VIEW: USING CLINICAL-ANATOMIC LOCALIZATION TO GUIDE THE IMAGING PROCESS

Clinical-anatomic localization is essential to making an accurate neuro-ophthalmic diagnosis. The clinician must use the details of the history and the examination findings to identify the anatomic region of interest, and then select the appropriate imaging study (**Table 1**). The diagnostic yield of neuroimaging depends not only on what imaging technique is chosen but also on whether one is looking in the right place!

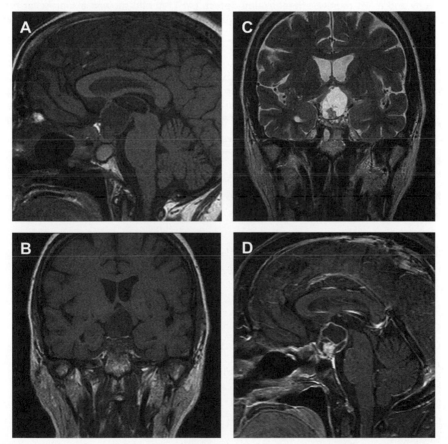

Fig. 9. In this patient with a craniopharyngiomas, (A) a sagittal and (B) coronal T1W MRI scans shows a lesion with hyper- and hypointense signal features arising from the sella with extension into the third ventricle. In the T2W coronal study (C) the lesion is hyperintense compared with surrounding brain. (D) Gadolinium-enhanced T1W sagittal imaging shows lesion enhancement.

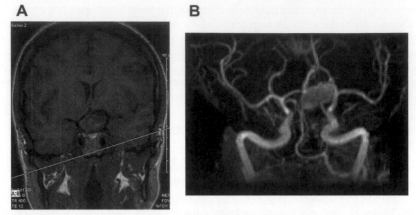

Fig. 10. A 38-year-old woman presented with a 6-month history of vision loss in the left eye. Visual acuity was 20/20 in the right eye and 20/100 in the left eye. There was left optic atrophy and a left relative afferent pupil defect. (*A*) T1W MRI showed a suprasellar mass with heterogeneous signal intensity. (*B*) MRA showed a large intracavernous segment internal carotid artery aneurysm.

Orbit

Orbital lesions may present with pain, proptosis, ophthalmoplegia, and vision loss. There are many potential causes of orbital dysfunction, including inflammation, infection, and tumor infiltration. US can be helpful in assessing vascular tumors and

---

Box 1
Lesions of the cavernous sinus

Meningioma

Invasive pituitary adenoma

Metastatic lesions

Intracavernous ICA aneurysm

Dural arteriovenous fistula

Schwannoma

Lymphoma

Cavernous hemangioma

Cavernous sinus thrombosis

Abscess

Cavernous sinusitis (Tolosa Hunt syndrome)

Nasopharyngeal carcinoma

Chordoma

Sarcoidosis

Tuberculoma

Data from Optic Neuritis Study Group. Multiple sclerosis risk after optic neuritis: final optic neuritis treatment trial follow-up. Arch Neurol 2008;65(6):727–32.

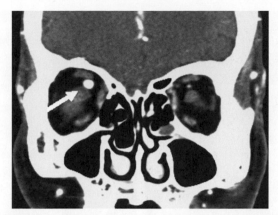

Fig. 11. An enhanced CT scan (coronal) shows an enlarged superior ophthalmic vein on the right (*arrow*) in a patient with a right dural carotid-cavernous sinus fistula.

malformations in the orbit. CT is often used to detect pathology in the anterior orbit; and the effects of trauma, foreign bodies, acute hemorrhage, and bony invasion are best visualized with this imaging modality (**Table 2**).[1] For lesions at or beyond the orbital apex, MRI is the imaging modality of choice, as fat-suppression techniques with gadolinium can help define the extent of soft tissue (extraocular muscles and lacrimal glands) and cavernous sinus involvement.[1] The imaging characteristics of various orbital lesions are presented in **Table 2**.

Optic Nerve

Patients with optic nerve damage often have diminished visual acuity, decreased color vision, a relative afferent pupil defect (RAPD), visual field loss, and ipsilateral optic disc

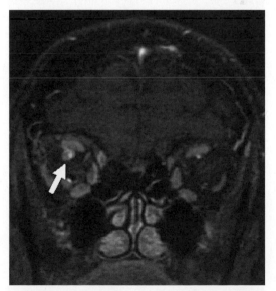

Fig. 12. T1W coronal MRI, with gadolinium enhancement and fat suppression, shows enlarged right superior ophthalmic vein in a patient with a right carotid-cavernous sinus fistula.

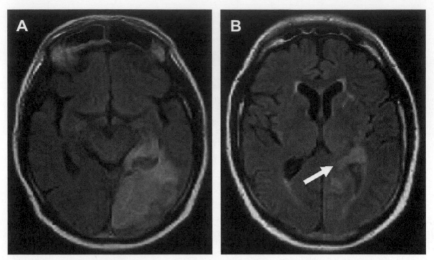

Fig. 13. A 65-year-old man with hypertension and diabetes presented with a right homonymous hemianopia. He was able to write but could not read (alexia without agraphia). FLAIR MRI images (axial) showed (*A*) a left posterior cerebral artery territory infarct, with (*B*) involvement of the splenium of the corpus callosum (*arrow*).

pallor. Damage to the optic nerve may occur along its intraorbital, intraosseous, and intracranial segments. Once it exits the eye behind the lamina cribrosa the optic nerve acquires myelin, and thus becomes vulnerable to demyelinating injury in its retrobulbar course (**Fig. 1**). In its intracanalicular segment the optic nerve exits the orbit through the optic foramen, which is the anterior opening of the optic canal in the orbital

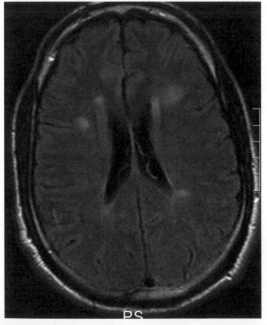

Fig. 14. A cranial MRI scan (FLAIR sequence, axial view) showing multifocal white matter lesions in a patient with multiple sclerosis.

apex. Because it is tightly fixed at this location, the optic nerve may suffer the effects of percussive forces transmitted from frontal skull trauma. Along its intracranial route, the gyrus recti of the frontal lobes are situated superiorly and the internal carotid arteries laterally to the optic nerves. In this region, the optic nerve can be directly compressed by mass lesions arising from contiguous brain and vascular structures (**Fig. 2**). In general, the best means of visualizing optic nerve pathology is with fat-suppressed, gadolinium-enhanced MRI views. Inflammatory optic neuropathies including idio-pathic retrobulbar optic neuritis (see **Fig. 1**), sarcoidosis, and tuberculosis cause a focal area of increased signal within the nerve on T2W and T1W, gadolinium-enhanced images.[1,21,22] Neoplasms such as optic nerve gliomas (**Fig. 3**) are well visu-alized with MRI and show a tubular or fusiform enlargement of the nerve, which appears kinked or tortuous.[1,23,24] The lesion appears isointense or hypointense to normal brain on T1W imaging and may enhance after gadolinium injection. Gliomas of the optic nerve may demonstrate the "pseudo CSF" sign, which refers to the increase in T2W signal around the optic nerve caused by perineural arachnoid glioma-tosis.[1,25] Optic nerve sheath meningiomas appear as a uniform or globular enlarge-ment of the optic nerve, and are isointense on T1W studies. MRI is especially useful in distinguishing optic nerve gliomas from meningiomas, by showing that in the latter the tumor is separate from the optic nerve on coronal views.[1,23,24] MRI also visualizes the intracanalicular and intracranial portion of the optic nerve and helps determine the extent of intracranial spread of optic nerve sheath meningiomas. CT can show peri-neural calcification or "tram tracking," which is virtually diagnostic of optic nerve sheath meningioma.[1] In addition, CT imaging may show also hyperostosis of adjacent bone (**Fig. 4**). Patients with papilledema can demonstrate subtle findings of raised intracranial pressure on MRI including flattening of the posterior sclera, enlargement of the prelaminar optic nerve, tortuosity and elongation of the optic nerve, distension of the perioptic subarachnoid space, and a partially empty sella sign (**Fig. 5**).[1,25] The imaging characteristics of optic nerve lesions are presented in **Table 3**.

Optic Chiasm

The optic chiasm is vulnerable to demyelinating, compressive, infectious (**Fig. 6**), and inflammatory lesions, which are best visualized with MRI. Pituitary tumors, craniophar-yngiomas, and meningiomas are common sources of optic chiasm compression, which can be detected with gadolinium-enhanced T1W and T2W MRI.[1] A pituitary

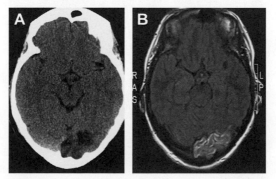

Fig. 15. A 46-year-old woman presented with sudden-onset vision loss. Examination showed a visual acuity of 20/20 in both eyes. There was a right homonymous visual field and no RAPD. The fundus examination was normal. (*A*) An unenhanced cranial CT scan (axial) showed a left occipital lobe infarct. (*B*) MRI (*flair*) showed parenchymal enhancement.

macroadenoma (**Fig. 7**) appears as a sellar mass without a separate identifiable pituitary gland.[29] On CT, pituitary macroadenomas are isodense with surrounding gray matter, and show inhomogeneous enhancement with contrast.[29] On MRI pituitary macroadenomas are isointense relative to surrounding brain on T1W studies; hyperintense on FLAIR imaging; and "bloom" if hemorrhage is present on T2-GRE studies.[29] In cases of pituitary apoplexy, CT shows a sellar mass with patchy or confluent hyperdense signal, and minimal to no enhancement with contrast.[29] If acute, pituitary apoplexy (**Fig. 8**) shows a lesion that appears isointense to hypointense relative to brain on T1W, whereas FLAIR imaging shows hyperintense signal change. MRI T2 GRE will show blooming if blood products are present.[29] With the administration of contrast, there is rim enhancement on T1W MRI.[29] Craniopharyngiomas (**Fig. 9**) show partial calcification, solid constituents, and high signal intensity on precontrast T1W

A

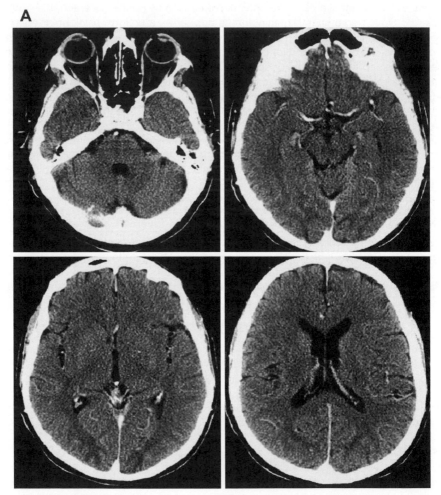

Fig. 16. (*A*) Contrast-enhanced CT scan in PRES showing hypodensity in bilateral occipital white matter without any significant mass effect; (*B*) T2W and FLAIR MRI shows hyperintense signal change in the parieto-occipital regions; (*C*) GRE, DWI and post-contrast T1W images show no hemorrhage, restriction of diffusion or enhancement.

B

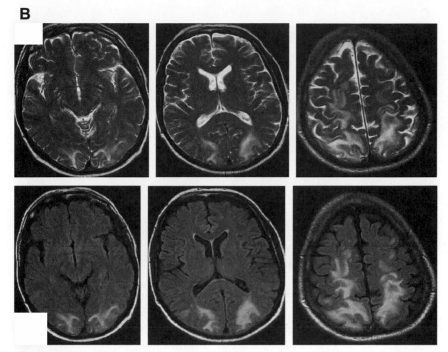

Fig. 16. (*continued*)

MRI studies. With contrast, 90% of craniopharyngiomas enhance.[29] Parasellar aneurysms (**Fig. 10**) are often smooth and lobular in shape. These vascular lesions have variable internal density and show heterogeneous enhancement after contrast.[29] Meningiomas in the region of the sella appear isodense to isointense on CT and MRI, respectively, and enhance with contrast administration.[29]

Cavernous Sinus

The oculomotor, trochlear, abducens, trigeminal (V1–2), and sympathetic nerves all course through the cavernous sinus. Therefore, the constellation of multiple cranial neuropathies and orbital signs implicates a lesion in this region, which may be inflammatory, vascular, or neoplastic in origin (**Box 1**).[30] Cavernous sinus lesions are best detected by gadolinium-enhanced MRI; and MRA can illustrate the relationship between cavernous sinus structures and the internal carotid artery (ICA) (see **Fig. 10**).[29] An asymmetric spherical flow void in this region is suggestive of an aneurysm or fistula,[1] and catheter angiography can be used to confirm the diagnosis. Enlargement of the superior ophthalmic vein, which occurs with carotid-cavernous sinus fistulas, can be seen with CT or MRI (**Figs. 11** and **12**). CT can be used to characterize lesions in the cavernous sinus and delineate the relationship to bony landmarks, including the sella and clivus. For this region, this imaging modality is useful in detecting aneurysms, which may invade bone.[29] Meningiomas of the cavernous sinus appear as dural-based enhancing masses, with associated hyperostosis of contiguous bone.[1,24] These lesions may also demonstrate tumoral calcifications and increased vascular markings. More than 95% of cavernous sinus meningiomas enhance homogeneously and intensely. CT shows a sharply circumscribed smooth

C

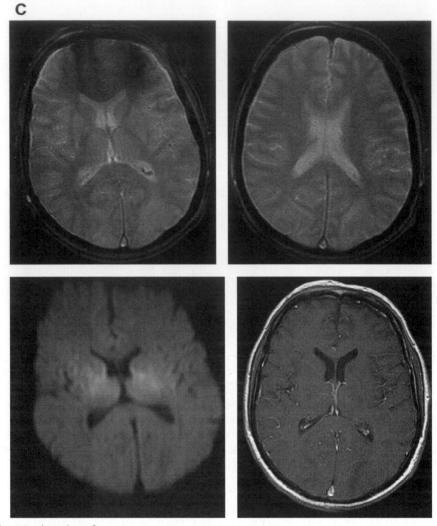

Fig. 16. (*continued*)

mass abutting the dura, with calcification in 20% to 25% of cases.[29] T1W MRI of meningiomas reveals lesions that are isointense to slightly hypointense relative to cortex. With FLAIR imaging, the lesions may show hyperintense peritumoral edema and a dural tail.[29]

Retrochiasmal Visual Pathways

Patients with retrochiasmal lesions in the afferent visual pathway present with homonymous visual field defects (**Fig. 13**), and in these cases the imaging modality of choice is MRI (including T1W, FLAIR, DTI, and T2W studies). Gadolinium can be used to help delineate neoplastic, meningeal, abscess, demyelination, and ischemic pathologies in this region of the central nervous system. Although retrochiasmal demyelinating lesions are less common than retrobulbar optic neuritis in patients with multiple sclerosis (MS), imaging of the brain parenchyma is important because focal or confluent abnormalities in white matter are found in more than 95% of cases **(Fig. 14)**.[31] Typical sites of demyelination include the periventricular white matter, corpus callosum, and middle cerebellar peduncle.[31–34] The perivenular extension of lesions seen on T2W and FLAIR MRI sequences is referred to as "Dawson's fingers." Gadolinium-enhanced T1W scans show transient enhancement during active demyelination. On rare occasions MS patients have large tumefactive lesions, measuring several centimeters in size. The long-term follow-up from the Optic Neuritis Treatment Trial (ONTT)[32] demonstrated that in patients with optic neuritis (ON), the baseline MRI scan was the most potent predictor for the diagnosis of clinically proven MS. After 15 years of follow-up, ONTT patients with one or more white matter lesions on their MRI had a 72% risk of MS, whereas patients with no lesions had a 25% risk of declaring this diagnosis.[32] The modified McDonald criteria[33,34] use MRI to establish dissemination in time and place, and are used to diagnose MS in the absence of a second clinical event. Dissemination in time of MR lesions requires one gadolinium-enhancing lesion at least 3 months after the onset of the clinical event; or a new T2W lesion compared with a reference scan done at least 30 days after onset of the clinical event. In the case of recurrent stereotyped clinical episodes at the same neurologic site, criteria for MRI dissemination in space include 3 of the following features: (1) 1 gadolinium-enhancing lesion or 9 T2W MRI lesions; (2) 1 or more infratentorial lesions; (3) 1 or more juxtacortical lesions; or (4) 3 or more periventricular lesions.[31,33,34] Acquired visual field defects due to ischemic lesions in the retrochiasmal pathways are best seen with DTI, which shows diffusion restriction.[1,29] On plain CT imaging, evidence of stroke may be accompanied by hyperdense vessel with acute loss of gray-white matter differentiation in 60% to 70% of patients.[29] CTA can be used to identify vessel occlusions and stenoses, and to characterize the status of collateral flow.[29] DWI shows hyperintense restriction from cytotoxic edema, and is sensitive to hyperacute stroke detection in 95% of cases **(Fig. 15)**.[29] MRI T1W scans show variable enhancement patterns in the subacute phase, after stroke. Hypertensive encephalopathy or posterior reversible encephalopathy syndrome (PRES) is a disorder of cerebrovascular autoregulation, which may be caused by hypertension **(Fig. 16)**. Neuroimaging features of this diagnosis include patchy, cortical, and subcortical posterior cerebral artery territory

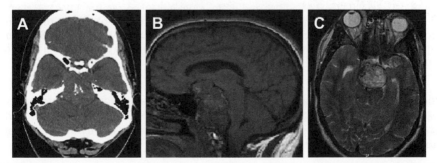

Fig. 17. A 23-year-old man presented for evaluation of bilateral vision loss. On examination he had count-fingers vision in the left eye and 20/50 vision in the right eye. Visual field testing showed a dense central scotoma in the left eye and a temporal hemifield defect in the right eye. The patient had a left relative afferent pupil defect and bilateral optic atrophy. (A) CT (axial) showed a large midline lesion that was isodense relative to surrounding brain structures. (B) T1W MRI sagittal and (C) axial views showed a large heterogeneous mass arising from the clivus. Subsequent biopsy showed the lesion to be a chordoma.

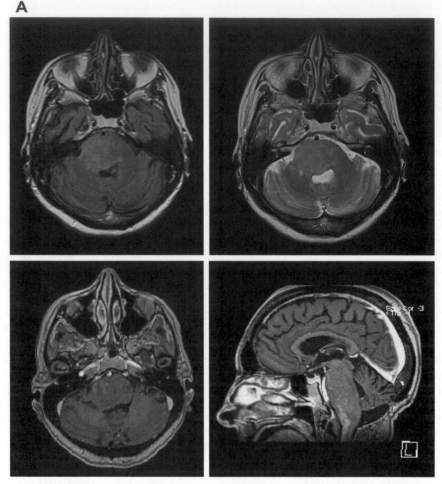

Fig. 18. (*A*) Axial T1W, FLAIR, T2W, and gadolinium-enhanced sagittal T1W MRI demonstrating diffuse enlargement of the brainstem with compression of the fourth ventricle secondary to a brainstem astrocytoma. (*B*) Sagittal T2W and FLAIR MRI of the posterior fossa and cervical spine showing hyperintense signal changes in the same patient with a brainstem astrocytoma.

lesions in a patient with severe acute to subacute hypertension.[29] Parieto-occipital FLAIR hyperintense signal changes occur in 95% of PRES cases, whereas DWI is usually normal.[29] On CT there may be bilateral hypodense foci in the posterior parietal, occipital, basal ganglia, and brainstem regions.[29]

Posterior Fossa

Lesions of the posterior fossa affect brainstem and cerebellar function, and may present with oscillopisa and diplopia. In keeping with the general theme, MRI is superior to CT in the evaluation of the cerebellum, brainstem, and craniocervical junction structures because there is no bone artifact. Hence, MRI is the imaging choice for patients presenting with nystagmus, gaze palsies, and cranial nerve deficits. MRI can aid in the visualization of the ocular motor cranial nerves, and may detect

B

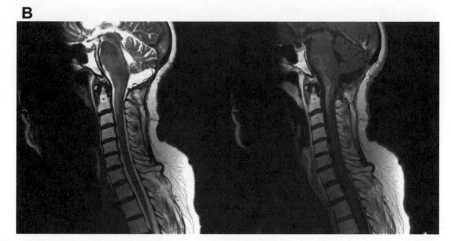

Fig. 18. (*continued*)

compressive and inflammatory lesions. MRI can also be used to detect ischemia, demyelination, and neoplastic lesions in the brainstem and contiguous structures (**Figs. 17** and **18**). Lesions of the craniocervical junction, such as Arnold Chiari malformation (**Fig. 19**), can present with downbeat nystagmus and are seen best with MRI. Patients with acquired intracranial hypotension show epidural and meningeal enhancement on MRI (**Fig. 20**). In addition, bilateral subdural fluid collections and downward displacement of cerebral structures may also be observed.[35] Brainstem gliomas (see **Fig. 18**) present with diffuse infiltration of the pons, which often increases the size of the brainstem. These lesions are associated with increased signal intensity

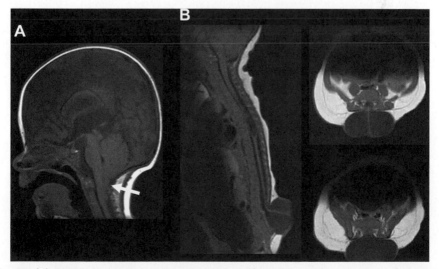

Fig. 19. (*A*) T1W MRI showing a Type 2 Chiari malformation with protrusion of the cerebellar tonsils into the foramen magnum (*arrow*), and (*B*) myelomeningocele.

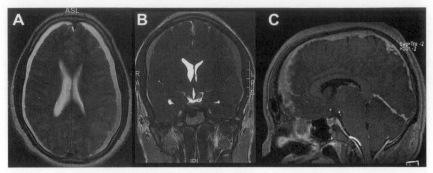

Fig. 20. A 42-year-old man presented with bilateral sixth nerve palsies and postural head-ache. (*A*) Axial, (*B*) coronal, and (*C*) sagittal MRI scans showed bilateral subdural fluid collec-tions over the convexities. The clinical presentation and MRI findings were consistent with spontaneous intracranial hypotension.

on T2W and reduced signal intensity on T1W imaging. Furthermore, brainstem gliomas usually do not show contrast enhancement.[36]

Vascular Imaging

Vascular abnormalities affect the afferent and efferent visual pathways in a myriad of ways, and can be evaluated by CTA, MRA, and conventional angiography. Transient monocular vision loss caused by carotid artery stenosis or dissection is often initially assessed with US. US signs of carotid dissection include an intramural hematoma, localized increased diameter of the artery, a narrowed or false lumen, an intimal flap, and pseudoaneurysm formation.[37–40] US has a sensitivity of 95% for the detec-tion of extracranial ICA dissection.[37–40] MRA may also be of value in evaluating the carotid artery, but may overestimate the extent of stenosis due to signal loss from turbulent flow, particularly at the level of the bifurcation and in areas of vessel

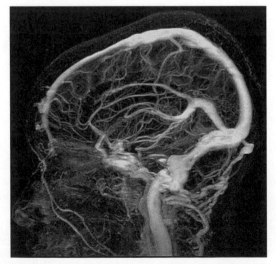

Fig. 21. Normal gadolinium-enhanced MR venogram showing detailed venous anatomy of the brain.

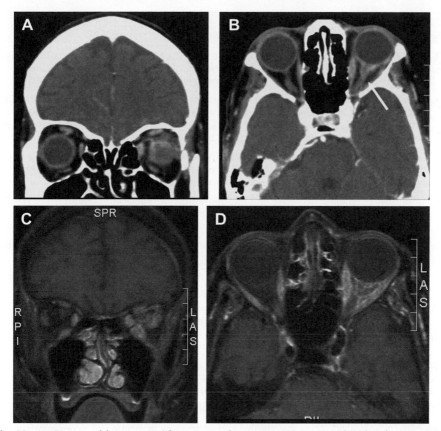

Fig. 22. An 83-year old woman with recurrent breast cancer presented with a frozen globe on the left. (*A*) Coronal and (*B*) axial orbital CT scans showed enlargement of the extraocular muscles and enhancement involving the optic nerve (*arrow*). Gadolinium-enhanced T1W MRI (*C*) coronal and (*D*) axial views showed "stringy" enhancement of the orbit with diffuse involvement of the extraocular muscles, orbital fat, and optic nerve in the left eye.

tortuosity.[1] An acute, painful Horner syndrome should be considered secondary to a carotid artery dissection until proven otherwise. In cases of cervical dissection, transcranial Doppler shows collateral supply from the anterior or posterior communicating arteries, and high-intensity transient signals suggestive of recurrent emboli.[41,42] Intracranial and extracranial stenoses of the anterior and posterior cerebrovascular circulation may also be evaluated with conventional angiography, but CT and MRA (TOF and gadolinium-enhanced techniques) are noninvasive alternatives to DSA.[1,43–46] Thrombo-occlusive disease in the central venous system can arise from external compression or central venous catheterization, and may present with manifestations of raised intracranial pressure. Abnormalities of venous patency can be visualized with CTV, magnetic resonance venography (MRV), US, and catheter venography (see **Fig. 19**). Contrast-enhanced CT may show the presence of an empty delta sign in cases of superior sagittal sinus thrombosis. Furthermore, there may be evidence of a hyperdense dural sinus, cortical and subcortical petechial hemorrhages, and edema. CTA can also show thrombus filling defects.[29] On MRI, acutely thrombosed blood appears hypointense, and becomes hyperintense with time.[29] Venous

---

Box 2
Guidelines for ordering imaging studies in ophthalmology

1. Decide whether a CT or MRI scan is indicated or not. The MRI scan is superior to CT for most neuro-ophthalmic indications, but CT is superior to MRI for calcification, bone, acute hemorrhage, if an emergent scan is needed, or if the patient cannot undergo an MRI scan.

2. Decide if contrast is needed. In most cases, contrast material should be ordered for both CT and MRI studies. Contrast may not be necessary in acute hemorrhage, thyroid eye disease, or in trauma cases. Caution is necessary for both iodinated contrast and gadolinium contrast in patients with renal failure, and contrast may be contraindicated in these settings.

3. Topographically localize the lesion clinically ("where is the lesion"), define the differential diagnosis ("what is the lesion"), establish the urgency of the imaging request, and then order the best study tailored to the lesion location (eg, head, orbit, or neck).

4. Order specific imaging sequences (eg, fat suppression for orbital postcontrast study, FLAIR for white matter lesions, gradient recall echo for hemorrhage, DWI for stroke or PRES) depending on clinical indication.

5. Order special imaging for specific vascular indications (eg, MRA or CTA, MRV, conventional angiography).

6. Call the radiologist if there is any doubt about localization, image study of choice, contrast selection, indications, or the final report.

7. If the imaging shows either no abnormality or an abnormality that does not match the clinical localization then call the radiologist or, better yet, review the films directly with them. Ask the radiologist if the area of interest has been adequately imaged, if artifact might be obscuring the lesion, or if additional studies might show the lesion.

8. If the clinical picture suggests a specific lesion or localization and initial imaging is "normal," consider repeating the imaging with thinner slices and higher magnification of the area of interest, especially if the clinical signs and symptoms are progressive.

9. Recognize that the lack of an imaging abnormality does not exclude pathology.

Modified from Lee AG, Brazis PW, Garrity J, et al. Imaging in orbital and neuro-ophthalmic disease. Am J Ophthalmol 2004;138:852–62; with permission.

---

infarcts may show mass effect with hyperintense signals on MRI in adjacent parenchyma. On FLAIR imaging, venous thrombus appears hyperintense, as do venous infarcts. In cases of venous thrombosis, MRI T2W GRE shows blooming.[29] MRV shows absence of flow in the occluded sinus on 2D TOF MRV, and there may be a "frayed" or "shaggy" appearance to the venous sinus.[29] Contrast-enhanced MRV has a high degree of sensitivity and specificity in detecting abnormalities of the cerebral venous system, and can be used to demonstrate collateral flow (**Fig. 21**).[47,48]

SUMMARY

As the neuro-ophthalmologist's arsenal of neuroimaging tools expands, the ability to visualize lesions of the afferent and efferent pathways continues to improve. Recent advances in US, MRI, CT, and angiography have allowed clinicians to obtain high-resolution, noninvasive images, with reduced risks and adverse side effects for patients. The expanding role of neuroimaging, however, does not obviate the role of clinical-anatomic localization. Rather, neuroimaging strategies should be viewed as an extension of, and not a substitute for, the clinical examination. The mechanism of injury and anatomic region of interest must already be established for the role of neuroimaging to be fully realized in the diagnostic process. Regardless of the imaging technique, the diagnostic yield will be low if the wrong imaging technique is chosen; or, alternatively, if the right imaging test is used to visualize the wrong anatomic site. Because neuroimaging strategies are constantly evolving, it is a reasonable to course of action for a neurologist or neuro-ophthalmologist to discuss his or her clinical impressions with a neuroradiologist. This approach (**Box 2**) will help in selecting the best imaging strategy, and enhance one's ability to care for the patients.

REFERENCES

1. Kline LB, Takhtani D, Cure JK. Neuroimaging. In: Levin LA, Arnold AC, editors. Neuro-ophthalmology the practical guide. New York, Stuttgart: Thieme Medical Publishers Inc; 2005. p. 445–58.
2. Jacobson JA. Principles of radiologic imaging. Available at: http://www.merck.com/mmpe/sec22/ch329/ch329d.html. Accessed July, 2008.
3. Souvik S. Magnetic resonance imaging in acute stroke. Available at: http://emedicine.medscape.com/article/1155506. Accessed July 15, 2009.
4. Gillard JH, Waldman AD, Barker PB, editors. Clinical MR neuroimaging: diffusion, perfusion, and spectroscopy. Cambridge (UK), New York, Port Melbourne, Cape Town, Madrid: Cambridge University Press; 2005. p. 229.
5. Bowen B. MR angiography versus CT angiography in the evaluation of neurovascular disease. Radiology 2007;245:357–61.
6. Bose S. Orbital tumors. In: Levin LA, Arnold AC, editors. Neuro-ophthalmology the practical guide. New York, Stuttgart: Thieme Medical Publishers Inc; 2005. p. 345–55.
7. Lien C. Dermoid tumor, CNS: imaging. Available at: http://emedicine.medscape.com/article/339797-imaging. Accessed February 5, 2010.
8. Paonessa A, Limbucci N, Gallucci M. Are bilateral cavernous hemangiomas of the orbit rare entities? The role of MRI in a retrospective study. Eur J Radiol 2008;66:282–6.
9. Jung WS, Ahn KJ, Park MR, et al. The radiological spectrum of orbital pathologies that involve the lacrimal gland and the lacrimal fossa. Korean J Radiol 2007;8(4):336–42.
10. Gündüz K, Shields CL, Günalp I, et al. Magnetic resonance imaging of unilateral lacrimal gland lesions. Graefes Arch Clin Exp Ophthalmol 2003;241(11):907–13.
11. Sohaib S, Moseley I, Wright J. Orbital rhabdomyosarcoma the radiological characteristics. Clin Radiol 1998;53:357–62.
12. Hogan N. Orbital inflammation and infection. In: Levin LA, Arnold AC, editors. Neuro-ophthalmology the practical guide. New York, Stuttgart: Thieme Medical Publishers Inc; 2005. p. 356–86.
13. Kirsch C. Orbit, infection. Available at: http://emedicine.medscape.com/article/383902. Accessed December 11, 2007.
14. Zafar MA, Waheed SS, Enam SA. Orbital *Aspergillus* infection mimicking a tumour: a case report. Cases J 2009;2:7860.
15. Amaral L, Murilo Maschietto M, Maschietto R, et al. Unusual manifestations of neurocysticercosis in MR imaging. Arq Neuropsiquiatr 2003;61:533–41.
16. Courcoutsakis NA, Langford CA, Sneller M. Orbital involvement in Wegener granulomatosis: MR findings in 12 patients. J Comput Assist Tomogr 1997;21:452–8.
17. Wein F. Thyroid-associated orbitopathy. In: Levin LA, Arnold AC, editors. Neuro-ophthalmology the practical guide. New York, Stuttgart: Thieme Medical Publishers Inc; 2005. p. 340–4.

18. Ing E. Thyroid ophthalmopathy: differential diagnoses and work up. Available at: http://emedicine.medscape.com/article/12188444. Accessed April 30, 2008.
19. Gottfried JS, Simbrunner J, Lechner H. Idiopathic sclerotic inflammation of the orbit with left optic nerve compression in a patient with multifocal fibrosclerosis. AJNR Am J Neuroradiol 2000;21:194–7.
20. Roh JH, Koh SB, Kim JH, et al. Orbital myositis in Behçet's disease: a case report with MRI findings. Eur Neurol 2006;56:44–5.
21. Levin LA, Arnold AC. Idiopathic optic neuritis. In: Levin LA, Arnold AC, editors. Neuro-ophthalmology the practical guide. New York, Stuttgart: Thieme Medical Publishers Inc; 2005. p. 198–201.
22. Frohman LP. Other inflammatory optic neuropathies. In: Levin LA, Arnold AC, editors. Neuro-ophthalmology the practical guide. New York, Stuttgart: Thieme Medical Publishers Inc; 2005. p. 202–16.
23. Miller NR. Optic nerve tumors. In: Levin LA, Arnold AC, editors. Neuro-ophthalmology the practical guide. New York, Stuttgart: Thieme Medical Publishers Inc; 2005. p. 253–62.
24. Girkin CA. Compressive optic neuropathy. In: Levin LA, Arnold AC, editors. Neuro-ophthalmology the practical guide. New York, Stuttgart: Thieme Medical Publishers Inc; 2005. p. 217–21.
25. Suzuki H, Takanashi J, Kobayashi K, et al. MR imaging of idiopathic intracranial hypertension. AJNR Am J Neuroradiol 2001;22:196–9.
26. Gossman MV. Pseudopapilledema: differential diagnoses and work up. Available at: http://emedicine.medscape.com/article/1217393. Accessed December 10, 2008.
27. Golnick KC. Congenital optic nerve anomalies. In: Levin LA, Arnold AC, editors. Neuro-ophthalmology the practical guide. New York, Stuttgart: Thieme Medical Publishers Inc; 2005. p. 222–30.
28. Rubin RM. Traumatic optic neuropathy. In: Levin LA, Arnold AC, editors. Neuro-ophthalmology the practical guide. New York, Stuttgart: Thieme Medical Publishers Inc; 2005. p. 246–52.
29. Osborne A, Blaser S, Salzman K. Diagnostic Imaging - Brain. Salt Lake city (Utah): Amirsys Inc; 2004.
30. Pless ML. Cavernous sinus disorders. In: Levin LA, Arnold AC, editors. Neuro-ophthalmology the practical guide. New York, Stuttgart: Thieme Medical Publishers Inc; 2005. p. 296–303.
31. Compston A, Coles A. Multiple sclerosis. Lancet 2008;372:1502–17.
32. Optic Neuritis Study Group. Multiple sclerosis risk after optic neuritis: final optic neuritis treatment trial follow-up. Arch Neurol 2008;65(6):727–32.
33. Polman CH, Reingold SC, Edan G, et al. Diagnostic criteria for multiple sclerosis: 2005 revisions to the "McDonald criteria". Ann Neurol 2005;58:840–6.
34. McDonald WI, Compston A, Edan G, et al. Recommended diagnostic criteria for multiple sclerosis: guidelines from the international panel on the diagnosis of multiple sclerosis. Ann Neurol 2001;50:121–7.
35. Buguet-Brown ML, Le Gulluche Y, Vichard A, et al. Spontaneous intracranial hypotension: a recent indication for epidural blood patch. Br J Anaesth 2006; 96(5):668–9.
36. Guillamo JS, Monjour A, Taillandier L, et al. Brainstem gliomas in adults: prognostic factors and classification. Brain 2001;124:2528–39.
37. Zohrabian D. Dissection, carotid artery. Available at: http://www.emedicine.com/emerg/TOPIC82. Accessed October 30, 2008.
38. Kidwell CS. Dissection syndromes. Available at: http://www.emedicine.com/neuro/topic99. Accessed September 12, 2007.

39. Arnold M, Baumgartner RW, Stapf C, et al. Ultrasound diagnosis of spontaneous carotid dissection with isolated Horner syndrome. Stroke 2008;39:82–6.
40. Gobin-Metteil MP, Oppenheim C, Domigo V, et al. Cervical arteries dissection: diagnostic color Doppler US criteria at the acute phase. J Radiol 2006;87:343–4.
41. Roy J, Akhtar N, Watson T, et al. Transcranial Doppler microembolic signal monitoring is useful in diagnosis and treatment of carotid artery dissection: two case reports. J Neuroimaging 2007;17:350–2.
42. Srinivasan J, Newell DW, Sturzenegger M, et al. Transcranial Doppler in the evaluation of internal carotid artery dissection. Stroke 1996;27:1226–30.
43. Bash S, Villablanca P, Jahan R, et al. Intracranial vascular stenosis and occlusive disease: evaluation with CT angiography, MR angiography, and digital subtraction angiography. AJNR Am J Neuroradiol 2005;26:1012–21.
44. Skutta B, Furst G, Eilers J, et al. Intracranial stenoocclusive disease: double-detector helical CT angiography versus digital subtraction angiography. AJNR Am J Neuroradiol 1999;20:791–9.
45. Hirai T, Korogi Y, Ono K, et al. Prospective evaluation for suspected stenoocclusive disease of the intracranial artery: combined MR angiography and CT angiography compared with digital subtraction angiography. AJNR Am J Neuroradiol 2002;23:93–101.
46. Khan S, Rich P, Clifton A, et al. Noninvasive detection of vertebral artery stenosis: a comparison of contrast-enhanced MR angiography, CT angiography, and ultrasound. Stroke 2009;40:3499–503.
47. Thornton MJ, Ryan R, Varghese JC, et al. A three dimensional gadolinium enhanced MR venography technique for imaging central veins. AJR Am J Roentgenol 1999;173:999–1003.
48. Rodallec MH, Krainik A, Feydy A, et al. Cerebral venous thrombosis and multidetector CT angiography: tips and tricks. Radiographics 2006;26(Suppl 1):S5–18.
49. Lee AG, Brazis PW, Garrity J, et al. Imaging in orbital and neuro-ophthalmic disease. Am J Ophthalmol 2004;138:852–62.

Functional Visual Loss

Beau B. Bruce, MD*, Nancy J. Newman, MD

KEYWORDS

• Functional visual loss • Nonorganic visual loss

Neurologists are frequently called on to evaluate patients complaining of vision loss. Similar to other areas of neurology, a significant proportion of these patients have nonorganic disease.[1–3] Nonorganic visual loss is frequently called functional visual loss.[4–6] The ability to differentiate between organic and functional visual loss has important clinical and medicolegal implications.[7,8]

NEURO-OPHTHALMOLOGY AND NONORGANIC DYSFUNCTION

One of the most common interactions between the neurologist and the ophthalmologist occurs over patients with nonorganic visual dysfunction. It is estimated that such cases constitute up to 5% of a general ophthalmologist's practice, frequently resulting in neurologic consultation after no ocular cause is identified.[9,10] Using objective measurements, one can identify nonphysiologic responses and can sometimes unequivocally prove the organic integrity of the visual system.[9,11–15]

Functional visual loss is never a diagnosis of exclusion; positive findings are required to make the diagnosis. Occasionally these positive findings may not be related to the patient's primary complaint. Furthermore, it is not enough to demonstrate that the patient's responses are nonphysiologic. This demonstration is a helpful adjunct and acts as confirmatory evidence in the diagnosis of a nonorganic disorder. However, organic and nonorganic disease can and do coexist. In reviews of 2 neuro-ophthalmologists' experiences, 53% of patients with evidence of functional visual loss

Support: This work was supported in part by a departmental grant (Department of Ophthalmology) from Research to Prevent Blindness Inc, New York, NY, USA, by core grant P30-EY06360 (Department of Ophthalmology) from the National Institutes of Health/National Eye Institute, and PHS Grant KL2-RR025009 (B.B.B.) from the Clinical and Translational Science Award Program, National Institutes of Health/National Center for Research Resources. B.B.B. was a recipient of the American Academy of Neurology Practice Research Fellowship. N.J.N. is a recipient of the Research to Prevent Blindness Lew R. Wasserman Merit Award.

This article is adapted from: Newman NJ. Neuro-ophthalmology and psychiatry. Gen Hosp Psych 1993;15(2):102–14; with permission.

Departments of Ophthalmology and Neurology, and Neurological Surgery, Emory University School of Medicine, 1365-B Clifton Road, NE, Atlanta, GA 30322, USA
* Corresponding author.
E-mail address: bbbruce@emory.edu

Neurol Clin 28 (2010) 789–802
doi:10.1016/j.ncl.2010.03.012 **neurologic.theclinics.com**

had coexistent organic disease.[14,16] In a recent study of a series of patients with idiopathic intracranial hypertension, 6% had concurrent functional visual loss, complicating the decision to proceed with surgical intervention.[17] A purely nonorganic disorder can only be diagnosed if the maneuvers used during examination prove normal function of the system being tested.

Patients with evidence of nonorganic visual dysfunction are typically described as having functional visual loss, in an attempt to avoid distinguishing between patients whose conditions are intentionally feigned and those whose conditions are thought to be outside the realm of the patient's consciousness. There are 3 major categories of functional disorders: (1) somatoform disorders (commonly referred to as hysteria), (2) factitious disorders, and (3) malingering.[18] In general, malingering implies purposeful feigning or exaggeration of symptoms usually for clear secondary gain, whereas somatoform disorders are thought to occur outside the patient's conscious awareness.[9,11,13–15] Factitious disorders are characterized by intentionally produced symptoms for the purpose of assuming a sick role.[18] Differentiating among these diagnostic categories remains difficult and within the psychiatrist's realm, demonstrating that the nonphysiologic nature of the complaint is in the neurologist's and neuro-ophthalmologist's realm.

Neurologists and neuro-ophthalmologists are particularly adept at demonstrating the organic or nonorganic nature of a symptom or sign because they evaluate an organ system that respects certain anatomic rules that are not intuitively understood by the patient. In addition, the visual system, more than other parts of the sensory system, is closely observable and measurable. Armed with the knowledge of neuroanatomy and neurophysiology, a working understanding of basic ophthalmologic tools, and a little sleight of hand, one can demonstrate the integrity of the visual system.

Like any evaluation of visual loss, one's approach begins by first differentiating monocular from binocular visual loss. This differentiation allows physicians to appropriately localize potential organic lesions and strategize the history and physical examination. Next, the physicians should further refine the examination by identifying whether the visual loss is primarily central (visual acuity loss) or peripheral (visual field loss) so that techniques tailored to each case can assist clinicians in determining whether the responses are nonphysiologic.

MONOCULAR VISUAL ACUITY LOSS

Loss of visual acuity is a common presenting complaint of the patient with functional visual loss. When it assumes a monocular pattern, the ideal testing situation is established. All these tests are designed to take advantage of the fact that in binocular vision it is difficult to separate out what each eye sees. Patients feigning monocular visual loss may try to close one eye or the other during the examination. The success of these tests depends on a skilled examiner, and each test can be described to the patient in a manner that obscures the true intent of the test for the purpose of detecting functional visual loss. One of the best tests available to the neurologist is a test of stereopsis, which requires good vision and good binocular fusion. The widely available and relatively inexpensive Titmus or Randot StereoTests (Stereo Optical Co, Inc, Chicago, IL, USA) are examples of tests for stereopsis. Presenting stereopsis as a test of how the eyes work together is usually successful. The degree of stereopsis in a set of standardized tests has been correlated with the minimum visual acuity required in each eye (**Table 1**).[19]

Colored lenses allow only similarly colored light to pass through. If a patient wears glasses with one green and one red lens while viewing an eye chart with alternate

Table 1	
Relationship of stereopsis to visual acuity	
Stereopsis (Arc Second)	Visual Acuity
40	20/20
43	20/25
52	20/30
61	20/40
78	20/50
94	20/70
124	20/100
160	20/200

Data from Levy NS, Glick EB. Stereoscopic perception and Snellen visual acuity. Am J Ophthalmol 1974;78(4):722–4.

green and red letters, the function and acuity of each eye can be individually assessed. This assessment can be presented to a patient as a color test. Similarly, the patient can be given polarized glasses with different axes in each lens and asked to read a polarized eye chart with some letters perceptible only to one eye or the other.

Another set of tests works on the principle of "fogging."[9,11,13–15] While the patient views the eye chart with both eyes open, the "good" eye is subtly fogged so that any useful binocular vision must be a result of "bad" eye function. Using the phoropter, an instrument of refraction, convex lenses of high strength are placed in front of the good eye so that binocular vision of 20/20 would prove to be 20/20 vision of the "bad eye." Unfortunately, this test relies on a piece of specialized equipment that is usually unavailable to the neurologist. All of these tests have the advantage of not only proving that the presumed bad eye has vision, but also documenting the amount of vision present, which is critical to demonstrating normal function and thereby proving pure functional loss.

Other less quantitative tests may be necessary to prove better vision than that claimed by the patient. These maneuvers are similar to those performed on the patient with severe binocular visual loss (see later in the article), except that the good eye in the monocular cases must be occluded during testing, with the following exceptions: First, in the patient claiming profound monocular visual loss, the absence of a relative afferent pupillary defect (Marcus Gunn pupil or swinging flashlight sign) makes functional visual loss, refractive error, or media opacity more likely. Second, one could also place a 4 diopter prism over the better-seeing eye of a patient complaining of substantial monocular visual loss. If the patient reports seeing 2 images when viewing an object that they previously claimed to be unable to see, one should suspect at least a degree of functional visual loss, because a patient with organic disease will only see 1 image.[20] There are other variations of this test, which uses a single prism, that require a minimal sleight of hand, but presumably have a reduced chance of being foiled by the astute malingerer.[21] Finally, binocular visual fields can be evaluated to see if the patient has sufficient vision in the affected eye to prohibit plotting of the physiologic blind spot of the normal eye. If the bad eye is truly nonseeing, the physiologic blind spot of the good eye should be plottable.

BINOCULAR VISUAL ACUITY LOSS

More difficult are the cases of binocular visual loss, where the level of expectation as communicated by the examiner becomes extremely important. The patient is asked to read the eye chart from the bottom upwards, obscuring the other lines and beginning with the smallest available line, usually 20/10. The examiner allows for significant time on each line, repeatedly encouraging the patients to make the best guesses, and explaining that they should be able to see the chart. By the time patients reach the 20/20 or 20/25 lines, frequently good vision is established; this may be particularly useful in the patient whose symptoms seem to be highly suggestive of functional visual loss rather than the obvious malingerer. Similarly, lenses that when combined are the equivalent of plain glass can be placed in front of the patient's refractive correction while the examiner suggests that these would magnify the letters on the chart. Another feature of patients with functional visual loss is that they frequently claim the same visual acuity when the distance from the eye chart is halved. The physiology of vision is such that if patients see the 20/100 line at 20 ft, they should be able to see the 20/50 line at 10 ft. This form of visual acuity testing has been shown to be highly specific and sensitive for functional visual loss.[22]

Less quantitative maneuvers that at least establish the presence of vision may be necessary in those patients with professed severe bilateral visual loss. In the mirror test, a large mirror is rotated back and forth in the vertical axis in front of the patient.[9,11,13] It is very difficult for a patient with normal vision to avoid following this moving image. Similarly, the optokinetic drum or tape elicits appropriate fast and slow phases of nystagmus in eyes that have at least 20/200 vision.[11,13] Under the guise of coordination tests, patients who report vision loss can be asked to wiggle their fingers, open and close their fists, and then perform a movement, while the examiner quickly performs another simple movement of the hands.[6] The patient with normal vision may mimic the new movement before realizing the slip. Simply observing the patient may be informative. The "blind" patient who easily maneuvers around physical obstacles in the examining room, or who flinches when an object or bright light is suddenly presented, is likely to have at least a component of functional visual loss. Additional findings confirming nonphysiologic tendencies include a failure to direct the eyes to look at one's own hand and an inability to touch the 2 index fingertips together when so instructed (**Fig. 1**); these tests of proprioception are easily passed by a truly blind person. Spasm of the near triad (purposeful convergence with associated pupillary miosis) may also be witnessed. It has been observed that patients with functional visual loss frequently wear sunglasses (46%) in the clinic, and yet have no ocular findings to provide an organic reason for this.[9,23]

VISUAL FIELD LOSS

Functional visual loss may assume the form of visual field loss. The most common visual field complaint is that of concentric loss of peripheral vision, such as "tunnel vision." The field may be constricted to 5° to 10° centrally, yet the patient has no difficulty maneuvering around objects in the periphery. The classic configuration on tangent screen testing is that of circular constriction that does not expand appropriately when the distance between the patient and the tangent screen is increased (**Fig. 2**).[9,11–15] This "tunnel field" can also be confirmed with confrontation testing at different distances. Visual fields performed kinetically on the Goldmann perimeter may show a similar constriction with nonphysiologic overlap of isopters (ie, the patient claims to see the smaller less bright object at the same place as the larger brighter test object). Alternatively, the patient with functional visual loss may plot out a continuous spiral or a jagged inconsistent star pattern (**Fig. 3**). It is not unusual for the patient with functional visual loss complaining of defects other than visual field loss to have visual fields plotted in these patterns. In those cases, the visual field abnormalities can act as

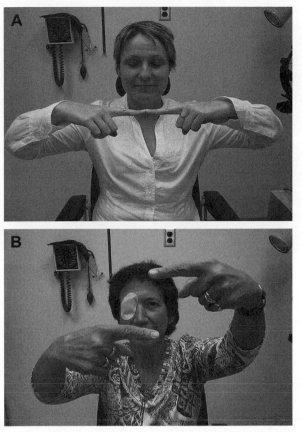

Fig. 1. (*A*) A person who is truly blind can touch the tips of the fingers properly. (*B*) A person with functional visual loss is often unable to touch the tips of the fingers properly. (*From* Biousse V, Newman NJ. Neuro-ophthalmology illustrated. New York: Thieme; 2009. p. 504; with permission.)

additional evidence of functional visual loss. Automated static perimetry is generally not helpful in the assessment of patients with suspected functional visual loss. Poor testing parameters and inconsistent responses do not differentiate between the patient with nonphysiologic visual dysfunction and the organic patient unable to adequately perform this test. Some have suggested that square or cloverleaf appearances are seen more frequently in cases of functional visual loss,[9] but this cannot be relied on as a diagnostic of functional visual loss (**Fig. 4**).

Other patterns of visual field loss are less common. Monocular hemianopia can often be proven functional by the patient's performance on binocular visual field testing. In the patient with organic disease, the good eye's visual field will compensate for most of the missing bad eye's field. With the patient with functional visual loss, the hemianopia may persist binocularly (**Fig. 5**).[12,13,24] Similarly, in the patient with professed severe monocular visual loss, a binocular visual field (with both eyes open) may reveal a nonphysiologic constriction or absence of the visual field on the side of the monocular loss, a region clearly seen on previous testing of the good eye alone (**Fig. 6**). Patients with true bitemporal hemianopia will not be able to see objects beyond the point of fixation because they will lie entirely within the missing

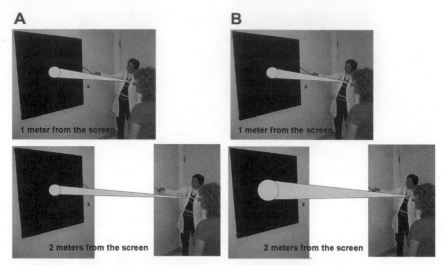

Fig. 2. (A) Nonorganic constriction of visual field on tangent screen test. The size of the visual field does not increase when the patient is moved farther away from the screen. (B) Organic constriction of visual field on tangent screen test. The size of the visual field increases when the patient is moved farther away from the screen. (*From* Biousse V, Newman NJ. Neuro-ophthalmology illustrated. New York: Thieme; 2009. p. 504; with permission.)

temporal fields of vision.[12,13,25] Patients with functional visual loss having bitemporal hemianopia are rarely medically sophisticated enough to demonstrate this. Central scotomas or arcuate defects are unlikely manifestations of functional visual loss and should prompt a careful search for true organic abnormality.[16]

ANCILLARY TESTING

A thorough neuro-ophthalmic evaluation, complete with appropriate special maneuvers specifically directed toward revealing nonphysiologic responses, are usually sufficient to not only establish the presence of nonorganic visual dysfunction but also prove normal function of the system. In those patients in whom completely normal function cannot be demonstrated, but a nonorganic cause is suspected, ancillary tests are occasionally useful. Visual evoked potentials of normal and symmetric amplitude and latency in a patient with profound monocular visual loss are confirmatory evidence of a functional loss of vision.[11] Although not widely available, multifocal visual evoked potentials may demonstrate normal electrophysiological responses in the region of purported visual loss.[26] However, an abnormal visual evoked response is less helpful. Voluntary alteration or obliteration of evoked potentials is not uncommon and may be unapparent even to a trained observer.[25,27] A similar situation exists with pattern and multifocal electroretinograms where a normal and symmetric response argues against the presence of severe organic disease, and an abnormal test is inconclusive.[28–30] The flash electroretinogram measures the function of predominantly the outer retinal layers of cells involved in vision. It should be abnormal in a patient with diffuse retinal dysfunction but will be normal in a patient with more distal organic disease such as optic neuropathy, chiasmal neuropathy, or retrochiasmal visual dysfunction. Neuroimaging may help rule out obvious compressive or vascular lesions, but negative studies do not establish the diagnosis of a functional disorder. Indeed, Moster and

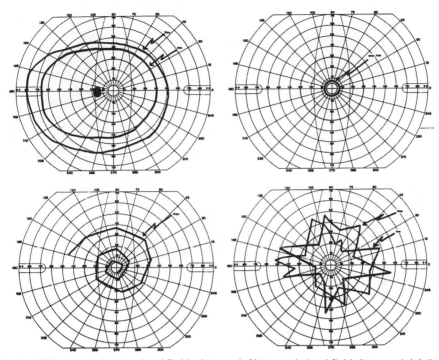

Fig. 3. Goldmann perimetry visual fields. (*Upper left*) Normal visual field. (*Upper right*) Constricted visual field of a patient with functional visual loss. Note that the constriction is to the same degree for 2 different-sized stimuli. (*Lower left*) Spiral visual field of a patient with functional visual loss. (*Lower right*) Star-pattern visual field with inconsistent responses in a patient with functional visual loss. (*From* Newman NJ. Neuro-ophthalmology and psychiatry. Gen Hosp Psych 1993;15:105; with permission.)

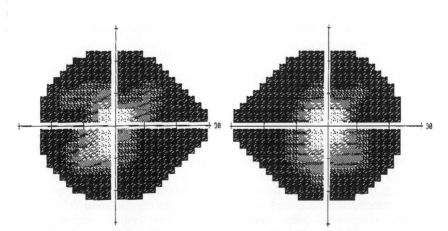

Fig. 4. Nonphysiologic static (Humphrey) perimetry. Note the box-like appearance of the right eye's visual field and the cloverleaf-like pattern of loss in the left eye's visual field in a patient claiming severe bilateral visual loss. Goldmann perimetry confirmed nonphysiologic visual field loss.

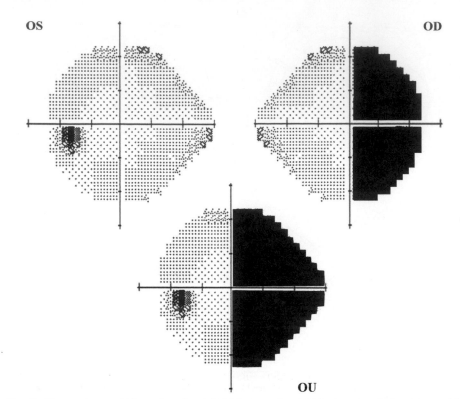

Fig. 5. Monocular and binocular visual field in a patient with functional visual loss with monocular hemianopia of the right eye. In the binocular field the hemianopia persists, whereas in organic disease the normal nasal visual field of the right eye compensates for the deficit in the temporal field of the left eye.

colleagues[31] found lesions on nuclear medicine imaging studies (single photon emission computed tomography and positron emission tomography) while evaluating 2 patients with suspected functional visual loss. A functional disturbance must never be a diagnosis of exclusion.

FUNCTIONAL VISUAL LOSS: A MARKER OF PSYCHIATRIC DISEASE?

Evidence of a functional visual disturbance may be seen in a range of patients, from the "deliberate malingerer" to the "indifferent hysteric" to the "suggestible innocent."[15] Patients vary in their degree of awareness, fraud, and suggestibility. Few, if any, of the maneuvers outlined in the previous sections distinguish between these underlying differences in motive and cause. As a result the prognosis, management, and therapy for these patients differ markedly.

As a group, patients with functional visual disturbances may not have an incidence of true psychiatric disease as high as had been previously assumed.[10,14,15,32,33] Krill and Newell[34] claimed "no uniform psychological factors" in their group of 59 patients with functional visual loss. Similarly, Van Balen and Slijper[35] found no difference on psychological testing between 43 children with functional visual loss and age-matched controls. Older studies report the incidence of psychiatric disease in patients presenting with functional visual loss as ranging from 70% to 100%.[10,36–39] However,

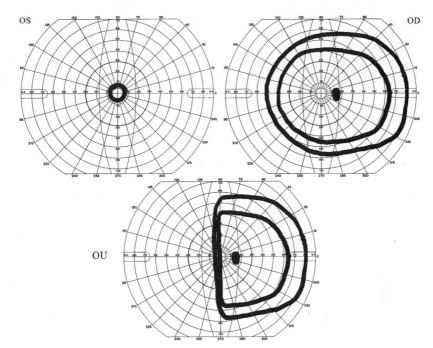

Fig. 6. Goldmann visual fields in a patient claiming severe monocular visual loss in the left eye. The right eye is normal and the left eye shows severe tubular constriction. In the binocular visual field, there is nonphysiologic constriction to the left side, a region clearly seen by the patient previously when testing the right eye alone.

many of these patients were given diagnoses including headache, mixed psychoneurosis, tension state, fatigue, vertigo, cardiovascular spasm, convulsion, hysteria, psychosis, low intellect, overly dependent, compulsiveness, anxiousness, and overly independent, all of which are not accepted under the current classification of psychiatric disorders.[10] A recent series of 140 patients reported by Lim and colleagues[40] found that 39% of adults and 18% of children had an underlying history of psychiatric disease, and that a significant proportion of both adults and children reported concomitant psychosocial events (36%). These events were more likely to be related to trauma in adults and to social causes in children. In another series of 71 consecutive children with functional visual loss, 27% had previously diagnosed psychiatric disturbances, 31% had significant home or school stress, 23% wanted glasses, and 14% of the patients had no identifiable cause.[41] However, both of these studies were limited by retrospective nonsystematic screening for psychiatric disease.

Review of the literature also led Kathol and colleagues[10] to conclude that psychiatric disease is far from being uniformly present, and that many patients with functional visual loss do not appear to have psychiatric syndromes or personality disorders.[32,33] The investigators reexamined 42 of their own patients with functional visual loss at an average of 4 years after the initial diagnosis: 22 were diagnosed with a psychiatric disorder based on the criteria mentioned in the *Diagnostic and Statistical Manual of Mental Disorders*, Third Edition (DSM-III) and/or personality disorder at some time during the course of their observation, 23 had persistent findings of nonphysiologic visual disturbances at follow-up, but only 8 of these 23 patients had a diagnosed psychiatric disorder and few were either socially or economically impaired. One criticism of this study is that patients were included as examples of functional visual loss even if the abnormalities were incidentally discovered. It is not surprising that patients such as these would not be assigned a DSM-III–based psychiatric diagnosis. The investigators concluded that some patients with functional visual loss are merely suggestible. This theory is not new, because Babinski[42] postulated in 1909 that isolated "hysterical" symptoms were a product of the patient's suggestibility.

The reemergence of the idea of suggestibility has led several investigators to emphasize the role of simple reassurance in the treatment of many patients with functional visual disturbances.[13,15,32,33,40] In some cases, patients may be convinced that their symptoms are not signs of serious illness, are commonly seen by the examiner, and are likely to improve with time. This form of therapy can begin in the clinician's office and may be sufficient to preclude further psychiatric management. It is generally unhelpful to directly confront patients who are malingering; indeed, the explanation to the patient on why the findings are nonphysiologic may merely educate them on how to better evade detection in the future.

Differences in underlying motive and cause may help explain the generally poor response of functional visual loss to a wide range of treatments including psychotherapy.[10,15,32,33,40] Kathol and colleagues[10] retrospectively reviewed the response of patients with nonorganic visual dysfunction to a variety of therapies including hypnosis, behavior modification, psychotherapy, and nonspecific treatments such as special glasses, eye drops, placebos, surgery, prayer, sham lumbar puncture, and electroconvulsive therapy. No treatment was more beneficial than another, and there was no significant difference in the outcome of those receiving psychiatric treatment and those not. In Lim and colleagues'[40] series, 11% of the patients were referred for counseling and the remainder only needed reassurance. However, patients with functional visual loss may have a wide variety of underlying psychiatric and nonpsychiatric diagnoses. It is obvious that prospective randomized studies that attempt to separate patients by underlying diagnoses are necessary before conclusions can be drawn regarding the success of specific therapies.

ORGANIC DYSFUNCTION MIMICKING FUNCTIONAL VISUAL LOSS

Some organic disorders can present with visual loss combined with symptoms and signs of psychiatric disease that may lead the clinician to falsely presume that the visual loss is functional in nature.[40,43–46] Early recognition of these disorders may aid in the timely evaluation and institution of appropriate therapy. In several of these disorders, the neuro-ophthalmologic examination may provide evidence of organic disorder and suggest the location and nature of the underlying problem, allowing subsequent directed evaluation and management.

Neoplasms involving the central nervous system, especially in the pituitary-hypothalamic region and frontal lobes, may cause visual loss associated with psychiatric features. Up to 50% of patients with intracranial mass lesions will develop psychiatric symptoms and occasionally these will be the presenting manifestation.[46] Patients with pituitary tumors, especially those that secrete adrenocorticotropic hormone or those that cause panhypopituitarism, may present with depression.[47,48] Similarly, mass lesions involving the hypothalamic region, including craniopharyngioma and neurosarcoidosis, may result in personality changes and frank psychiatric symptoms.[49–52]

Examination of the visual system may show evidence of compression of the optic nerves or chiasm on visual field testing and ophthalmoscopic examination. Central scotomas, arcuate defects, and subtle bitemporal defects are likely to be manifestations of organic disease. Unrecognized tumors of the frontal lobes may result in papilledema and visual loss associated with apathy, depression, and personality changes. Without adequate fundoscopic examination, the visual complaints might be attributed to functional visual loss.[46] A paraneoplastic photoreceptor degeneration can result in rapid visual loss, initially misdiagnosed as nonorganic in origin.[53–55] Ophthalmoscopic examination combined with electroretinography will ultimately result in correct diagnosis.

Strokes may occasionally mimic functional visual loss. For example, top-of-the-basilar infarction can present with visual disturbances and behavioral alterations.[56] Careful examination may reveal abnormalities of vertical gaze and visual field defects suggestive of occipital lobe ischemia. The posterior form of Alzheimer disease can also present with visual complaints and psychiatric/cognitive disturbances that are not infrequently thought to represent functional complaints. Signs can include prominent visual agnosia, visual-spatial difficulties, and even frank visual field defects.[57,58] Multiple sclerosis is another disorder in which visual complaints are often combined with unusual conditions that may at first appear to be the symptoms of nonorganic disease. The neuro-ophthalmologic history and examination can be useful in revealing clinical evidence of demyelination involving the afferent and efferent visual systems.

The clinician must also be cautious while evaluating patients with known psychiatric disease to not quickly dismiss complaints of visual loss as functional. Some of the visual complaints in a patient with psychiatric disorders may be a direct result of psychiatric medications.[59,60] The classic example is pigmentary retinopathy caused by thioridazine (Mellaril),[61,62] but this is much less frequent because the largest manufacturers of the drug discontinued its production in 2005. Early complaints include difficulties with night vision and a brownish tinge to vision. Chlorpromazine (Thorazine) remains on the market and can also cause pigmentary retinopathy, but usually only at high doses.[63] Retinal screening examinations may reveal abnormalities prior to symptoms. Phenothiazines can also cause opacities of the cornea or lens. Ocular surface disease is a frequent cause of decreased vision and can result from antidopaminergic drug–induced pseudoparkinsonism, resulting in decreased blink and consequent corneal surface symptoms. Anticholinergics can also contribute to ocular surface disease through decreased tear production. Other anticholinergic effects that affect vision are decreased accommodative ability and aggravation of narrow-angle glaucoma.

SUMMARY

The neurologist frequently interacts with the ophthalmologist regarding patients with suspected functional visual loss. Simple examination techniques combined with the judicious use of ancillary testing can confirm the nonphysiologic nature of the visual complaints and often prove normal visual function. A neurologist who has a patient with visual loss should always seek consultation with an ophthalmologist to ensure that there is no underlying ophthalmic explanation. Similarly, if hysteria or malingering is suspected in a patient without overt visual system involvement, ophthalmologic examination may reveal confirmatory signs of nonorganic dysfunction or instead may discover findings supporting an organic neurologic cause. Communication between the neurologist and ophthalmologist regarding the specific questions to be addressed can help to focus the examination and allow the ophthalmologist to aid in the diagnosis of functional visual loss with some of their specialized tools. If uncertainty remains, consultation with a neuro-ophthalmologist is likely appropriate, because many of the tests are beyond the scope of those usually performed by a general ophthalmologist, and require significant patience and time on the part of the examiner.

REFERENCES

1. Berlin RM, Ronthal M, Bixler EO, et al. Psychiatric symptomatology in an outpatient neurology clinic. J Clin Psychiatry 1983;44(6):204–6.
2. Kirk C, Saunders M. Primary psychiatric illness in a neurological out-patient department in North East England. An assessment of symptomatology. Acta Psychiatr Scand 1977;56(4):294–302.
3. Kirk CA, Saunders M. Psychiatric illness in a neurological out-patient department in North East England. Use of the General Health Questionnaire in the prospective study of neurological out-patients. Acta Psychiatr Scand 1979; 60(5):427–37.
4. Biousse V, Newman NJ. Nonorganic neuro-ophthalmic symptoms and signs. Neuro-ophthalmology illustrated. New York: Thieme; 2009:501–10.
5. Miller NR. Neuro-ophthalmologic manifestations of nonorganic disease. In: Miller NR, Newman NJ, editors. Walsh and Hoyt's clinical neuro-ophthalmology, vol. 2. 6th edition. Philadelphia: Lippincott William & Wilkins; 2005. p. 1315–34.
6. Newman NJ. Neuro-ophthalmology and psychiatry. Gen Hosp Psychiatry 1993; 15(2):102–14.
7. Wasfy IA, Wasfy E, Aly TA, et al. Ophthalmic medicolegal cases in Upper Egypt. Int Arch Med 2009;2(1):1.
8. Mavrakanas NA, Schutz JS. Feigned visual loss misdiagnosed as occult traumatic optic neuropathy: diagnostic guidelines and medical-legal issues. Surv Ophthalmol 2009;54(3):412–6.
9. Miller BW. A review of practical tests for ocular malingering and hysteria. Surv Ophthalmol 1973;17(4):241–6.
10. Kathol RG, Cox TA, Corbett JJ, et al. Functional visual loss: I. A true psychiatric disorder? Psychol Med 1983;13(2):307–14.
11. Kramer KK, La Piana FG, Appleton B. Ocular malingering and hysteria: diagnosis and management. Surv Ophthalmol 1979;24(2):89–96.
12. Keane JR. Neuro-ophthalmic signs and symptoms of hysteria. Neurology 1982; 32(7):757–62.
13. Smith CH, Beck RW, Mills RP. Functional disease in neuro-ophthalmology. Neurol Clin 1983;1(4):955–71.
14. Keltner JL, May WN, Johnson CA, et al. The California syndrome. Functional visual complaints with potential economic impact. Ophthalmology 1985;92(3): 427–35.
15. Thompson HS. Functional visual loss. Am J Ophthalmol 1985;100(1):209–13.
16. Scott JA, Egan RA. Prevalence of organic neuro-ophthalmologic disease in patients with functional visual loss. Am J Ophthalmol 2003;135(5):670–5.
17. Ney JJ, Volpe NJ, Liu GT, et al. Functional visual loss in idiopathic intracranial hypertension. Ophthalmology 2009;116(9):1808–13, e1801.
18. American Psychiatric Association. Diagnostic and statistical manual of mental disorders: DSM-IV-TR. 4th edition. Washington, DC: American Psychiatric Association; 2000.
19. Levy NS, Glick EB. Stereoscopic perception and Snellen visual acuity. Am J Ophthalmol 1974;78(4):722–4.
20. Golnik KC, Lee AG, Eggenberger ER. The monocular vertical prism dissociation test. Am J Ophthalmol 2004;137(1):135–7.
21. Chen CS, Lee AW, Karagiannis A, et al. Practical clinical approaches to functional visual loss. J Clin Neurosci 2007;14(1):1–7.

22. Zinkernagel SM, Mojon DS. Distance doubling visual acuity test: a reliable test for nonorganic visual loss. Graefes Arch Clin Exp Ophthalmol 2009;247(6): 855–8.

23. Bengtzen R, Woodward M, Lynn MJ, et al. The "sunglasses sign" predicts nonorganic visual loss in neuro-ophthalmologic practice. Neurology 2008;70(3): 218–21.

24. Keane JR. Hysterical hemianopia. The 'missing half' field defect. Arch Ophthalmol 1979;97(5):865–6.

25. Mills RP, Glaser JS. Hysterical bitemporal hemianopia. Arch Ophthalmol 1981; 99(11):2053.

26. Massicotte EC, Semela L, Hedges TR 3rd. Multifocal visual evoked potential in nonorganic visual field loss. Arch Ophthalmol 2005;123(3):364–7.

27. Bumgartner J, Epstein CM. Voluntary alteration of visual evoked potentials. Ann Neurol 1982;12(5):475–8.

28. Reiss AB, Biousse V, Yin H, et al. Voluntary alteration of full-field electroretinogram. Am J Ophthalmol 2005;139(3):571–2.

29. Rover J, Bach M. Pattern electroretinogram plus visual evoked potential: a decisive test in patients suspected of malingering. Doc Ophthalmol 1987;66(3): 245–51.

30. Vrabec TR, Affel EL, Gaughan JP, et al. Voluntary suppression of the multifocal electroretinogram. Ophthalmology 2004;111(1):169–76.

31. Moster ML, Galetta SL, Schatz NJ. Physiologic functional imaging in "functional" visual loss. Surv Ophthalmol 1996;40(5):395–9.

32. Kathol RG, Cox TA, Corbett JJ, et al. Functional visual loss: II. Psychiatric aspects in 42 patients followed for 4 years. Psychol Med 1983;13(2):315–24.

33. Kathol RG, Cox TA, Corbett JJ, et al. Functional visual loss. Follow-up of 42 cases. Arch Ophthalmol 1983;101(5):729–35.

34. Krill AE, Newell FW. The diagnosis of ocular conversion reaction involving visual function. Arch Ophthalmol 1968;79(3).254–61.

35. van Balen AT, Slijper FE. Psychogenic amblyopia in children. J Pediatr Ophthalmol Strabismus 1978;15(3):164–7.

36. Linhart WO. Field findings in functional disease; report of 63 cases. Am J Ophthalmol 1956;42(1):75–84.

37. Friesen H, Mann WA. Follow-up study of hysterical amblyopia. Am J Ophthalmol 1966;62(6):1106–15.

38. Rada RT, Meyer GG, Krill AE. Visual conversion reaction in children. I. Diagnosis. Psychosomatics 1969;10(1):23–8.

39. Gross MP, Sloan SH. Patients with eye symptoms and no organic illness: an interdisciplinary study. Psychiatry Med 1971;2(4):298–307.

40. Lim SA, Siatkowski RM, Farris BK. Functional visual loss in adults and children patient characteristics, management, and outcomes. Ophthalmology 2005; 112(10):1821–8.

41. Taich A, Crowe S, Kosmorsky GS, et al. Prevalence of psychosocial disturbances in children with nonorganic visual loss. J AAPOS 2004;8(5):457–61.

42. Babinski J. Demembrement de l'hysterie traditionnelle: pithiatisme. La Semaine Medicale 1909;29:3–8 [in French].

43. Hall RCW. Psychiatric presentations of medical illness: somatopsychic disorders. Springer (NY): Scientific & Medical Books; 1980.

44. Hayes JR, Butler NE, Martin CR. Misunderstood somatopsychic concomitants of medical disorders. Psychosomatics 1986;27(2):128–30, 133.

45. Cummings JL. Organic psychosis. Psychosomatics 1988;29(1):16–26.

46. Binder RL. Neurologically silent brain tumors in psychiatric hospital admissions: three cases and a review. J Clin Psychiatry 1983;44(3):94–7.
47. Cohen SI. Cushing's syndrome: a psychiatric study of 29 patients. Br J Psychiatry 1980;136:120–4.
48. Kelly WF, Checkley SA, Bender DA, et al. Cushing's syndrome and depression—a prospective study of 26 patients. Br J Psychiatry 1983;142:16–9.
49. Baskin DS, Wilson CB. Surgical management of craniopharyngiomas. A review of 74 cases. J Neurosurg 1986;65(1):22–7.
50. Delaney P. Neurologic manifestations in sarcoidosis: review of the literature, with a report of 23 cases. Ann Intern Med 1977;87(3):336–45.
51. Stern BJ, Krumholz A, Johns C, et al. Sarcoidosis and its neurological manifestations. Arch Neurol 1985;42(9):909–17.
52. Heffernan A, Cullen M, Towers R, et al. Sarcoidosis of the hypothalamus. A case report with a review of the literature. Hormones 1971;2(1):1–12.
53. Sawyer RA, Selhorst JB, Zimmerman LE, et al. Blindness caused by photoreceptor degeneration as a remote effect of cancer. Am J Ophthalmol 1976; 81(5):606–13.
54. Thirkill CE, Roth AM, Keltner JL. Cancer-associated retinopathy. Arch Ophthalmol 1987;105(3):372–5.
55. Thirkill CE, FitzGerald P, Sergott RC, et al. Cancer-associated retinopathy (CAR syndrome) with antibodies reacting with retinal, optic-nerve, and cancer cells. N Engl J Med 1989;321(23):1589–94.
56. Caplan LR. "Top of the basilar" syndrome. Neurology 1980;30(1):72–9.
57. Katz B, Rimmer S. Ophthalmologic manifestations of Alzheimer's disease. Surv Ophthalmol 1989;34(1):31–43.
58. Mendez MF, Mendez MA, Martin R, et al. Complex visual disturbances in Alzheimer's disease. Neurology 1990;40(3 Pt 1):439–43.
59. Fraunfelder FT, Meyer SM. Ocular toxicology. In: Duane TD, editor. Clinical ophthalmology, vol. 5. Philadelphia: J.B. Lippincott; 1988.
60. Grant WM. Toxicology of the eye. Springfield (IL): Charles C. Thomas; 1986.
61. May RH, Selymes P, Weekley RD, et al. Thioridazine therapy: results and complications. J Nerv Ment Dis 1960;130:230.
62. Meredith TA, Aaberg TM, Willerson WD. Progressive chorioretinopathy after receiving thioridazine. Arch Ophthalmol 1978;96(7):1172–6.
63. Li J, Tripathi RC, Tripathi BJ. Drug-induced ocular disorders. Drug Saf 2008; 31(2):127–41.

Paralytic Strabismus: Third, Fourth, and Sixth Nerve Palsy

Sashank Prasad, MD[a],*, Nicholas J. Volpe, MD[b]

KEYWORDS

• Paralytic strabismus • Nerve palsy • Ocular motor nerves
• Eye movement abnormalities

ANATOMY

Eye movements are subserved by the ocular motor nerves (cranial nerves 3, 4, and 6), which innervate the 6 extraocular muscles of each eye (**Fig. 1**). The oculomotor (third) nerve innervates the medial rectus, inferior rectus, superior rectus, and inferior oblique muscles, as well as the levator palpebrae. The trochlear (fourth) nerve innervates the superior oblique muscle, and the abducens (sixth) nerve innervates the lateral rectus muscle.

The nuclear complex of the third nerve lies in the dorsal midbrain, anterior to the cerebral aqueduct. It consists of multiple subnuclei that give rise to distinct sets of fibers destined for the muscles targeted by the third nerve. In general, the axons arising from these subnuclei travel in the ipsilateral nerve, except axons arising from the superior rectus subnucleus that travel through the contralateral third nerve complex to join the third nerve on that side.[1] In addition, a single central caudate nucleus issues fibers that join both third nerves to innervate the levator palpebrae muscles bilaterally.[2] The preganglionic cholinergic fibers that innervate the pupillary constrictor arise from the paired Edinger-Westphal nuclei. On exiting the nuclear complex, the third nerve fascicles travel ventrally, traversing the red nucleus and the cerebral peduncles, before exiting the midbrain into the interpeduncular fossa. The proximal portion of the nerve passes between the superior cerebellar and posterior cerebral arteries.[3] The axons are topographically arranged, with fibers for the inferior rectus, medial rectus, superior rectus, and inferior oblique arranged along the

Dr Prasad is supported by a Clinical Research Training Grant from the American Academy of Neurology.
[a] Division of Neuro-Ophthalmology, Department of Neurology, Brigham and Women's Hospital, Harvard Medical School, 75 Francis Street, Boston, MA 02115, USA
[b] Division of Neuro-Ophthalmology, Scheie Eye Institute, University of Pennsylvania, 51 North 39th Street, Philadelphia, PA 19104, USA
* Corresponding author.
E-mail address: sashank.prasad@uphs.upenn.edu

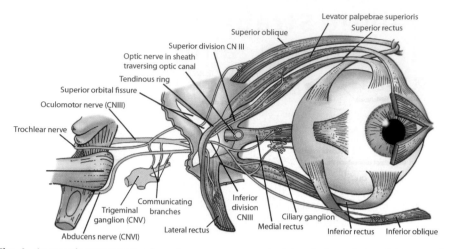

Levator palpebrae superioris
Superior rectus
Superior oblique
Superior division CN III
Optic nerve in sheath
traversing optic canal
Tendinous ring
Superior orbital fissure
Oculomotor nerve (CNIII)
Trochlear nerve
Trigeminal
ganglion (CNV)
Communicating
branches
Inferior
division
CNIII
Ciliary ganglion
Lateral rectus
Medial rectus
Inferior rectus   Inferior oblique
Abducens nerve (CNVI)

Fig. 1. Anatomic structures subserving eye movements: lateral view of the right eye. The oculomotor nerve (CN III), trochlear nerve (CN IV), and abducens nerve (CN VI) arise from the brainstem. After passing through the subarachnoid space and cavernous sinus, they enter the orbit through the superior orbital fissure. The oculomotor nerve divides into superior and inferior divisions, and ultimately innervates the superior rectus, inferior rectus, medial rectus, inferior oblique (shown cut), and levator palpebrae muscles. In addition, parasympathetic fibers of the third nerve synapse in the ciliary ganglion then innervate the pupillary constrictor muscle. The trochlear nerve innervates the superior oblique muscle. The abducens nerve innervates the lateral rectus muscle (shown cut). (*Adapted from* Agur AMR, Dalley AF. Grant's atlas of anatomy. 12th edition. Philadelphia: Lippincott, Williams & Wilkins; 2009; with permission.)

medial-to-lateral axis. Pupillary fibers are generally located superficially, in the superior and medial portion of the nerve.

The trochlear (fourth) nucleus is situated in the pontomesencephalic junction, ventral to the cerebral aqueduct. Unlike all other cranial nerves, these axons exit the brainstem dorsally. They then decussate within the anterior medullary velum (beneath the inferior colliculi), and ultimately innervate the contralateral superior oblique muscle.

The abducens (sixth) nucleus lies in the dorsal pons, in close proximity to the facial (seventh) nerve fascicle. The sixth nerve fascicle travels ventrally, through the corticospinal tracts, before exiting anterolaterally at the pontomedullary junction.

The 3 ocular motor nerves pass through the subarachnoid space before piercing the dura and arriving at the cavernous sinus (**Fig. 2**). Although the third and fourth nerves are situated along the lateral wall of the cavernous sinus, the abducens nerve has a more medial position, just lateral to the internal carotid artery. The third nerve splits into superior and inferior divisions within the anterior cavernous sinus. The superior division innervates the levator palpebrae and the superior rectus muscles, whereas the inferior division innervates the remaining third nerve muscles (the medial rectus, inferior rectus, inferior oblique, and the pupillary constrictor). All 3 ocular motor nerves exit the cavernous sinus via the superior orbital fissure, and then pass through the orbital apex to reach their target muscles.

The blood supply to the third, fourth, and sixth nerves has multiple sources that feed a vasa nervorum capillary network.[4] In the subarachnoid space, the third nerve is supplied by small thalamomesenchephalic branches from the basilar artery and posterior ciliary artery (PCA); in the cavernous sinus, it is supplied by branches of

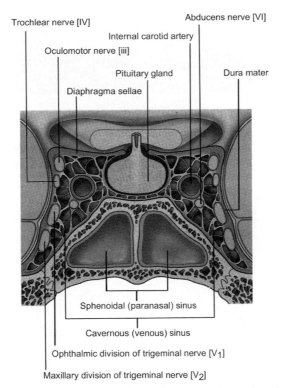

Trochlear nerve [IV]

Abducens nerve [VI]

Internal carotid artery

Oculomotor nerve [iii]

Pituitary gland

Dura mater

Diaphragma sellae

Sphenoidal (paranasal) sinus

Cavernous (venous) sinus

Ophthalmic division of trigeminal nerve [V₁]

Maxillary division of trigeminal nerve [V₂]

Fig. 2. The cavernous sinus, coronal view. The oculomotor nerve and trochlear nerve are situated on the lateral wall of the cavernous sinus (along with the ophthalmic and maxillary divisions of the trigeminal nerve). The abducens nerve floats freely within the cavernous sinus. The internal carotid artery is located medially in the cavernous sinus, and the pituitary gland is within the sella turcica in the midline. (*Reprinted from* Drake R, Vogl W, Mitchell A. Gray's anatomy for students. 2nd edition. London: Churchill Livingstone; 2010; with permission.)

the intracavernous carotid, and within the orbit its supply arises from recurrent branches of the ophthalmic artery. A watershed zone may exist between the subarachnoid and intracavernous portions of this blood supply.[5] In the subarachnoid segment, the blood supply of the fourth nerve comprises branches from the superior cerebellar artery (SCA), and that of the sixth nerve arises from branches of the PCA and SCA.[4] In the cavernous sinus and the orbit, the blood supply to both of these nerves arises from the same vessels that supply the third nerve.

THIRD NERVE PALSY
Clinical Features

Complete, isolated third nerve palsy causes ipsilateral weakness of elevation, depression, and adduction of the globe, in combination with ptosis and mydriasis. Depending on the specific cause, complete third nerve palsy may involve the pupil (causing mydriasis) or spare the pupil (**Figs. 3** and **4**). In partial third nerve palsy, different patterns of impaired motility may occur with or without pupillary involvement. The motility deficit may be subtle, and a reduced duction may not be easily observed. In this case, more detailed assessment of alignment, with alternate cover or Maddox rod testing, will

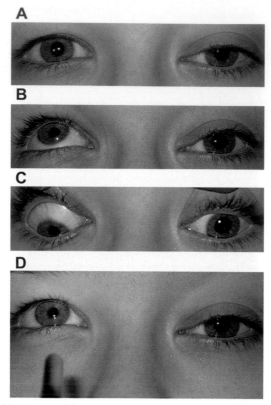

Fig. 3. A 32-year-old woman with traumatic complete left third nerve palsy, showing right hypertropia in upgaze that becomes left hypertropia in downgaze. (*A*) Left ptosis, mydriasis, exotropia, and right hypertropia in primary gaze. (*B*) Absent left elevation. (*C*) Reduced left depression. (*D*) The left pupil shows minimal consensual response to light, with greater anisocoria.

show an incomitant pattern of ocular misalignment supporting the diagnosis of partial third nerve palsy. A characteristic feature is that the affected eye is hypotropic in upgaze but hypertropic in downgaze, because of the combined weakness of the superior and inferior rectus muscles.

As opposed to lesions of the third nerve fascicle or nerve, a lesion of the third nerve nucleus will cause bilateral abnormalities. Specifically, there is bilateral ptosis (because the central caudal nucleus supplies both levator palpebrae muscles) and a bilateral elevation deficit (because the superior rectus subnucleus sends fibers through the contralateral third nerve nucleus to join the opposite nerve) (**Fig. 5**).[1,6,7] Therefore, the classic clinical picture of unilateral nuclear third nerve palsy is ipsilateral mydriasis; ipsilateral weakness of the medial rectus, inferior rectus, and inferior oblique muscles; bilateral ptosis; and bilateral superior rectus weakness.

As the third nerve fascicle travels ventrally through the midbrain, it is vulnerable to an intraparenchymal lesion. Partial deficits are possible, in keeping with the topographic arrangement of fibers within the nerve fascicle.[2,8–10] In these cases, other neurologic deficits often accompany the third nerve palsy. For example, a lesion also affecting the corticospinal tracts in the cerebral peduncle will cause contralateral hemiparesis (Weber syndrome), a lesion involving the red nucleus will cause contralateral limb

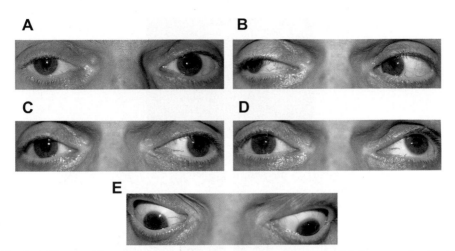

Fig. 4. A 55-year-old woman with a microvasculopathic partial right third nerve palsy due to diabetes and hypertension. Magnetic resonance imaging and magnetic resonance angiography were normal. (*A*) Right ptosis without mydriasis in primary position. Mild physiologic anisocoria was present. (*B*) Normal right gaze. (*C*) Decreased right adduction on left gaze. (*D*) Decreased right elevation on upgaze. (*E*) Decreased right depression on downgaze. The motility became normal within 8 weeks.

tremor (Benedikt syndrome), and a lesion involving the brachium conjunctivum (involving the crossing dentatorubrothalamic fibers of the superior cerebellar peduncle) will cause contralateral ataxia (Claude syndrome).[11] Rarely, fascicular third nerve palsy may occur in isolation.[6]

Given the segregation of the third nerve into superior and inferior divisions, a lesion of the anterior cavernous sinus or orbit may cause selective impairments. Disruption of the superior division causes ptosis and impaired elevation, whereas disruption of the inferior division causes impaired depression, adduction, and mydriasis (**Figs. 6** and **7**).[12] However, in rare cases, more proximal lesions (ie, intraparenchymal fascicular lesions or subarachnoid lesions) may mimic a divisional palsy.[10,13–16]

Aberrant regeneration refers to miswiring of third nerve innervated structures, leading to patterns of co-contraction (ie, synkinesis).[17] Common manifestations are contraction of the levator palpebrae on adduction or depression of the eye, or miosis of a dilated pupil during adduction (**Fig. 8**). This phenomenon occurs in primary and secondary forms. Primary aberrant regeneration suggests chronic compression, typically due to an expanding cavernous sinus lesion such as a meningioma, aneurysm, tumor, or other mass.[18–20] Secondary aberrant regeneration occurs in the recovery phase following acute third nerve palsy, commonly after trauma but also after ophthalmoplegic migraine, pituitary apoplexy, or inflammation. Aberrant regeneration does not occur after vasculopathic third nerve palsy.

Differential Diagnosis

Nuclear or fascicular third nerve palsy is typically due to midbrain infarction from occlusion of a small penetrating artery from the proximal PCA. Other possible causes of midbrain disease include tumors, vascular malformations, abscesses, demyelination, and inflammatory disorders.

In the subarachnoid space, an expanding aneurysm of the posterior communicating artery (PComm) is an important cause of third nerve palsy. More than 90% of patients

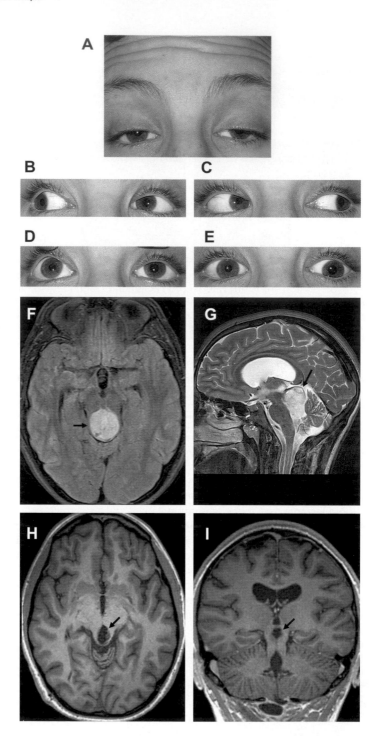

with subarachnoid hemorrhage from a PComm aneurysm initially present with a third nerve palsy.[21,22] These aneurysms commonly project posterolaterally to compress the third nerve and involve the pupillary fibers in most cases. When the motility deficits are complete, pupillary involvement is virtually always present. If the motility deficit is partial, then the pupil may initially be spared.[23] Sparing of pupillomotor fibers may occur because they are resistant to evenly distributed compression, or because they are positioned dorsally, and in some cases compression is limited to the inferior aspect of the nerve.[24] A PComm aneurysm presenting acutely as a third nerve palsy represents a true neurosurgical emergency and may be treated by surgical clipping or endovascular coiling.[25]

Microvascular third nerve palsy is commonly associated with risk factors including hypertension, diabetes, hyperlipidemia, advanced age, and smoking (see **Fig. 4**). This disorder results from impairment of microcirculation leading to circumscribed, ischemic demyelination of axons at the core of the nerve, typically in the cavernous sinus portion where a watershed territory exists.[5,26] Most of these patients exhibit pupillary sparing, because the pupillary fibers are located peripherally, closest to the blood supply provided by the surrounding vasa nervorum. However, some pupillary involvement may occur, typically with less than 1 mm (up to a maximum of 2.5 mm) of anisocoria found in approximately 40% of cases.[27] A microvascular third nerve palsy is frequently associated with orbital pain, which can be severe. Although it remains uncertain, the pain may result from ischemia of trigeminal sensory fibers that join the third nerve within the cavernous sinus.[28] There is an excellent prognosis for recovery of motility deficits from microvascular third nerve palsy, typically in 8 to 12 weeks.[29]

Severe trauma is another common cause of third nerve palsies, involving traction at the skull base or fracture of the bones of the orbit or skull base (**Fig. 9**).[30,31] A third nerve palsy that follows minor head trauma may indicate an underlying structural lesion.[32,33] Although there is good prognosis for recovery following traumatic third nerve palsy, there is a high incidence of secondary aberrant regeneration.

Slowly progressive third nerve palsies occasionally occur due to growth of a primary tumor of the nerve or nerve sheath. These lesions include neurinomas, neurofibromas, neurilemmomas, and schwannomas.[34] Neuroimaging will identify an enlarged, enhancing nerve in these cases. Uncommonly, a malignant meningioma, glioblastoma multiforme, or lymphoma may directly affect the third nerve.[35]

Uncal herniation can cause direct compression of the third nerve against the free edge of the tentorium. In addition to third nerve deficits, these patients will have depressed mental status among other prominent neurologic deficits. In this situation, isolated pupil dilation may be the earliest manifestation of third nerve dysfunction. However, an isolated dilated pupil is never a manifestation of third nerve dysfunction in an awake and alert patient.

Fig. 5. A 15-year-old boy with bilateral nuclear third nerve palsies following resection of a midline juvenile pilocytic astrocytoma. (*A*) Severe bilateral ptosis in primary gaze. Note compensatory contraction of the frontalis muscle. (*B*) Reduced left adduction. Mydriasis of the left pupil is observed. (*C*) Slightly reduced right adduction. (*D*) Severe elevation limitation on attempted upgaze. The vertical gaze limitation was not overcome by the oculocephalic maneuver. (*E*) Bilateral depression deficit, greater on the right than on the left. Preoperative axial fluid-attenuated inversion-recovery (FLAIR) (*F*) and sagittal T2-weighted brain MRI (*G*) revealed a large heterogeneous midline mass (*arrow*) compressing the dorsal midbrain and causing hydrocephalus. Axial (*H*) and coronal MRI (*I*) 2 years following surgical resection showing focal volume loss in the dorsal midbrain (*arrow*).

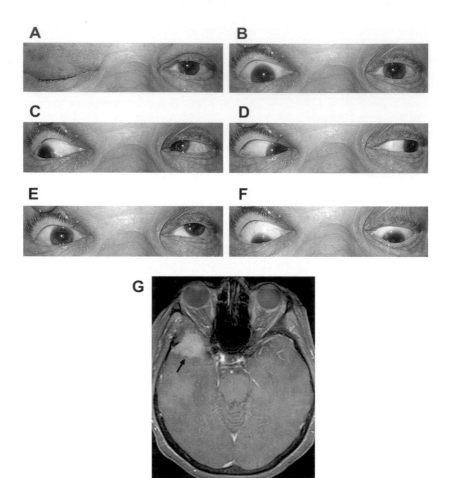

Fig. 6. 63-year-old woman with right superior divisional third nerve palsy following resection of right sphenoid wing meningioma, causing isolated dysfunction of the levator palpebrae and superior rectus muscles. (*A*) Complete right ptosis. (*B*) Slight right hypotropia in primary gaze. (*C*) Right hypotropia in right gaze. (*D*) Slight right hypotropia in left gaze. (*E*) Markedly reduced elevation of the right eye. (*F*) Normal downgaze. (*G*) Preoperative postcontrast T1-weighted brain MRI showing right sphenoid wing meningioma (*arrow*).

In the pediatric population, ophthalmoplegic migraine may cause transient isolated third nerve palsy. This rare form of complicated migraine typically presents before the age of 10 years.[36] Ispilateral headache and nausea often accompany abnormal eye movements. For unclear reasons, third nerve involvement is most common, occurring in 95% of cases. The cause may relate to transient ischemia or compression of the nerve within the cavernous sinus by an edematous, dilated carotid artery.[37,38] This condition is a diagnosis of exclusion, after a workup including imaging, blood work, and often lumbar puncture are unrevealing. Ophthalmoplegic migraine should be considered extremely unlikely in an adult without prior history of similar episodes in childhood.

Isolated persistent third nerve palsy in childhood is commonly a congenital defect.[39] These cases are believed to result from aplasia or maldevelopment of the structures of the ocular motor nucleus due to in utero insult.[40] The motility deficit and ptosis is

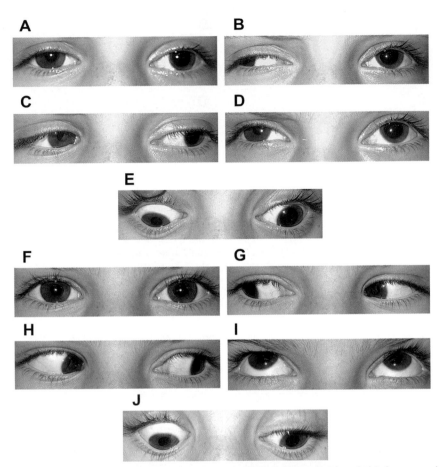

Fig. 7. An 8-year-old girl with idiopathic postviral left inferior divisional third nerve palsy, causing isolated dysfunction of the medial rectus, inferior rectus, and pupillary constrictor muscles. Brain MRI and spinal fluid constituents were normal. (*A*) Left mydriasis and exotropia. (*B*) Complete left adduction deficit on right gaze. (*C*) Normal left gaze. (*D*) Normal upgaze bilaterally (not fully seen in this photograph). (*E*) Left depression deficit. (*F*) At 3-month follow-up, there was marked improvement of the motility deficit, with residual left mydriasis (anisocoria greatest in light). (*G*) Left adduction deficit has resolved. (*H*) Left gaze remains normal. (*I*) Upgaze remains normal. (*J*) Slight left depression deficit persists.

typically accompanied by miosis, rather than mydriasis, which probably results from anomalous innervation of the pupillary constrictor. Cyclic oculomotor spasms may occur, which are characterized by brief (10–30 seconds), involuntary contractions of third nerve innervated structures, causing periods of adduction, lid elevation, and miosis.[41] This condition rarely occurs with acquired third nerve palsy, typically due to a compressive lesion.

Third nerve palsy frequently occurs in combination with other cranial nerve deficits. The disorders capable of affecting multiple cranial nerves include cavernous sinus lesions, neoplasms of the base of the skull, carcinomatous meningitis, sinus mucoceles, infections, and inflammatory conditions. These conditions are discussed later in this article.

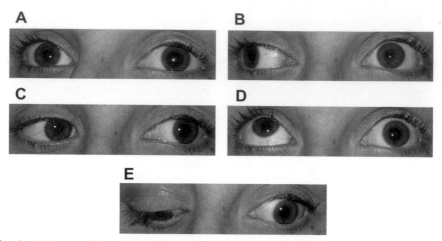

Fig. 8. A 45-year-old woman with aberrant regeneration following traumatic left third nerve palsy. (*A*) Left mydriasis, exotropia, and right hypertropia in primary position. (*B*) Reduced left adduction with synkinetic left pupillary constriction and left lid elevation. (*C*) Complete left gaze (not fully shown in this photograph). (*D*) Reduced left elevation. (*E*) Reduced left depression with abnormal lid elevation due to synkinesis.

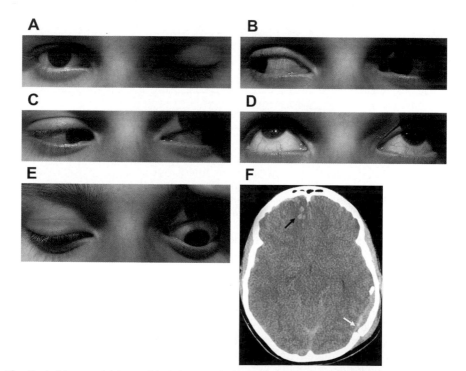

Fig. 9. A 14-year-old boy with left partial third nerve palsy following head trauma. (*A*) Complete left ptosis. (*B*) Reduced left adduction. No mydriasis is evident. (*C*) Complete left gaze. (*D*) Reduced left elevation. (*E*) Normal depression. (*F*) Noncontrast head computed tomography (CT) revealed frontal contusions (*black arrow*), occipital fracture, and epidural hematoma (*white arrow*). The motility deficit recovered completely within 3 months, without aberrant regeneration.

Diagnostic Testing

The appropriate workup for a patient with third nerve palsy depends on the patient's age and pupil function. In adults with acquired, isolated, complete, or partial third nerve palsy that involves the pupil, there is no controversy to the workup: these patients need urgent imaging to exclude a PComm aneurysm or other mass.[42,43] Computed tomography angiography (CTA) and magnetic resonance angiography are useful, but the exact sensitivity and availability of these tests vary across institutions.[44] Nevertheless, if these tests are negative, a catheter angiogram often remains necessary in these patients because small aneurysms are potentially missed on noninvasive imaging studies.

For patients with complete, pupil-sparing third nerve palsy who are more than 50 years of age and have vascular risk factors, clinical observation may be reasonable. If these patients fail to spontaneously recover within 12 weeks, then detailed neuroimaging is necessary. However, the appropriate threshold for obtaining imaging in this patient population remains an ongoing source of controversy. There are a growing number of reports of lesions diagnosed by magnetic resonance imaging (MRI) in patients who mimicked microvasculopathic third nerve palsy.[43] Therefore, in clinical practice it may be prudent to obtain imaging studies to exclude vascular lesions in these patients.

In patients with partial, pupil-sparing third nerve palsies, the threshold to obtain imaging is also low. Historically, it would have been reasonable to observe these patients for several days; in cases of evolving acute third nerve palsy due to aneurysm, mydriasis would occur in almost all cases within that time period.[23] If mydriasis develops, urgent imaging becomes necessary. If the motility deficit remains unaccompanied by pupillary abnormalities after 1 week, then a microvasculopathic cause is most likely. In the modern era, given the high risks of missing the diagnosis of an aneurysm and the increased availability of magnetic resonance (MR) or computed tomography (CT) imaging, it has become an appropriate strategy to obtain imaging in these patients earlier.

Consideration of imaging should also be given to patients with third nerve palsy due to trauma, especially if the extent of trauma was minor, because of the incidence of underlying mass lesions (including aneurysms). Imaging these patients will also evaluate for muscle entrapment due to fracture of the orbital wall.

In cases in which an infectious, inflammatory, or neoplastic cause is suspected, and MRI is negative or nonspecific, additional workup may include serologies for Lyme disease, syphilis, and an erythrocyte sedimentation rate to exclude temporal arteritis. Cerebrospinal fluid (CSF) analysis including cell counts, protein, glucose, cytology, and Lyme and Venereal Disease Reference Laboratory (VDRL) titers may be required.

Treatment

The treatment of diplopia due to acute third nerve palsy may include monocular patching or prisms. If the third nerve palsy is improving quickly over several weeks, prisms may be unnecessary and difficult to use successfully. If the misalignment remains fairly stable, then prisms may reduce diplopia in primary gaze. However, given the incomitance of these deviations, prisms are unlikely to alleviate diplopia in eccentric gaze, and patient satisfaction may vary.

Once ocular misalignment from third nerve palsy has been stable for 6 to 12 months, surgical correction can be considered. The complexity of these cases depends on whether the third nerve palsy is complete or partial. Complete third nerve palsy presents a highly incomitant deviation in the horizontal and vertical planes. The ultimate goal for surgery in these cases is to establish single binocular vision in the primary position.[45] Exodeviation in the primary position may be reduced by performing a supramaximal lateral rectus recession (a weakening procedure that completely abolishes abduction), potentially in combination with a medial rectus resection (a tightening procedure to augment the muscle's action). A medial rectus resection alone often becomes ineffective in these cases. Other strategies include transposition of the horizontal muscles to facilitate vertical eye movements and transposition of the superior oblique tendon to create an adducting force.

For patients with partial third nerve palsy, the surgical plan is tailored to the specific pattern of misalignment. In general, a combination of procedures is used to achieve better alignment. These include resection of the partially paretic muscle and recession or posterior fixation suture of the contralateral yoke muscle. A posterior fixation suture creates a mild limitation of eye movement without affecting primary position. A recession procedure can be done with adjustable sutures so that the realignment can be fine-tuned based on the awake patient's subjective experience.[46] For instance, a patient with partial third nerve palsy causing isolated impairment of elevation or depression can be treated with a resection of the involved vertical muscle combined with an adjustable recession (or posterior fixation suture) of the contralateral yoke muscle, producing an improved field of single binocular vision.

The risks of surgery should be weighed carefully in the decision to treat patients with third nerve palsy. Patients should be warned that more disabling diplopia may occur following strabismus surgery, as the images from each eye become perceived much closer together. Correction of ptosis accompanying third nerve palsy is usually easily accomplished but carries some risk of corneal exposure.

FOURTH NERVE PALSY
Clinical Features

Fourth nerve palsy presents with vertical diplopia and is commonly accompanied by compensatory contralateral head tilt.[47] Identification of a fourth nerve palsy in a patient with vertical diplopia involves application of the Parks-Bielchowsky three-step test. First, hypertropia suggests weakness of the ipsilateral superior oblique, ipsilateral inferior rectus, contralateral inferior oblique, or contralateral superior rectus muscle. Second, increased hypertropia in contralateral gaze narrows the possibilities to the weakness of the ipsilateral superior oblique or contralateral superior rectus muscles. Third, increased hypertropia on ipsilateral head tilt further reduces the possibilities, ultimately identifying ipsilateral superior oblique weakness.

Although the abnormal ductions may be detected by direct observation, in many cases, patients with vertical misalignment to have no visible impairment in ocular motility (**Fig. 10**). Therefore, assessment of alignment using alternate cover or Maddox rod testing can be particularly useful to show the characteristic pattern of impaired motility.

The reason that hypertropia is exacerbated in contralateral gaze is that superior oblique palsy causes weakness of depression in adduction (in long-standing cases, the hypertropia in adduction is further enhanced by overaction of the ipsilateral inferior oblique). The reason hypertropia is worse with ipsilateral head tilt is that the ocular counterroll reflex stimulates ipsilateral intorters (superior oblique and superior rectus) and contralateral extorters (inferior oblique and inferior rectus); when the superior oblique is weak, this reflex causes a compensatory increase in ipsilateral superior rectus action, resulting in additional hypertropia (because the superior rectus is an elevator).

Torsional diplopia, which results from ocular cyclotorsion, often accompanies vertical diplopia in acquired fourth nerve palsy. This condition can be quickly assessed by having the patient view a horizontal straight line, such as the edge of a door. A patient with cyclotorsion from unilateral fourth nerve palsy will see a horizontal line

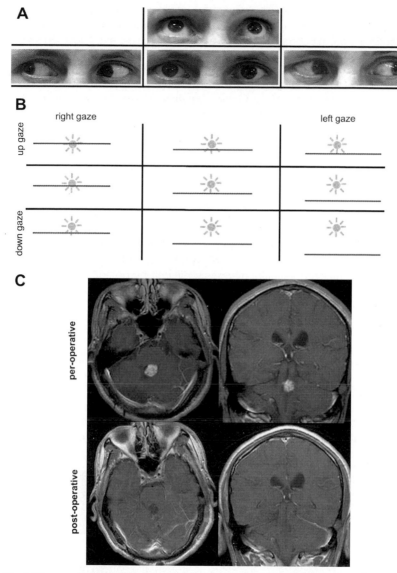

Fig. 10. A 36-year-old man with right fourth nerve palsy following resection of cerebellar he-
mangioblastoma. (*A*) Essentially normal ductions, with small right hypertropia in primary gaze
and upgaze, increased in left gaze. (*B*) Simulation of patient's view through Maddox rod in
each direction of gaze. Note greatest vertical separation in down-and-left gaze. (*C*) Pre- and
postoperative gadolinium-enhanced T1-weighted MRI scans, showing fourth ventricle he-
mangioblastoma. (*Reprinted from* Prasad S, Volpe NJ, Tamhankar MA. Clinical reasoning:
a 36-year-old man with vertical diplopia. Neurology 2009;72:e93–9; with permission.)

and a second tilted line above or below it, intersecting on the side of the affected eye.
Cyclotorsion can also be evaluated with the double Maddox rod, which refracts a light
source into one red line (seen by the right eye) and one white line (seen by the left eye).
The degree of relative cyclotorsion is measured by rotating the filters until the subject
reports that the lines are parallel. Cyclotorsion can also be evaluated during dilated

fundus examination, by assessing the position of the macula with respect to the optic disc. Excyclotorsion of the hypertropic eye suggests fourth nerve palsy because of weakened intorsion; in contrast, intorsion of the hypertropic eye occurs in skew deviation, due to decreased stimulation of the inferior oblique subnucleus.

Assessing cyclotorsion and vertical misalignment in the upright and supine positions may be helpful in distinguishing a fourth nerve palsy from a skew deviation.[48] The misalignment remains fairly constant between these positions in fourth nerve palsy, whereas it is mitigated in the supine position in skew deviation, possibly because the utricular imbalance that causes a skew deviation becomes reduced.[48]

A final clue about the cause of vertical misalignment comes from the fusional amplitude (the ability to fuse disparate images), which suggests the chronicity of strabismus. The fusional amplitude is measured by asking the patient to report double vision while progressively increased prisms are placed over 1 eye. A vertical fusional capacity greater than 8 to 10 diopters suggests the presence of higher compensatory mechanisms that occur with long-standing misalignment, such as a congenital lesion.

Bilateral fourth nerve palsy, which most commonly results from trauma, is characterized by a unique constellation of findings.[49] Primary position vertical alignment may be fairly good because of the canceling effect from bilateral palsies. Esotropia may be present, making the initial diagnosis difficult by potentially suggesting sixth nerve palsies. However, with careful examination, bilateral fourth nerve palsies are readily identified. First, hyperdeviation alternates such that it is contralateral to the direction of gaze and ipsilateral to the side of head tilt. Second, there is esotropia greatest in downgaze (so-called V-pattern esotropia, with >15 prism diopters difference between upgaze and downgaze) because of weakened abduction in depression (the superior oblique acts as an abductor). Third, there is often a large angle of excyclotorsion (>10°), accompanied by prominent torsional diplopia. Rarely, bilateral congenital fourth nerve palsy may occur (**Fig. 11**).

Identifying fourth nerve palsy in the setting of concomitant third nerve palsy can be difficult, because the failure of adduction prevents complete testing of superior oblique function. In this setting, the superior oblique can be evaluated by assessing its

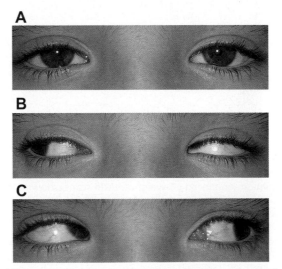

Fig. 11. A 7-year-old girl with bilateral congenital fourth nerve palsy. Brain MRI was normal. (*A*) Normal alignment in primary gaze. (*B*) Left hypertropia in right gaze, with left inferior oblique overaction. (*C*) Right hypertropia in left gaze, with right inferior oblique overaction.

secondary function: intorsion of the abducted eye on attempted downgaze. The torsional movement that indicates intact superior oblique function is best appreciated by observing a conjunctival vessel (**Fig. 12**).

Differential Diagnosis

The most common cause of acquired fourth nerve palsy is trauma.[31,49,50] The trochlear nerve is the longest and thinnest of all the cranial nerves, coursing along the free edge of the tentorium through the prepontine cistern, where it is vulnerable to crush or shearing injury. Fracture of the base of the skull is an alternative cause. In cases of bilateral traumatic fourth nerve palsies, both nerves are often injured at the anterior medullary vellum, where they decussate.[49] Traumatic fourth nerve palsies may occur after minor head injuries without loss of consciousness or skull fractures.

Decompensated congenital fourth nerve palsy is also common and may present in adulthood. There is often a long-standing head tilt, which may be observed on inspection of prior photographs, and an insidious onset of intermittent vertical diplopia. Characteristic features of congenital fourth nerve palsy include inferior oblique overaction, large vertical fusional amplitude, and minimal torsional diplopia. The precise cause of congenital fourth nerve palsy is unclear but may include hypoplasia of the nucleus, birth trauma, anomalous muscle insertion, muscle fibrosis, structural abnormalities of the tendon, or inferior oblique muscle abnormalities.[51] Decompensation later in life probably relates to breakdown of vertical fusion leading to symptomatic diplopia, rather than progressive superior oblique dysfunction.[52]

Microvascular ischemia may cause fourth nerve palsy, typically in patients more than 50 years of age with vascular risk factors. There is often periorbital aching pain on presentation, which can be severe. There is an excellent chance of spontaneous recovery within several months.

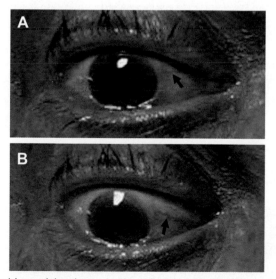

Fig. 12. A 75-year-old man (also shown in **Fig. 20**) with right third nerve palsy from pituitary apoplexy with spared superior oblique function. (*A*) A conjunctival vessel is observed (*arrow*) in primary gaze. (*B*) On attempted downgaze, the conjunctival vessel is observed to move from the 2 o'clock position to the 3 o'clock position (*arrow*), showing intorsion of the eye by an intact superior oblique muscle.

Superior oblique myokymia is a microtremor that causes characteristic episodes of monocular tortional oscillopsia or transient diplopia.[53] It may occur in the primary position or with movements opposite the superior oblique direction of action. It may follow superior oblique palsy or occur spontaneously. Some cases may be due to compression of the fourth nerve by an overlying blood vessel.

Less-frequent causes of fourth nerve palsy include midbrain hemorrhage, infarction, or demyelination.[54,55] Given the proximity to other structures in the midbrain, a lesion of the fourth nerve nucleus or proximal fascicle may cause contralateral superior oblique weakness in association with ipsilateral Horner syndrome,[56] ipsilateral internuclear ophthalmoplegia,[57] or contralateral relative afferent pupillary defect without visual loss (by affecting the brachium of the superior colliculus).[58]

Other causes of fourth nerve palsy include schwannoma, aneurysmal compression, meningitis, hydrocephalus, and herpes zoster ophthalmicus. Inflammatory, infectious, and neoplastic processes that may affect the fourth nerve in the subarachnoid space often cause multiple cranial nerve deficits and are discussed later. When ancillary testing fails to support a definitive cause, a diagnosis of idiopathic acquired fourth nerve palsy can be made.

Management

There are several treatment options for the patient with fourth nerve palsy. Occlusion of the affected eye (or, if diplopia occurs only in down-and-contralateral gaze, occlusion of the lower half of the lens over the affected eye) can serve as a temporary measure when spontaneous recovery is expected. Alternatively, base-down prism over the affected,

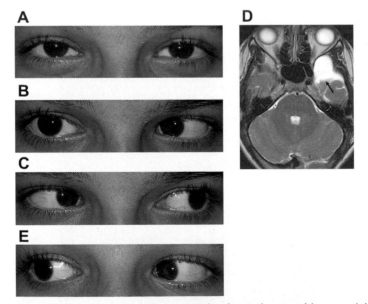

Fig. 13. 15-year-old boy with right sixth nerve palsy due to increased intracranial pressure (54 cm H_2O) in association with an arachnoid cyst. (*A*) Primary position. (*B*) Right gaze, showing right abduction deficit. (*C*) Normal left gaze. (*D*) T2-weighted MRI revealing a left middle temporal fossa arachnoid cyst (*arrow*). (*E*) Two months after surgical decompression of the arachnoid cyst, the right sixth nerve palsy had improved considerably, with a slight residual abduction deficit.

hypertropic eye may be effective. Prisms are generally effective for patients with congenital palsies because they have large fusional amplitudes. However, torsional diplopia cannot be corrected by prisms, and may limit the patient's satisfaction.

Surgery may be necessary for persistent symptomatic fourth nerve palsy when conservative measures fail, as long as the misalignment has been stable for several months. Patients with decompensated congenital fourth nerve palsy generally have a better prognosis after surgery than patients with acquired fourth nerve palsy, because they often have increased vertical fusional amplitude that reduces the likelihood of postoperative diplopia.[59] Selection of the optimal surgical strategy depends

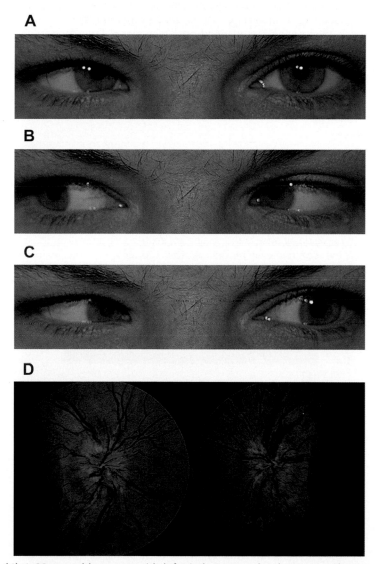

Fig. 14. (*A*) A 29-year-old woman with left sixth nerve palsy due to pseudotumor cerebri following pregnancy. Brain MRI, MR venogram, and CSF constituents were normal. Opening pressure was 35 cm H20. (*A*) Esotropia in primary gaze. (*B*) Normal right gaze. (*C*) Left abduction deficit with intact right adduction.

on the amplitude of deviation and the presence of associated features such as inferior oblique overaction, superior rectus contracture, or superior oblique tendon laxity.[60] In a patient with less than 10 diopters of deviation, recession of 1 muscle may be sufficient. If the inferior oblique shows overaction, it should be selected. However, if the deviation is greater than 15 diopters, then a second muscle should also be recessed. For this purpose, the contralateral inferior rectus or the ipsilateral superior rectus may be selected.[60] Unless superior rectus contracture needs to be addressed, recession of the contralateral inferior rectus may be the superior procedure because it can be performed with adjustable sutures.[46]

The approach outlined earlier can be effective at reducing vertical diplopia. Surgery directly on the superior oblique should generally be avoided in this situation because it carries the risk of iatrogenic Brown syndrome (superior oblique tendon sheath insufficiency). However, with bilateral palsies, or with unilateral palsy causing significant torsional diplopia, the Harado-Ito procedure may be required, in which the anterior portion of the superior oblique is advanced toward the lateral rectus.

SIXTH NERVE PALSY
Clinical Features

Weakness of the lateral rectus due to sixth nerve palsy leads to horizontal diplopia, worse to the affected side and at distance. Often, the abnormal duction is easily observed, but in subtle cases, an incomitant esotropia must be shown by testing binocular alignment.

Differential Diagnosis

Nuclear sixth nerve palsy affects the ipsilateral sixth nerve as well as the interneurons destined for the contralateral medial rectus subnucleus. This lesion causes an

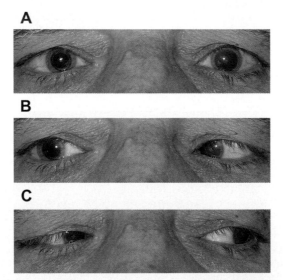

Fig. 15. A 70-year-old man with horizontal binocular diplopia and periorbital aching pain due to microvasculopathic right sixth nerve palsy. Brain MRI and erythrocyte sedimentation rate were normal. (A) Slight esotropia in primary gaze. The pupils were pharmacologically dilated. (B) Right abduction deficit. (C) Normal left gaze. The abduction deficit resolved within 2 months.

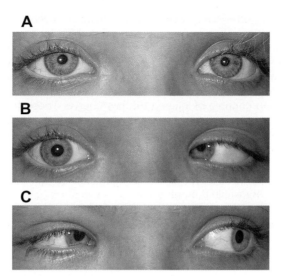

Fig. 16. A 5-year-old girl with right Duane syndrome, type 1. (*A*) Normal alignment in primary position. (*B*) Severe right abduction deficit. (*C*) Full ductions on left gaze, with retraction of the right globe and narrowing of the palpebral fissure.

abduction deficit of the ipisilateral eye as well as an adduction deficit of the contralateral eye; together, this is a conjugate gaze palsy. In contrast, a lesion affecting the sixth nerve fascicle or nerve will produce an ipsilateral abduction deficit but spare adduction of the contralateral eye. Because of the proximity between the seventh nerve fascicle and the sixth nerve nucleus (within the facial colliculus), a single lesion at that location will typically produce ipsilateral gaze palsy and upper and lower facial weakness. A lesion more ventral in the pons may affect the sixth nerve fascicle and the descending corticospinal tract, producing an ipsilateral abduction deficit with contralateral hemiparesis or in isolation. These pontine lesions are commonly ischemic, due to occlusion of a paramedian penetrating branch from the basilar artery, but the differential diagnosis also includes a vascular malformation, demyelination, or neoplasm.[61]

At the base of the skull, as the sixth nerve rises along the clivus over the petrous ligament into Dorello's canal, it is vulnerable to injury from downward mass effect due to

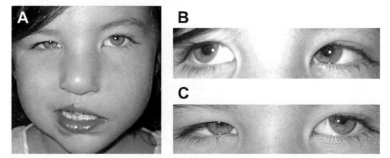

Fig. 17. A 4-year-old girl with bilateral gaze paresis and facial diplegia. (*A*) Upper and lower facial weakness, worse on the left than the right. (*B*) Partial right gaze palsy. (*C*) Marked left gaze palsy.

increased intracranial pressure. Therefore, unilateral or bilateral sixth nerve palsies may occur in the setting of a supratentorial mass (**Fig. 13**), sinus venous thrombosis,[62] hydrocephalus, or pseudotumor cerebri (**Fig. 14**). Conversely, a sixth nerve palsy can also arise in cases of low intracranial pressure, as may occur with a CSF leak.[63] Sixth nerve palsies in these situations tend to improve soon after normal intracranial pressure is restored. Masses growing at the base of the skull, such as meningiomas or chordomas, are also capable of injuring the sixth nerve. These tumors occasionally present with a sixth nerve palsy that has shown spontaneous resolution.[64]

Microvascular ischemia is another common cause of sixth nerve palsies, especially in an elderly patient with vascular risk factors (**Fig. 15**). Similar to other microvasculopathic palsies, these may present with substantial periorbital aching pain. Progression of the abduction deficit in the first week is not uncommon.[65] There is an excellent prognosis for recovery within 3 months.

Severe head trauma is another cause of sixth nerve palsy, which may occur due to shearing forces or fracture of the base of the skull or orbital bones.[31] Gradenigo syndrome refers to sixth nerve palsy in combination with ipsilateral hearing loss and facial pain, which occurs when infectious mastoiditis involves the structures of the

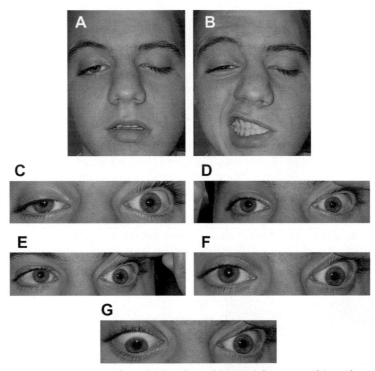

Fig. 18. A 15-year-old boy with multiple idiopathic cranial neuropathies who presented with 3 days of diplopia and facial weakness. There was hyporeflexia and mild ataxia in the arms. Brain MRI was normal and spinal fluid revealed 1 leukocyte and normal protein (55 mg/dL). Anti-GQ1b antibody was negative. (*A*) Bilateral ptosis and facial weakness. (*B*) Upper and lower facial weakness, left greater than right. (*C*) Slight exotropia in primary gaze. (*D*) Severely reduced right abduction and left adduction on attempted right gaze. (*E*) Reduced left abduction and right adduction on attempted left gaze. (*F*) Severely reduced elevation bilaterally on attempted upgaze. (*G*) Reduced depression, left greater than right, on attempted downgaze. Complete resolution occurred within 2 months.

petrous apex.[66] In children, a benign, recurring form of idiopathic sixth nerve palsy may occur, in which esotropia lasts for days to months.[67,68] The diagnostic workup in these cases, including MRI and CSF analysis, is unrevealing.

Congenital abnormalities of the sixth nerve include Duane retraction syndrome and Mobius syndrome. There are 3 varieties of Duane syndrome, which have in common a paradoxic co-contraction of the lateral and medial rectus muscles (**Fig. 16**). This condition causes a visible retraction of the globe and narrowing of the palpebral fissure on attempted adduction. In Duane type 1, abduction is impaired with essentially full adduction; in type 2, adduction is impaired with normal abduction; in type 3, adduction and abduction are reduced.[69] The abduction deficit in types 1 and 3 cause the patient to be esotropic on lateral gaze to the affected side, but these patients can be distinguished from those with acquired abduction deficits because they have normal alignment (rather than esotropia) in primary gaze. Pathologic studies of patients with Duane syndrome show hypoplasia of the sixth nerve nucleus and abnormalities of the fascicle, with branches of the third nerve supplying the lateral rectus muscle.[70,71] Most cases of Duane syndrome are sporadic but, in rare familial cases, defects of the CHN1 gene on chromosome 2 have been identified.[72] Surgical treatment is not necessary for most patients with Duane syndrome, but it can be helpful in rare cases such as those with misalignment in primary position, abnormal head turn, or significant up- or downshoots.[73]

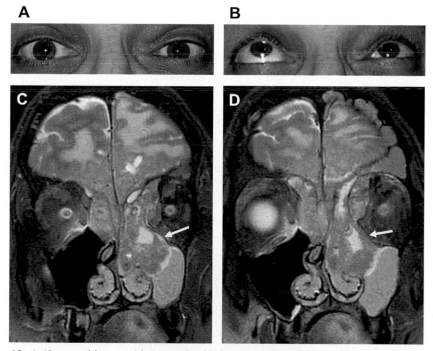

Fig. 19. A 49-year-old man with 1 month of left periorbital swelling and vertical diplopia in upgaze. (*A*) Normal alignment in the primary position, with 5 mm proptosis of the left globe. (*B*) Limited elevation of the left eye in upgaze. (*C, D*) T2-weighted MRI revealing a large mass arising from the left facial sinuses and invading the left orbit supralaterally (*arrow*). Pathologic analysis revealed a highly infiltrating, poorly differentiated epithelial tumor with neuroendocrine features.

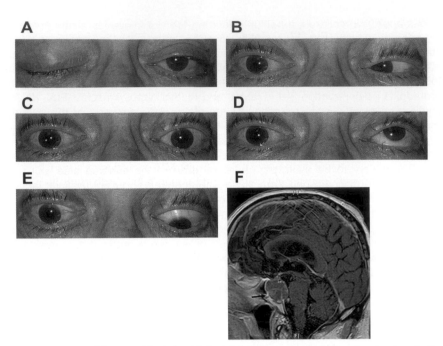

Fig. 20. A 75-year-old man with right third, right sixth, and left sixth palsy due to pituitary apoplexy. (*A*) Complete right ptosis. (*B*) Dilated right pupil and right abduction deficit. (*C*) Complete left abduction deficit and right adduction deficit on attempted left gaze. (*D*) Right elevation deficit. (*E*) Right depression deficit. (*F*) Sagittal postcontrast T1-weighted MRI reveals a heterogeneous mass in the pituitary sella, suggesting pituitary macroadenoma and apoplexy (*arrow*).

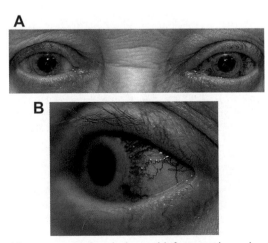

Fig. 21. A 70-year-old woman with headache and left eye redness due to a low-flow (indirect) CCF. (*A*) Left proptosis, periorbital edema, and arteriolization of episcleral vessels. The pupils are pharmacologically dilated. (*B*) Corkscrew arteriolization of episcleral vessels extending to the limbus.

Mobius syndrome describes congenital facial diplegia that is frequently associated with sixth nerve palsy (**Fig. 17**).[74] Conjugate gaze paresis may be present, typically in cases with more severe abduction deficit. Other abnormalities such as complete external ophthalmoplegia, third nerve palsy, or ptosis occur less frequently. The cause of these deficits is believed to be hypoplasia of the relevant brainstem structures.

Other inflammatory, infectious, and neoplastic processes that may affect the sixth nerve in the subarachnoid space are the same as those that can cause third and fourth nerve palsies and other cranial nerve deficits, and are discussed later.

Diagnostic Testing

Many patients with acute sixth nerve palsy require MRI to exclude structural, inflammatory, or neoplastic causes. All children and young adults with sixth nerve palsy should undergo imaging because of a higher prevalence of tumors and demyelinating

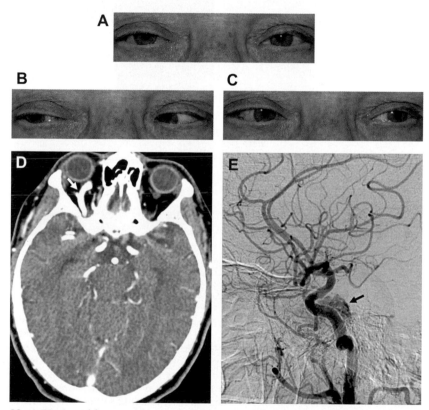

Fig. 22. A 75-year-old man with right CCF who presented with several months of left retroorbital headache and 2 days of horizontal binocular diplopia. (*A*) Slight esotropia in primary gaze. (*B*) Normal right gaze. (*C*) Limited left abduction. (*D*) CT angiogram revealed dilation and tortuosity of the right superior ophthalmic vein (*arrow*). Catheter angiography revealed a cavernous sinus dural arteriovenous fistula (type D indirect CCF) supplied by bilateral internal and external carotid artery branches (*arrow*) with dominant venous drainage through the right superior ophthalmic vein. The right external carotid supply (via an accessory meningeal artery) was successfully embolized with Onyx 18. Other supplying branches were not amenable to embolization.

lesions.[43,75] However, in a patient in whom a microvasculopathic cause is strongly considered, observation for spontaneous improvement over several weeks may prevent the need for imaging. Additional workup in selected patients with sixth nerve palsy may include serologies and CSF analysis.

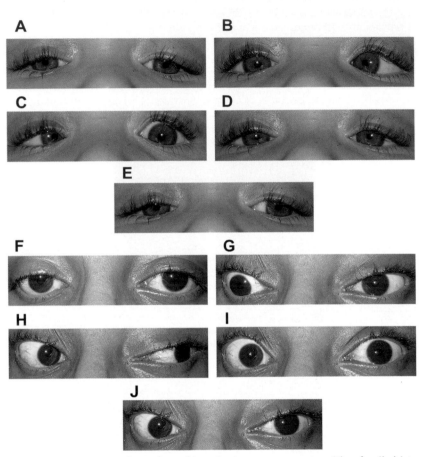

Fig. 23. A 3-year-old boy with ptosis and impaired eye movements, with a family history of similar abnormalities. Sequence analysis of the CFEOM1/KIF21A gene revealed a heterozygous, missense mutation 2821C>T in exon 21, which is a pathogenic mutation associated with congenital fibrosis of the extraocular muscles. He had received prior ptosis surgery. (*A*) Bilateral ptosis, esotropia, and head tilt in primary position. (*B*) Right gaze, revealing right abduction deficit. (*C*) Left gaze, revealing left abduction deficit. (*D*) Severe impairment bilaterally on attempted upgaze. (*E*) Downgaze. (*F*) The patient's father, who had also had surgery for ptosis, in primary gaze with a mild right hypertropia and exotropia. (*G*) Right gaze, showing reduced abduction and adduction. (*H*) Left gaze, showing slight impairments of abduction and adduction. (*I*) Severe bilateral impairments on attempted upgaze. (*J*) Severe bilateral impairments on attempted downgaze. (*K*) The patient's grandfather, with complete right ptosis. (*L*) Right gaze, showing left hypertropia and reduced left adduction. (*M*) Left gaze, showing right hypertropia and mild right adduction deficit. (*N*) Attempted upgaze, revealing severe bilateral impairments with left hypertropia. (*O*) Attempted downgaze, revealing left hypertropia with reduced left infraduction. (*P*) The family tree of the patient (*arrow*) reveals an autosomal dominant inheritance pattern through 5 generations.

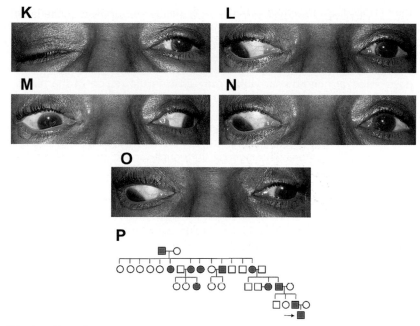

Fig. 23. (*continued*)

Treatment

As with any type of binocular diplopia, the horizontal diplopia resulting from acute sixth nerve palsy may be managed with occlusion or prism. Prism may be helpful to alleviate the compensatory head turn to the affected side. Ultimately, once the amount of eso-deviation has been stable for 6 to 12 months, surgical correction can be considered. Treatment of partial sixth nerve palsy may include a combined medial rectus recession and lateral rectus resection on the affected side. In addition, surgery on the contralateral horizontal rectus muscles may further expand the field of binocular single vision. In cases of complete sixth nerve palsy, the affected lateral rectus is typically left intact to preserve anterior segment circulation. Restoration of abduction on the affected side may be attempted by transposition procedures that aim to move the vertically acting rectus muscles into the horizontal plane. Of these, a full tendon transposition with posterior fixation suture seems to be the most effective, durable procedure.

COMBINED THIRD, FOURTH, AND SIXTH NERVE PALSY

As mentioned earlier, diseases of the subarachnoid space that may affect multiple cranial nerves include infectious, inflammatory, and neoplastic processes. Infectious processes include viral,[76] fungal, or bacterial infection (including tuberculosis, syphilis, and Lyme disease). Inflammatory diseases include sarcoidosis and idiopathic pachymeningitis. Neoplastic processes include carcinomatous and lymphomatous meningitis. Peripheral demyelinating disorders including Guillain-Barre syndrome, the Miller Fisher variant, chronic inflammatory demyelinating polyneuropathy, and idiopathic cranial neuropathies (**Fig. 18**) are other considerations when multiple ocular motor nerves are involved. Patients with myasthenia gravis may present with complex patterns of limited eye movements that closely mimic cranial nerve dysfunction, but these patients are often distinguished by the presence of normal pupillary responses.

Expanding masses at the base of the skull can cause compression of multiple ocular motor nerves. One consideration is meningioma of the sphenoid wing (causing ophthalmoplegia, proptosis, and hyperostosis of the temporal bone) or clivus. Other rare possibilities are chordoma, which may arise in the region of the clivus from remnants of the embryologic notochord, or chondrosarcoma, which arises from cartilage in bone.

A process involving the cavernous sinus may affect any combination of the third, fourth, or sixth nerves and cause dysfunction of the first and second divisions of the trigeminal nerve. The differential diagnosis of a superior orbital fissure process and a cavernous sinus process is similar, with the main clinical distinction that the second division of the trigeminal nerve is spared in the former. The differential diagnosis for these syndromes includes neoplastic, infectious, inflammatory, and vascular diseases.[77]

Neoplastic considerations include meningiomas, lymphoma, pituitary adenoma, metastases, trigeminal neuromas, chordomas, chondrosarcomas, and nasopharyngeal carcinomas (**Fig. 19**). Although the slow growth of a pituitary adenoma makes it less likely to involve the ocular motor nerves, the rapid onset of headache and ophthalmoplegia strongly suggests pituitary apoplexy (**Fig. 20**).[78] The third nerve is the most commonly affected by apoplexy, followed by the sixth nerve and lastly the fourth nerve.[79]

Infectious considerations include herpes zoster ophthalmicus, may lead to ophthalmoplegia on the basis of secondary vasculitis or direct inflammation of the ocular motor nerves.[80] Mucormycosis or aspergillosis may spread from the sinuses into the cavernous sinus or orbit, particularly in immunocompromised patients. Tolosa-Hunt is an idiopathic inflammation of the cavernous sinus or superior orbital fissure that causes painful ophthalmoplegia.[81]

Vascular lesions of the cavernous sinus include aneurysms and carotid cavernous fistulas (CCF). Carotid aneurysms may present with pain and diplopia due to involvement of any of the ocular motor nerves, most frequently the sixth nerve. CCFs are characterized as being high flow (direct) or low flow (indirect) based on the source of the feeder vessel and the rate of flow. Most high-flow CCFs result from severe head trauma, but, less frequently, these may arise spontaneously. In some cases, a spontaneous high-flow CCF arises from rupture of a preexisting aneurysm in the cavernous sinus, and in other cases it may occur in the setting of a systemic connective tissue disorder. Patients with a high-flow CCF present with headache, diplopia, proptosis, and severe chemosis. The episcleral veins become dilated and tortuous, extending to the limbus. A bruit may be detected by auscultating over a closed eyelid or, if the CCF drains posteriorly, over the mastoid. Diplopia may occur in these patients because of ocular motor palsy, restrictive myopathy secondary to congestion, or both. An isolated abduction deficit is common, perhaps because the sixth nerve floats freely within the cavernous sinus, near the carotid artery. Other ocular motor palsies may result from direct compression by the expanding fistula or by ischemia due to altered hemodynamics.

In contrast, low-flow CCFs (or dural arteriovenous malformations) are abnormal connections between the cavernous sinus and arteries supplying the dura mater. They are more frequent in elderly women or in association with pregnancy, hypertension, connective tissue disease, or head trauma. The symptoms they produce depend on the route of venous drainage, but are often similar to those produced by a high-flow CCF, including diplopia, proptosis, and chemosis (**Figs. 21** and **22**). However, in a low-flow CCF, these symptoms often have a more insidious onset.

Congenital fibrosis syndromes present with ptosis and a complex pattern of restrictive ophthalmoparesis (**Fig. 23**). Autosomal dominant inheritance is typical and the different clinical forms of congenital fibrosis of the extraocular muscles have recently been linked to specific gene mutations.[82] Surgery can be useful to correct abnormal head position. However, corrective ptosis surgery may lead to corneal exposure, and this risk must be weighed carefully.

SUMMARY

This article discusses the important clinical features that help to distinguish third, fourth, and sixth nerve palsies. These lesions occur in isolation and among other deficits in a host of neurologic disorders. Detailed observations help to ascertain whether a given ocular motor nerve is partially or completely involved, and to determine the topical localization and chronicity of a lesion. These principles guide the formation of an appropriate differential diagnosis, rational clinical decision making, and, ultimately, effective therapies for this group of patients.

ACKNOWLEDGMENTS

The authors are grateful to the patients described in this article and to their colleagues, Drs Steven Galetta, Grant Liu, Laura Balcer, and Robert Avery, by whom many of these patients were seen.

REFERENCES

1. Kwon JH, Kwon SU, Ahn HS, et al. Isolated superior rectus palsy due to contralateral midbrain infarction. Arch Neurol 2003;60:1633–5.
2. Saeki N, Yamaura A, Sunami K. Bilateral ptosis with pupil sparing because of a discrete midbrain lesion: magnetic resonance imaging evidence of topographic arrangement within the oculomotor nerve. J Neuroophthalmol 2000;20: 130–4.
3. Uz A, Tekdemir I. Relationship between the posterior cerebral artery and the cisternal segment of the oculomotor nerve. J Clin Neurosci 2006;13:1019–22.
4. Krisht A, Barnett DW, Barrow DL, et al. The blood supply of the intracavernous cranial nerves: an anatomic study. Neurosurgery 1994;34:275–9 [discussion: 279].
5. Asbury AK, Aldredge H, Hershberg R, et al. Oculomotor palsy in diabetes mellitus: a clinico-pathological study. Brain 1970;93:555–66.
6. Bogousslavsky J, Maeder P, Regli F, et al. Pure midbrain infarction: clinical syndromes, MRI, and etiologic patterns. Neurology 1994;44:2032–40.
7. Kim JS, Kim J. Pure midbrain infarction: clinical, radiologic, and pathophysiologic findings. Neurology 2005;64:1227–32.
8. Chen L, Maclaurin W, Gerraty RP. Isolated unilateral ptosis and mydriasis from ventral midbrain infarction. J Neurol 2009;256:1164–5.
9. Ksiazek SM, Slamovits TL, Rosen CE, et al. Fascicular arrangement in partial oculomotor paresis. Am J Ophthalmol 1994;118:97–103.
10. Castro O, Johnson LN, Mamourian AC. Isolated inferior oblique paresis from brain-stem infarction. Perspective on oculomotor fascicular organization in the ventral midbrain tegmentum. Arch Neurol 1990;47:235–7.
11. Liu GT, Crenner CW, Logigian EL, et al. Midbrain syndromes of Benedikt, Claude, and Nothnagel: setting the record straight. Neurology 1992;42:1820–2.

12. Celebisoy N, Celebisoy M, Tokucoglu F, et al. Superior division paresis of the oculomotor nerve: Report of four cases. Eur Neurol 2006;56:50–3.

13. Bhatti MT, Eisenschenk S, Roper SN, et al. Superior divisional third cranial nerve paresis: clinical and anatomical observations of 2 unique cases. Arch Neurol 2006;63:771–6.

14. Ksiazek SM, Repka MX, Maguire A, et al. Divisional oculomotor nerve paresis caused by intrinsic brainstem disease. Ann Neurol 1989;26:714–8.

15. Guy JR, Day AL. Intracranial aneurysms with superior division paresis of the oculomotor nerve. Ophthalmology 1989;96:1071–6.

16. Chotmongkol V, Sawanyawisuth K, Limpawattana P, et al. Superior divisional oculomotor nerve palsy caused by midbrain neurocysticercosis. Parasitol Int 2006;55:223–5.

17. Shuttleworth GN, Steel DH, Silverman BW, et al. Patterns of III nerve synkinesis. Strabismus 1998;6:181–90.

18. Boghen D, Chartrand JP, Laflamme P, et al. Primary aberrant third nerve regeneration. Ann Neurol 1979;6:415–8.

19. Lepore FE, Glaser JS. Misdirection revisited. A critical appraisal of acquired oculomotor nerve synkinesis. Arch Ophthalmol 1980;98:2206–9.

20. Grunwald L, Sund NJ, Volpe NJ. Pupillary sparing and aberrant regeneration in chronic third nerve palsy secondary to a posterior communicating artery aneurysm. Br J Ophthalmol 2008;92:715–6.

21. Locksley HB. Natural history of subarachnoid hemorrhage, intracranial aneurysms and arteriovenous malformations. J Neurosurg 1966;25:321–68.

22. Okawara SH. Warning signs prior to rupture of an intracranial aneurysm. J Neurosurg 1973;38:575–80.

23. Kissel JT, Burde RM, Klingele TG, et al. Pupil-sparing oculomotor palsies with internal carotid-posterior communicating artery aneurysms. Ann Neurol 1983;13:149–54.

24. Nadeau SE, Trobe JD. Pupil sparing in oculomotor palsy: a brief review. Ann Neurol 1983;13:143–8.

25. Chen PR, Amin-Hanjani S, Albuquerque FC, et al. Outcome of oculomotor nerve palsy from posterior communicating artery aneurysms: comparison of clipping and coiling. Neurosurgery 2006;58:1040–6 [discussion: 1040–6].

26. Weber RB, Daroff RB, Mackey EA. Pathology of oculomotor nerve palsy in diabetics. Neurology 1970;20:835–8.

27. Jacobson DM. Pupil involvement in patients with diabetes-associated oculomotor nerve palsy. Arch Ophthalmol 1998;116:723–7.

28. Bortolami R, D'Alessandro R, Manni E. The origin of pain in 'ischemic-diabetic' third-nerve palsy. Arch Neurol 1993;50:795.

29. Capo H, Warren F, Kupersmith MJ. Evolution of oculomotor nerve palsies. J Clin Neuroophthalmol 1992;12:21–5.

30. Lepore FE. Disorders of ocular motility following head trauma. Arch Neurol 1995; 52:924–6.

31. Baker RS, Epstein AD. Ocular motor abnormalities from head trauma. Surv Ophthalmol 1991;35:245–67.

32. Walter KA, Newman NJ, Lessell S. Oculomotor palsy from minor head trauma: initial sign of intracranial aneurysm. Neurology 1994;44:148–50.

33. Eyster EF, Hoyt WF, Wilson CB. Oculomotor palsy from minor head trauma. An initial sign of basal intracranial tumor. JAMA 1972;220:1083–6.

34. Tanriover N, Kemerdere R, Kafadar AM, et al. Oculomotor nerve schwannoma located in the oculomotor cistern. Surg Neurol 2007;67:83–8 [discussion: 88].

35. Kozic D, Nagulic M, Ostojic J, et al. Malignant peripheral nerve sheath tumor of the oculomotor nerve. Acta Radiol 2006;47:595–8.
36. Friedman AP, Harter DH, Merritt HH. Ophthalmoplegic migraine. Arch Neurol 1962;7:320–7.
37. Vanpelt W. On the early onset of ophthalmoplegic migraine. Am J Dis Child 1964; 107:628–31.
38. Walsh JP, O'Doherty DS. A possible explanation of the mechanism of ophthalmoplegic migraine. Neurology 1960;10:1079–84.
39. Miller NR. Solitary oculomotor nerve palsy in childhood. Am J Ophthalmol 1977; 83:106–11.
40. Prats JM, Monzon MJ, Zuazo E, et al. Congenital nuclear syndrome of oculomotor nerve. Pediatr Neurol 1993;9:476–8.
41. Friedman DI, Wright KW, Sadun AA. Oculomotor palsy with cyclic spasms. Neurology 1989;39:1263–4.
42. Schultz KL, Lee AG. Diagnostic yield of the evaluation of isolated third nerve palsy in adults. Can J Ophthalmol 2007;42:110–5.
43. Chou KL, Galetta SL, Liu GT, et al. Acute ocular motor mononeuropathies: prospective study of the roles of neuroimaging and clinical assessment. J Neurol Sci 2004;219:35–9.
44. Vaphiades MS, Cure J, Kline L. Management of intracranial aneurysm causing a third cranial nerve palsy: MRA, CTA or DSA? Semin Ophthalmol 2008;23: 143–50.
45. Noonan CP, O'Connor M. Surgical management of third nerve palsy. Br J Ophthalmol 1995;79:431–4.
46. Jampolsky A. Current techniques of adjustable strabismus surgery. Am J Ophthalmol 1979;88:406–18.
47. Prasad S, Volpe NJ, Tamhankar MA. Clinical reasoning: a 36-year-old man with vertical diplopia. Neurology 2009;72:e93–9.
48. Parulekar MV, Dai S, Buncic JR, et al. Head position-dependent changes in ocular torsion and vertical misalignment in skew deviation. Arch Ophthalmol 2008;126:899–905.
49. von Noorden GK, Murray E, Wong SY. Superior oblique paralysis. A review of 270 cases. Arch Ophthalmol 1986;104:1771–6.
50. Dhaliwal A, West AL, Trobe JD, et al. Third, fourth, and sixth cranial nerve palsies following closed head injury. J Neuroophthalmol 2006;26:4–10.
51. Helveston EM, Krach D, Plager DA, et al. A new classification of superior oblique palsy based on congenital variations in the tendon. Ophthalmology 1992;99: 1609–15.
52. Mansour AM, Reinecke RD. Central trochlear palsy. Surv Ophthalmol 1986;30: 279–97.
53. Brazis PW, Miller NR, Henderer JD, et al. The natural history and results of treatment of superior oblique myokymia. Arch Ophthalmol 1994;112:1063–7.
54. Keane JR. Trochlear nerve pareses with brainstem lesions. J Clin Neuroophthalmol 1986;6:242–6.
55. Keane JR. Tectal fourth nerve palsy due to infarction. Arch Neurol 2004;61: 280.
56. Muri RM, Baumgartner RW. Horner's syndrome and contralateral trochlear nerve palsy. Neuroophthalmology 1995;15:161.
57. Vanooteghem P, Dehaene I, Van Zandycke M, et al. Combined trochlear nerve palsy and internuclear ophthalmoplegia. Arch Neurol 1992;49:108–9.

58. Elliot D, Cunningham JE Jr, Miller NR. Fourth nerve paresis and ipsilateral relative afferent pupillary defect without visual sensory disturbance: a sign of contralateral dorsal midbrain disease. J Clin Neuroophthalmol 1991;11:169–72.

59. Maruo T, Iwashige H, Kubota N, et al. Long-term results of surgery for superior oblique palsy. Jpn J Ophthalmol 1996;40:235–8.

60. Plager DA. Superior oblique palsy and superior oblique myokymia. In: Rosenbaum AL, Santiago AP, editors. Clinical strabismus management: principles and surgical techniques. Philadelphia: WB Saunders; 1999. p. 219–29.

61. Thomke F. Isolated abducens palsies due to pontine lesions. Neuroophthalmology 1998;20:91–100.

62. Prasad S, Liu GT, Abend NS, et al. Images in paediatrics: sinovenous thrombosis due to mastoiditis. Arch Dis Child 2007;92:749.

63. Thomke F, Mika-Gruttner A, Visbeck A, et al. The risk of abducens palsy after diagnostic lumbar puncture. Neurology 2000;54:768–9.

64. Volpe NJ, Lessell S. Remitting sixth nerve palsy in skull base tumors. Arch Ophthalmol 1993;111:1391–5.

65. Jacobson DM. Progressive ophthalmoplegia with acute ischemic abducens nerve palsies. Am J Ophthalmol 1996;122:278–9.

66. Dave AV, Diaz-Marchan PJ, Lee AG. Clinical and magnetic resonance imaging features of Gradenigo syndrome. Am J Ophthalmol 1997;124:568–70.

67. Afifi AK, Bell WE, Bale JF, et al. Recurrent lateral rectus palsy in childhood. Pediatr Neurol 1990;6:315–8.

68. Mahoney NR, Liu GT. Benign recurrent sixth (abducens) nerve palsies in children. Arch Dis Child 2009;94:394–6.

69. Duane A. Congenital deficiency of abduction, associated with impairment of adduction, retraction movements, contraction of the palpebral fissure and oblique movements of the eye. 1905. Arch Ophthalmol 1996;114:1255–6 [discussion: 1257].

70. Hotchkiss MG, Miller NR, Clark AW, et al. Bilateral Duane's retraction syndrome. A clinical-pathologic case report. Arch Ophthalmol 1980;98:870–4.

71. Miller NR, Kiel SM, Green WR, et al. Unilateral Duane's retraction syndrome (type 1). Arch Ophthalmol 1982;100:1468–72.

72. Miyake N, Chilton J, Psatha M, et al. Human CHN1 mutations hyperactivate alpha2-chimaerin and cause Duane's retraction syndrome. Science 2008;321: 839–43.

73. Pressman SH, Scott WE. Surgical treatment of Duane's syndrome. Ophthalmology 1986;93:29–38.

74. Ghabrial R, Versace P, Kourt G, et al. Mobius' syndrome: features and etiology. J Pediatr Ophthalmol Strabismus 1998;35:304–11 [quiz: 327–8].

75. Moster ML, Savino PJ, Sergott RC, et al. Isolated sixth-nerve palsies in younger adults. Arch Ophthalmol 1984;102:1328–30.

76. Prasad S, Brown MJ, Galetta SL. Transient downbeat nystagmus from West Nile virus encephalomyelitis. Neurology 2006;66:1599–600.

77. Keane JR. Cavernous sinus syndrome. Analysis of 151 cases. Arch Neurol 1996; 53:967–71.

78. Reid RL, Quigley ME, Yen SS. Pituitary apoplexy. A review. Arch Neurol 1985;42: 712–9.

79. Seyer H, Erbguth F, Kompf D, et al. [Acute hemorrhage and ischemic necroses in hypophyseal tumors: hypophyseal apoplexy]. Fortschr Neurol Psychiatr 1989;57: 474–88 [in German].

80. Marsh RJ, Dulley B, Kelly V. External ocular motor palsies in ophthalmic zoster: a review. Br J Ophthalmol 1977;61:677–82.
81. Kline LB. The Tolosa-Hunt syndrome. Surv Ophthalmol 1982;27:79–95.
82. Nakano M, Yamada K, Fain J, et al. Homozygous mutations in ARIX(PHOX2A) result in congenital fibrosis of the extraocular muscles type 2. Nat Genet 2001; 29:315–20.

Index

Note: Page numbers of article titles are in **boldface** type.

Neurol Clin 28 (2010) 835–844
doi:10.1016/S0733-8619(10)00076-9
0733-8619/10/$ – see front matter © 2010 Elsevier Inc. All rights reserved.

Moving?

Make sure your subscription moves with you!

To notify us of your new address, find your **Clinics Account Number** (located on your mailing label above your name), and contact customer service at:

Email: **journalscustomerservice-usa@elsevier.com**

800-654-2452 (subscribers in the U.S. & Canada)
314-447-8871 (subscribers outside of the U.S. & Canada)

Fax number: **314-447-8029**

Elsevier Health Sciences Division
Subscription Customer Service
3251 Riverport Lane
Maryland Heights, MO 63043

*To ensure uninterrupted delivery of your subscription, please notify us at least 4 weeks in advance of move.